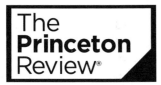

The
Princeton
Review®

MCAT®
Workout
Revised 3rd Edition

The Staff of The Princeton Review

Penguin
Random
House

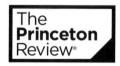

The Princeton Review
110 East 42nd St, 7th Floor
New York, NY 10017
E-mail: editorialsupport@review.com

Published in the United States by Penguin Random
House LLC, New York, and in Canada by Random House
of Canada, a division of Penguin Random House Ltd.,
Toronto.

Terms of Service: The Princeton Review Online
Companion Tools ["Student Tools"] for retail books
are available for only the two most recent editions of
that book. Student Tools may be activated only once
per eligible book purchased for a total of 24 months
of access. Activation of Student Tools more than once
per book is in direct violation of these Terms of Service
and may result in discontinuation of access to Student
Tools Services.

This book is the third edition of ISSN 1937-6375. Some
material in this book was previously published as *The
Princeton Review MCAT*, 2nd Edition, and *MCAT Critical
Analysis and Reasoning Skills Review*, 2nd Edition, both
trade paperbacks published by Penguin Random House
LLC in 2016.

ISBN: 978-0-525-57008-0
ISSN: 1937-6375

MCAT is a registered trademark of the Association of
American Medical Colleges.

The Princeton Review is not affiliated with
Princeton University.

Editor: Meave Shelton
Production Artist: Deborah Weber
Production Editor: Liz Dacey

Printed in the United States of America.

10 9 8 7 6 5 4 3 2 1

3rd Edition

Editorial

Rob Franek, Editor-in-Chief
David Soto, Director of Content Development
Stephen Koch, Student Survey Manager
Deborah Weber, Director of Production
Gabriel Berlin, Production Design Manager
Selena Coppock, Managing Editor
Aaron Riccio, Senior Editor
Meave Shelton, Senior Editor
Chris Chimera, Editor
Eleanor Green, Editor
Orion McBean, Editor
Brian Saladino, Editor

Penguin Random House Publishing Team

Tom Russell, VP, Publisher
Alison Stoltzfus, Publishing Director
Amanda Yee, Associate Managing Editor
Ellen Reed, Production Manager
Suzanne Lee, Designer

CONTRIBUTORS

TPR MCAT Biology and Biochemistry Development Team:
Jessica Adams, Ph.D.
Andrew D. Snyder, M.D.
Jenkang Tao, B.S., B.A.
Judene Wright, M.S., M.A.Ed., Senior Editor, Lead Developer
Sarah Woodruff, B.S., B.A.

TPR MCAT CARS Development Team:
Gina Granter, M.A.
Christopher Hinkle, Th.D.
Jennifer S. Wooddell, Senior Editor, Lead Developer

TPR MCAT General Chemistry Development Team:
Bethany Blackwell, M.S., Senior Editor, Lead Developer
William Ewing, Ph.D.
Chris Fortenbach, B.S.

Edited for Production by:
Judene Wright, M.S., M.A.Ed.
      National Content Director, MCAT Program,
      The Princeton Review

TPR MCAT Organic Chemistry Development Team:
Bethany Blackwell, M.S.
William Ewing, Ph.D.
Brandon Kelley, Ph.D.
Jason Osman, Ph.D., Senior Editor, Lead Developer

TPR MCAT Physics Development Team:
Jon Fowler, M.A., Senior Editor, Lead Developer
Chris Pentzell, M.S.
Carolyn J. Shiau, M.D.
Felicia Tam, Ph.D.

TPR MCAT Psychology and Sociology Development Team:
Matthew Dempsey, M.A.
Kevin Keogh
Anthony Krupp, Ph.D.
Tomislav Kurtovic, M.A., Senior Editor, Lead Developer

The Princeton Review would like to thank the following people for their contributions to this book :
Elizabeth Aamot (Fatith), Rizwan Ahmad, M.A., Kashif Anwar, M.D., M.M.S., Farhad Aziz, B.S., John Bahling, M.D., Gary Bedford, Kendra Bowman, Ph.D., Kristen Brunson, Ph.D., Jessica Burstrem, M.A., Brian Butts, B.S., B.A., Argun Can, Phil Carpenter, Ph.D., Erika C. Castro, B.A., Brian Cato, Khawar Chaudry, B.S., Nita Chauhan, H.BSc, MSc, Dan Cho, M.P.H., Maria S. Chushak, M.S., Alix Claps, M.A., Doug Couchman, Cynthia Cowan, B.A., Glenn E. Croston, Ph.D., Sara Daniel, B.S., Douglas S. Daniels, Ph.D., Nathan Deal, M.D., Guenevieve O. del Mundo, B.A., B.S., C.C.S., Ian Denham, B.Sc., B.Ed., Joshua Dilworth, M.D., Ph.D., Annie Dude, Amanda Edward, H.BSc., H.BEd., Cory Eicher, B.A., Rob Fong, M.D., Ph.D., Chris Fortenbach, B.S., Michelle E. Fox, B.S., Kirsten Frank, Ph.D., (James) Ben Gill, Jacqueline R. Giordano, Carlos Guzman, Corinne Harol, Alison Howard, James Hudson, M.A., Isabel L. Jackson, B.S., Adam Johnson, Nadia Johnson, M.A., M.S., Ryan Katchky, Jason N. Kennedy, M.S., Erik Kildebeck, Omair Adil Khan, Paul Kugelmass, George Kyriazis, Ph.D., Ali Landreau, B.A., Steven A. Leduc, M.S., Ben Lee, Jay Lee, Heather Liwanag, Ph.D., Brendan Lloyd, B.Sc., M.Sc., Stefan Loren, Ph.D., Travis Mackoy, B.S., Rohit Madani, B.S., Neil Maluste, B.S., Joey Mancuso, M.S., D.O., Chris Manuel, M.P.H., Ashley Manzoor, Ph.D., Janet Marshall, Ph.D., Douglas K. McLemore, B.S., Alan Marchand, Ph.D., Evan Martow, BMSc, Mike Matera, B.A., Jennifer A. McDevitt, M.A., Marion-Vincent L. Mempin, B.S., Donna Memran, Ashleigh Menhadji, Al Mercado, Brian Mikolasko, M.D., M.BA, Katherine Miller, Ph.D., Abhisehk Mohapatra, B.A., Katherine Montgomery, Christopher Moriates, M.D., Paola A. Munoz, M.A., Stephen L. Nelson, Jr., Ph.D., Tenaya Newkirk, Ph.D., Don Osborne, Daniel J. Pallin, M.D., Gina Passante, Rupal Patel, B.S., Vivek Patel, Tyler Peikes, Bikem Ayse Polat, Mary Qiu, Chris Rabbat, Ph.D., Steven Rines, Ph.D., Ina C. Roy, M.D., Jayson Sack, M.D., M.S., Karen Salazar, Ph.D., Will Sanderson, Jeanine Seitz-Partridge, M.S., Maryam Shambayati, M.S., Sina Shahbaz, B.S., Shalom Shapiro, Mark Shew, H.BSc., Gillian Shiau, M.D., Oktay Shuminov, B.S., Andrew D. Snyder, M.S., Angela Song, Kate Speiker, Teri Stewart, B.S.E., David Stoll, Dylan Sweeney, Preston Swirnoff, Ph.D., M.S., Jonathan Swirsky, Neil Thornton, Lara Tubelle de Gonzales, Rhead Uddin, Danish Vaiyani, Christopher Volpe, Ph.D., Betsy Walli, M.S., Ph.D., Jia Wang, Tom Watts, B.A., David Weiskopf, M.A., Barry Weliver, Chelsea K. Wise, M.S., Hesham Zakaria.

Periodic Table of the Elements

1 H 1.0																	2 He 4.0
3 Li 6.9	4 Be 9.0											5 B 10.8	6 C 12.0	7 N 14.0	8 O 16.0	9 F 19.0	10 Ne 20.2
11 Na 23.0	12 Mg 24.3											13 Al 27.0	14 Si 28.1	15 P 31.0	16 S 32.1	17 Cl 35.5	18 Ar 39.9
19 K 39.1	20 Ca 40.1	21 Sc 45.0	22 Ti 47.9	23 V 50.9	24 Cr 52.0	25 Mn 54.9	26 Fe 55.8	27 Co 58.9	28 Ni 58.7	29 Cu 63.5	30 Zn 65.4	31 Ga 69.7	32 Ge 72.6	33 As 74.9	34 Se 79.0	35 Br 79.9	36 Kr 83.8
37 Rb 85.5	38 Sr 87.6	39 Y 88.9	40 Zr 91.2	41 Nb 92.9	42 Mo 95.9	43 Tc (98)	44 Ru 101.1	45 Rh 102.9	46 Pd 106.4	47 Ag 107.9	48 Cd 112.4	49 In 114.8	50 Sn 118.7	51 Sb 121.8	52 Te 127.6	53 I 126.9	54 Xe 131.3
55 Cs 132.9	56 Ba 137.3	57 *La 138.9	72 Hf 178.5	73 Ta 180.9	74 W 183.9	75 Re 186.2	76 Os 190.2	77 Ir 192.2	78 Pt 195.1	79 Au 197.0	80 Hg 200.6	81 Tl 204.4	82 Pb 207.2	83 Bi 209.0	84 Po (209)	85 At (210)	86 Rn (222)
87 Fr (223)	88 Ra 226.0	89 †Ac 227.0	104 Rf (261)	105 Db (262)	106 Sg (266)	107 Bh (264)	108 Hs (277)	109 Mt (268)	110 Ds (281)	111 Rg (272)	112 Cn (285)	113 Uut (286)	114 Fl (289)	115 Uup (288)	116 Lv (293)	117 Uus (294)	118 Uuo (294)

*Lanthanide Series:

58 Ce 140.1	59 Pr 140.9	60 Nd 144.2	61 Pm (145)	62 Sm 150.4	63 Eu 152.0	64 Gd 157.3	65 Tb 158.9	66 Dy 162.5	67 Ho 164.9	68 Er 167.3	69 Tm 168.9	70 Yb 173.0	71 Lu 175.0

†Actinide Series:

90 Th 232.0	91 Pa (231)	92 U 238.0	93 Np (237)	94 Pu (244)	95 Am (243)	96 Cm (247)	97 Bk (247)	98 Cf (251)	99 Es (252)	100 Fm (257)	101 Md (258)	102 No (259)	103 Lr (260)

TABLE OF CONTENTS

Get More (Free) Content

at **PrincetonReview.com/cracking**

As easy as 1·2·3

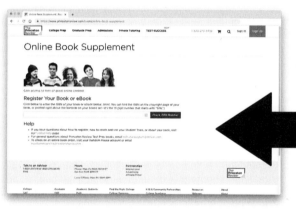

1 Go to PrincetonReview.com/cracking and enter the following ISBN for your book: 9780525570080

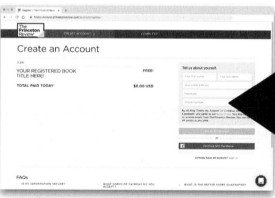

2 Answer a few simple questions to set up an exclusive Princeton Review account. *(If you already have one, you can just log in.)*

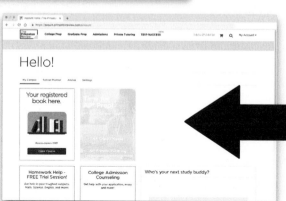

3 Enjoy access to your **FREE** content!

Once you've registered, you can...

- Find useful information about taking the MCAT and applying to medical school

- Check to see if there have been any corrections or updates to this edition

- Get our take on any recent or pending updates to the MCAT

Need to report a potential **content** issue?

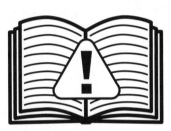

Contact **EditorialSupport@review.com** and include:

- full title of the book
- ISBN
- page number

Need to report a **technical** issue?

Contact **TPRStudentTech@review.com** and provide:

- your full name
- email address used to register the book
- full book title and ISBN
- Operating system (Mac/PC) and browser (Firefox, Safari, etc.)

Part 1

MCAT Overview

Chapter 1
MCAT Basics

WHAT IS THE MCAT...REALLY?

Most test-takers approach the MCAT as though it were a typical college science test, one in which facts and knowledge simply need to be regurgitated in order to do well. They study for the MCAT the same way they did for their college tests, by memorizing facts and details, formulas and equations. And when they get to the MCAT they are surprised...and disappointed.

It's a myth that the MCAT is purely a content-knowledge test. If medical school admission committees want to see what you know, all they have to do is look at your transcripts. What they really want to see, though, is how you *think*. Especially, how you think under pressure. And *that's* what your MCAT score will tell them.

The MCAT is really a test of your ability to apply basic knowledge to different, possibly new, situations. It's a test of your ability to reason out and evaluate arguments. Do you still need to know your science content? Absolutely. But not at the level that most test-takers think they need to know it. Furthermore, your science knowledge won't help you on the Critical Analysis and Reasoning Skills (CARS) section. So how do you study for a test like this?

You study for the science sections by reviewing the basics and then applying them to MCAT practice questions. You study for the CARS section by learning how to adapt your existing reading and analytical skills to the nature of the test.

MCAT Workout provides ample opportunities to tackle challenging practice problems until you know the exam back to front—and probably sideways too. With hundreds of realistic questions and passages designed to make you think about the material in a deeper way, along with detailed solutions to clarify the logical thought process needed to get to the answer, this book is a deep dive into the intensive prep you'll need to score well on this test.

> For a comprehensive review of the content on the MCAT, with specific strategies for each section, check out *The Princeton Review MCAT*.

MCAT NUTS AND BOLTS

Overview

The MCAT is a computer-based test (CBT) that is *not* adaptive. Adaptive tests base your next question on whether or not you've answered the current question correctly. The MCAT is *linear*, or *fixed-form*, meaning that the questions are in a predetermined order and do not change based on your answers. However, there are many versions of the test, so that on a given test day, different people will see different versions. The following table highlights the features of the MCAT exam.

Registration	Online via www.aamc.org. Begins as early as six months prior to test date; available up until week of test (subject to seat availability).
Testing Centers	Administered at small, secure, climate-controlled computer testing rooms.
Security	Photo ID with signature, electronic fingerprint, electronic signature verification, assigned seat.
Proctoring	None. Test administrator checks examinee in and assigns seat at computer. All testing instructions are given on the computer.
Frequency of Test	Many times per year distributed over January, April, May, June, July, August, and September.
Format	Exclusively computer-based. NOT an adaptive test.
Length of Test Day	7.5 hours
Breaks	Optional 10-minute breaks between sections, with a 30-minute break for lunch.
Section Names	1. Chemical and Physical Foundations of Biological Systems (Chem/Phys) 2. Critical Analysis and Reasoning Skills (CARS) 3. Biological and Biochemical Foundations of Living Systems (Bio/Biochem) 4. Psychological, Social, and Biological Foundations of Behavior (Psych/Soc)
Number of Questions and Timing	59 Chem/Phys questions, 95 minutes 53 CARS questions, 90 minutes 59 Bio/Biochem questions, 95 minutes 59 Psych/Soc questions, 95 minutes
Scoring	Test is scaled. Several forms per administration.
Allowed/ Not allowed	No timers/watches. Noise reduction headphones available. Noteboard booklet and wet-erase marker given at start of test and taken at end of test. Locker or secure area provided for personal items.
Results: Timing and Delivery	Approximately 30 days. Electronic scores only, available online through AAMC login. Examinees can print official score reports.
Maximum Number of Retakes	The test can be taken a maximum of three times in one year, four times over two years, and seven times over the lifetime of the examinee. An examinee can be registered for only one date at a time.

Registration

Registration for the exam is completed online at https://students-residents.aamc.org/applying-medical-school/taking-mcat-exam/register-mcat-exam. The AAMC opens registration for a given test date at least two months in advance of the date, often earlier. It's a good idea to register well in advance of your desired test date to make sure that you get a seat.

Sections

There are four sections on the MCAT exam: Chemical and Physical Foundations of Biological Systems (Chem/Phys), Critical Analysis and Reasoning Skills (CARS), Biological and Biochemical Foundations of Living Systems (Bio/Biochem), and Psychological, Social, and Biological Foundations of Behavior (Psych/Soc). All sections consist of multiple-choice questions.

Section	Concepts Tested	Number of Questions and Timing
Chemical and Physical Foundations of Biological Systems	Basic concepts in chemical and physical sciences, scientific inquiry, reasoning, research, and statistics skills	59 questions in 95 minutes
Critical Analysis and Reasoning Skills	Critical analysis of information drawn from a wide range of social science and humanities disciplines	53 questions in 90 minutes
Biological and Biochemical Foundations of Living Systems	Basic concepts in biology and biochemistry, scientific inquiry, reasoning, research, and statistics skills	59 questions in 95 minutes
Psychological, Social, and Biological Foundations of Behavior	Basic concepts in psychology, sociology, and biology, research methods, and statistics	59 questions in 95 minutes

Most questions on the MCAT (44 in each of the science sections, all 53 in the CARS section) are passage-based. The science sections each have 10 passages with 4–6 questions per passage and 15 freestanding questions (more on that below). The CARS section has 9 passages with 5–7 questions per passage. A passage consists of a few paragraphs of information on which several following questions are based. In the science sections, passages often include equations or reactions, tables, graphs, figures, and experiments to analyze. CARS passages come from literature in social sciences, humanities, ethics, philosophy, cultural studies, and population health, and they do not test content knowledge in any way.

Some questions in the science sections are *freestanding questions* (FSQs). These questions are independent of any passage information. These questions appear in several groups of about four to five questions, and they are interspersed throughout the passages. About 1/4 (15 of 59) of the questions in the science sections are freestanding, and the remainder are passage-based.

Each section on the MCAT is separated by either a 10-minute break or a 30-minute lunch break.

Section	Time
Test Center Check-In	Variable, can take up to 40 minutes if center is busy.
Tutorial	10 minutes
Chemical and Physical Foundations of Biological Systems	95 minutes
Break	10 minutes
Critical Analysis and Reasoning Skills	90 minutes
Lunch Break	30 minutes
Biological and Biochemical Foundations of Living Systems	95 minutes
Break	10 minutes
Psychological, Social, and Biological Foundations of Behavior	95 minutes
Void Option	5 minutes
Survey	5 minutes

The survey includes questions about your satisfaction with the overall MCAT experience, including registration, check-in, etc., as well as questions about how you prepared for the test.

Scoring

The MCAT is a scaled exam, meaning that your raw score will be converted into a scaled score that takes into account the difficulty of the questions. There is no guessing penalty. All sections are scored from 118–132, with a total scaled score range of 472–528. Because different versions of the test have varying levels of difficulty, the scale will be different from one exam to the next. Thus, there is no "magic number" of questions to get right in order to get a particular score. Plus, some of the questions on the test are considered "experimental" and do not count toward your score; they are just there to be evaluated for possible future inclusion in a test.

At the end of the test (after you complete the Psychological, Social, and Biological Foundations of Behavior section), you will be asked to choose one of the following two options, "I wish to have my MCAT exam scored" or "I wish to VOID my MCAT exam." You have five minutes to make a decision, and if you do not select one of the options in that time, the test will automatically be scored. If you choose the VOID option, your test will not be scored (you will not now, or ever, get a numerical score for this test), medical schools will not know you took the test, and no refunds will be granted. You cannot "unvoid" your scores at a later time.

So, what's a good score? The AAMC is centering the scale at 500 (i.e., 500 will be the 50th percentile) and recommends that application committees consider applicants near the center of the range. To be on the safe side, aim for a total score of 506–508. And remember that if your GPA is on the low side, you'll need higher MCAT scores to compensate, and if you have a strong GPA, you can get away with lower MCAT scores. But the reality is that your chances of acceptance depend on a lot more than just your MCAT scores. It's a combination of your GPA, your MCAT scores, your undergraduate coursework, letters of recommendation, experience related to the medical field (such as volunteer work or research), extracurricular activities, your personal statement, etc. Medical schools are looking for a complete package, not just good scores and a good GPA.

GENERAL LAYOUT, TEST TOOLS, AND PACING

Layout of the Test

In each section of the test, the computer screen is divided vertically, with the passage on the left and the range of questions for that passage indicated above (e.g., "Passage 1 Questions 1–5"). The scroll bar for the passage text appears in the middle of the screen. Each question appears on the right, and you need to click "Next" to move to each subsequent question.

In the science sections, the freestanding questions are found in groups of 4–5, interspersed with the passages. The screen is still divided vertically; on the left is the statement "Questions [X–XX] do not refer to a passage and are independent of each other," and each question appears on the right, as described above.

CBT Tools

There are a number of tools available on the test, including highlighting, strike-outs, the Flag for Review button, the Navigation and Review Screen buttons, the Periodic Table button, and of course, the noteboard booklet. All tools are available with both mouse control (buttons to click) or keyboard commands (Alt+ a letter). As everyone has different preferences, you should practice with both types of tools (mouse and keyboard) to see which is more comfortable for you personally. The following is a brief description of each tool.

1) **Highlighting:** This is done in the passage text (including table entries and some equations, but excluding figures and molecular structures), in the question stems, and in the answer choices (including Roman numerals). Select the words you wish to highlight (left-click and drag the cursor across the words), and in the upper left corner click the "Highlight" button to highlight the selected text yellow. Alternatively, press "Alt+H" to highlight the words. Highlighting can be removed by selecting the words again and in the upper left corner clicking the down arrow next to "Highlight." This will expand to show the "Remove Highlight" option; clicking this will remove the highlighting. Removing highlighting via the keyboard is cumbersome and is not recommended.

2) **Strike-outs:** This can be done on the answer choices, including Roman numeral statements, by selecting the text you want to strike out (left-click and drag the cursor across the text), then clicking the "Strikethrough" button in the upper left corner. Alternatively, press "Alt+S" to strikeout the words. The strike-out can be removed by repeating these actions. Figures or molecular structures cannot be struck out, however, the letter answer choice of those structures can.

3) **Flag for Review button:** This is available for each question and is found in the upper right corner. This allows you to flag the question as one you would like to review later if time permits. When clicked, the flag icon turns yellow. Click again to remove the flag. Alternatively, press "Alt+F."

4) **Navigation button:** This is found near the bottom of the screen and is only available on your first pass through the section. Clicking this button brings up a navigation table listing all questions and their statuses (unseen, incomplete, complete, flagged for review). You can also press "Alt+V" to bring up the screen. The questions can be sorted by their statuses, and clicking a question number takes you immediately to that question. Once you have reached the end of the section and viewed the Review screen (described below), the Navigation screen is no longer available.

5) **Review Screen button:** This button is found near the bottom of the screen after your first pass through the section, and when clicked, brings up a new screen showing all questions and their statuses (either incomplete, unseen, or flagged for review). Questions that are complete are assigned no additional status. You can then choose one of three options by clicking with the mouse or with keyboard shortcuts: Review All (Alt+A), Review Incomplete (Alt+I), or Review Flagged (Alt+R); alternatively, you can click a question number to go directly back to that question. You can also end the section from this screen.

6) **Periodic Table button:** Clicking this button will open a periodic table (or press "Alt+T"). Note that the periodic table is large, covering most of the screen. However, this window can be resized to see the questions and a portion of the periodic table at the same time. The table text will not decrease, but scroll bars will appear on the window so you can center the section of the table of interest in the window.

7) **Noteboard Booklet (Scratch Paper):** At the start of the test, you will be given a spiral-bound set of five laminated 8.5″ × 14″ sheets of paper and a wet-erase black marker to use as scratch paper. You can request a clean noteboard booklet at any time during the test; your original booklet will be collected. The noteboard is only useful if it is kept organized; do not give in to the tendency to write on the first available open space! Good organization will be very helpful when/if you wish to review a question. Indicate the passage number, the range of questions for that passage, and a topic in a box near the top of your scratch work, and indicate the question you are working on in a circle to the left of the notes for that question. Draw a line under your scratch work when you change passages to keep the work separate. Do not erase or scribble over any previous work. If you do not think it is correct, draw one line through the work and start again. You may have already done some useful work without realizing it.

Pacing

Since the MCAT is a timed test, you must keep an eye on the timer and adjust your pacing as necessary. It would be terrible to run out of time at the end and discover that the last few questions could have been easily answered in just a few seconds each.

In the science sections you will have about one minute and thirty-five seconds (1:35) per question, and in the CARS section you will have about one minute and forty seconds per question (1:40).

Section	# of Questions in passage	Approximate time (including reading the passage)
Chem/Phys, Bio/Biochem, and Psych/Soc	4	6.5 minutes
	5	8 minutes
	6	9.5 minutes
CARS	5	8.5 minutes
	6	10 minutes
	7	11.5 minutes

When starting a passage in the science sections, make note of how much time you will allot for it and the starting time on the timer. Jot down on your noteboard what the timer should say at the end of the passage. Then just keep an eye on it as you work through the questions. If you are near the end of the time for that passage, guess on any remaining questions, make some notes on your noteboard, Flag the questions, and move on. Come back to those questions if you have time.

For the CARS section, keep in mind that many people will maximize their score by *not* trying to complete every question or every passage in the section. A good strategy for test-takers who cannot achieve a high level of accuracy on all nine passages is to randomly guess on at least one passage in the section and spend your time getting a high percentage of the other questions right. To complete all nine CARS passages, you have about ten minutes per passage. To complete eight of the nine, you have about 11 minutes per passage.

TESTING TIPS

Before Test Day

- Take a trip to the test center a day or two before your actual test date so that you can easily find the building and room on test day. This will also allow you to gauge traffic and see if you need money for parking or anything like that. Knowing this type of information ahead of time will greatly reduce your stress on the day of your test.
- Don't do any heavy studying the day before the test. Try to get a good amount of sleep during the nights leading up to the test.
- Eat well. Try to avoid excessive caffeine and sugar. Ideally, in the weeks leading up to the actual test, you should experiment a little bit with foods and practice tests to see which foods give you the most endurance. Aim for steady blood sugar levels during the test: sports drinks, peanut-butter crackers, trail mix, etc. make good snacks for your breaks and lunch.

General Test Day Info and Tips

- On the day of the test, arrive at the test center at least a half hour prior to the start time of your test.
- Examinees will be checked in to the center in the order in which they arrive.
- You will be assigned a locker or secure area in which to put your personal items. Textbooks and study notes are not allowed, so there is no need to bring them with you to the test center.
- Your ID will be checked, your palm vein will be scanned, and you will be asked to sign in.
- You will be given your noteboard booklet and wet-erase marker, and the test center administrator will take you to the computer on which you will complete the test. You may not choose a computer; you must use the computer assigned to you.
- Nothing is allowed at the computer station except your photo ID, your locker key (if provided), and a factory sealed packet of ear plugs; not even your watch.
- If you choose to leave the testing room at the breaks, you will have your palm vein scanned again, and you will have to sign in and out.
- You are allowed to access the items in your locker, except for notes and cell phones. (Check your test center's policy on cell phones ahead of time; some centers do not even allow them to be kept in your locker.)
- Don't forget to bring the snack foods and lunch you experimented with in your practice tests.
- At the end of the test, the test administrator will collect your noteboard.
- Definitely take the breaks! Get up and walk around. It's a good way to clear your head between sections and get the blood (and oxygen!) flowing to your brain.
- Ask for a clean noteboard at the breaks if you use up all the space, or if you just want a fresh one for the next section.

Chapter 2
Overview and Strategy of the Science Sections

This chapter is designed to present you with an overview of the types of passages and questions that will appear in the science sections of the MCAT and to give you some general strategies for dealing with them. For more in-depth information on strategy for both the science and CARS sections, check out our comprehensive resource, *The Princeton Review MCAT*.

2.1   SCIENCE SECTIONS OVERVIEW

There are three science sections on the MCAT.

- Chemical and Physical Foundations of Biological Systems
- Biological and Biochemical Foundations of Living Systems
- Psychological, Social, and Biological Foundations of Behavior

The Chemical and Physical Foundations of Biological Systems section (Chem/Phys) is the first section on the test. It includes questions from General Chemistry (about 35%), Physics (about 25%), Organic Chemistry (about 15%), and Biochemistry (about 25%). Further, the questions often test chemical and physical concepts within a biological setting: for example, pressure and fluid flow in blood vessels. A solid grasp of math fundamentals is required (arithmetic, algebra, graphs, trigonometry, vectors, proportions, and logarithms); however, there are no calculus-based questions.

The Biological and Biochemical Foundations of Living Systems section (Bio/Biochem) is the third section on the test. Approximately 65% of the questions in this section come from biology, approximately 25% come from biochemistry, and approximately 10% come from Organic and General Chemistry. Math calculations are generally not required on this section of the test; however, a basic understanding of statistics as used in biological research is helpful.

The Psychological, Social, and Biological Foundations of Behavior section (Psych/Soc) is the fourth and final section on the test. About 65% of the questions will be drawn from Psychology (and about 5% of these will be biologically-based), about 30% from Sociology, and about 5% from Biology. As with the Bio/Biochem section, calculations are generally not required, however, a basic understanding of statistics as used in research is helpful.

Most of the questions in the science sections (44 of the 59) are passage-based, and each section has ten passages. Passages consist of a few paragraphs of information and include equations, reactions, graphs, figures, tables, experiments, and data. Four to six questions will be associated with each passage.

The remaining 25% of the questions (15 of 59) in each science section are freestanding questions (FSQs). These questions appear in approximately four groups interspersed between the passages. Each group contains four to five questions.

95 minutes are allotted to each of the science sections. This breaks down to approximately one minute and 35 seconds per question.

2.2 PASSAGES VS. FSQS: WHAT TO START WITH

Passages vs. FSQs in the Science Sections: What to Start With

Since the questions are displayed on separate screens, it is awkward and time consuming to click through all of the questions up front to find the FSQs. Therefore, go through the section on a first pass and decide whether to do the passage now or to save it for later, basing your decision on the passage text and the first question. Tackle the FSQs as you come upon them. More details are below.

Here is an outline of the procedure:

1) For each passage, write a heading on your noteboard with the passage number, the general topic, and its range of questions (e.g., "Passage 1, thermodynamics, Q 1–5" or "Passage 2, enzymes, Q 6–9). The passage numbers do not currently appear in the Navigation or Review screens, thus having the question numbers on your noteboard will allow you to move through the section more efficiently.

2) Skim the text and decide if you want to do the passage now or later. If a passage is a "Now," complete it before moving on to the next passage (also see "Attacking the Questions" below). If it is a "Later" passage, first write "SKIPPED" in block letters under the passage heading on your noteboard and leave room for your work when you come back to complete that passage. (Note that the specific passages you skip will be unique to you; in the Bio/Biochem section, you might choose to do all Biology passages first, then come back for Biochemistry. Or in Chem/Phys you might choose to skip experiment-based or analytical passages…know ahead of time what type of passage you are going to skip and follow your plan.)

3) Next, click on the "Navigation" button at the bottom to get to the Navigation screen. Click on the first question of the next passage; you'll be able to identify it because you know the range of questions from the passage you just skipped. This will take you to the next passage, where you will repeat steps 1–3.

4) Once you have completed your first pass through the section, go to the Review screen and click the first question for the first passage you skipped. Answer the questions and continue going back to the Review screen and repeating this procedure for other passages you have skipped.

Attacking the Questions

As you work through the questions, if you encounter a particularly lengthy question, or a question that requires a lot of analysis, you may choose to skip it. This is a wise strategy because it ensures you will tackle all the easier questions first, the ones you are more likely to get right. If you choose to skip the question (or if you attempt it but get stuck), write down the question number and the word "SKIP" on your noteboard and move on to the next question. At the end of the passage, click "Previous" to move back through the set of questions and complete any that you skipped over the first time through. Make sure that you have filled in an answer for every question.

2.3   SCIENCE PASSAGE TYPES

The passages in the science sections fall into one of three main categories: Information and/or Situation Presentation, Experiment/Research Presentation, or Persuasive Reasoning.

Information and/or Situation Presentation

These passages either present straightforward scientific information or they describe a particular event or occurrence. Generally, questions associated with these passages test basic science facts or ask you to predict outcomes given new variables or new information. Here is an example of an Information/Situation Presentation passage:

Figure 1 shows a portion of the inner mechanism of a typical home smoke detector. It consists of a pair of capacitor plates which are charged by a 9-volt battery (not shown). The capacitor plates (electrodes) are connected to a sensor device, D; the resistor, R, denotes the internal resistance of the sensor. Normally, air acts as an insulator and no current would flow in the circuit shown. However, inside the smoke detector is a small sample of an artificially produced radioactive element, americium-241, which decays primarily by emitting alpha particles, with a half-life of approximately 430 years. The daughter nucleus of the decay has a half-life in excess of two million years and therefore poses virtually no biohazard.

The decay products (alpha particles and gamma rays) from the 241Am sample ionize air molecules between the plates and thus provide a conducting pathway which allows current to flow in the circuit shown in Figure 1. A steady-state current is quickly established and remains as long as the battery continues to maintain a 9-volt potential difference between its terminals. However, if smoke particles enter the space between the capacitor plates and thereby interrupt the flow, the current is reduced, and the sensor responds to this change by triggering the alarm. (Furthermore, as the battery starts to "die out," the resulting drop in current is also detected to alert the homeowner to replace the battery.)

$$C = \varepsilon_0 \frac{A}{d}$$

Equation 1

where ε_0 is the universal permittivity constant, equal to 8.85×10^{-12} C^2/(N m^2). Since the area A of each capacitor plate in the smoke detector is 20 cm^2 and the plates are separated by a distance d of 5 mm, the capacitance is 3.5×10^{-12} F = 3.5 pF.

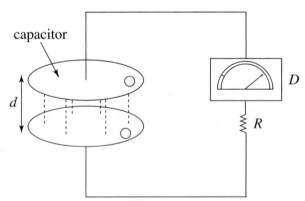

Figure 1   Smoke detector mechanism

Experiment/Research Presentation

These passages present the details of experiments and research procedures. They often include data tables and graphs. Generally, questions associated with these passages ask you to interpret data, draw conclusions, and make inferences. Here is an example of an Experiment/Research Presentation passage:

The development of sexual characteristics depends upon various factors, the most important of which are hormonal control, environmental stimuli, and the genetic makeup of the individual. The hormones that contribute to the development include the steroid hormones estrogen, progesterone, and testosterone, as well as the pituitary hormones FSH (follicle-stimulating hormone) and LH (luteinizing hormone).

To study the mechanism by which estrogen exerts its effects, a researcher performed the following experiments using cell culture assays.

Experiment 1:

Human embryonic placental mesenchyme (HEPM) cells were grown for 48 hours in Dulbecco's Modified Eagle Medium (DMEM), with media change every 12 hours. Upon confluent growth, cells were exposed to a 10 mg per mL solution of green fluorescent-labeled estrogen for 1 hour. Cells were rinsed with DMEM and observed under confocal fluorescent microscopy.

Experiment 2:

HEPM cells were grown to confluence as in Experiment 1. Cells were exposed to Pesticide A for 1 hour, followed by the 10 mg/mL solution of labeled estrogen, rinsed as in Experiment 1, and observed under confocal fluorescent microscopy.

Experiment 3:

Experiment 1 was repeated with Chinese Hamster Ovary (CHO) cells instead of HEPM cells.

Experiment 4:

CHO cells injected with cytoplasmic extracts of HEPM cells were grown to confluence, exposed to the 10 mg/mL solution of labeled estrogen for 1 hour, and observed under confocal fluorescent microscopy.

The results of these experiments are given in Table 1.

Experiment	Media	Cytoplasm	Nucleus
1	+	+	+
2	+	+	+
3	+	+	+
4	+	+	+

Table 1 Detection of Estrogen (+ indicates presence of estrogen)

After observing the cells in each experiment, the researcher bathed the cells in a solution containing 10 mg per mL of a red fluorescent probe that binds specifically to the estrogen receptor only when its active site is occupied. After 1 hour, the cells were rinsed with DMEM and observed under confocal fluorescent microscopy. The results are presented in Table 2. The researcher also repeated Experiment 2 using Pesticide B, an estrogen analog, instead of Pesticide A. Results from other researchers had shown that Pesticide B binds to the active site of the cytosolic estrogen receptor (with an affinity 10,000 times greater than that of estrogen) and causes increased transcription of mRNA.

Experiment	Media	Cytoplasm	Nucleus	Estrogen effects observed?
1	G only	G and R	G and R	Yes
2	G only	G only	G only	No
3	G only	G only	G only	No
4	G only	G and R	G and R	Yes

Table 2 Observed Fluorescence and Estrogen Effects (G = green, R = red)

Based on these results, the researcher determined that estrogen had no effect when not bound to a cytosolic, estrogen-specific receptor.

Persuasive Reasoning

These passages typically present a scientific phenomenon along with a hypothesis that explains the phenomenon, and may include counter-arguments as well. Questions associated with these passages ask you to evaluate the hypothesis or arguments. Persuasive Reasoning passages in the science sections of the MCAT tend to be less common than Information Presentation or Experiment-based passages. Here is an example of a Persuasive Reasoning passage:

Two theoretical chemists attempted to explain the observed trends of acidity by applying two interpretations of molecular orbital theory. Consider the pK_a values of some common acids listed along with their conjugate bases:

acid	pK_a	conjugate base
H_2SO_4	< 0	HSO_4^-
H_2CrO_4	5.0	$HCrO_4^-$
H_2PO_4	2.1	$H_2PO_4^-$
HF	3.9	F^-
HOCl	7.8	ClO^-
HCN	9.5	CN^-
HIO_3	1.2	IO_3^-

Recall that acids with a $pK_a < 0$ are called strong acids, and those with a $pK_a > 0$ are called weak acids. The arguments of the chemists are given below.

Chemist #1:

"The acidity of a compound is proportional to the polarization of the H—X bond, where X is some nonmetal element. Complex acids, such as H_2SO_4, $HClO_4$, and HNO_3, are strong acids because the H—O bonding electrons are strongly drawn toward the oxygen. It is generally true that a covalent bond weakens as its polarization increases. Therefore, one can conclude that the strength of an acid is proportional to the number of electronegative atoms in that acid."

Chemist #2:

"The acidity of a compound is proportional to the number of stable resonance structures of that acid's conjugate base. H_2SO_4, $HClO_4$, and HNO_3 are all strong acids because their respective conjugate bases exhibit a high degree of resonance stabilization."

A NOTE ABOUT PSYCH/SOC PASSAGES

Passages in the Psychology and Sociology section of the MCAT tend to be a blend of Information and Experiment Presentation passages. They often present data from recent research studies. For example, consider the following Psych/Soc passage:

Psychotic disorders—most notably schizophrenia and bipolar disorder with psychotic features—affect approximately 2% of Americans. These disorders are extremely manageable with psychotropic medications—to relieve symptoms such as hallucinations and delusions—and behavioral therapy, such as social skills training and hygiene maintenance.

However, individuals with psychotic disorders have the lowest level of medication compliance, as compared to individuals with mood or anxiety disorders. Antipsychotic medications can have extremely negative side effects, including uncontrollable twitching of the face or limbs, blurred vision, and weight gain, among others. They also must be taken frequently, and at high doses, in order to be effective. While relatively little is known about the reasons for noncompliance, studies do suggest that in schizophrenia, age of schizophrenia diagnosis and medication compliance is positively correlated. Evidence also suggests that medication noncompliance is disproportionally prevalent in individuals of a low socioeconomic status (SES) due to issues such as homelessness, lack of insurance benefits, and lack of familial or social support.

Researchers were interested to see how drug education might affect compliance or noncompliance with psychotropic medications based on patient socioeconomic status. In a study of 1200 mentally ill individuals in the Los Angeles metro area, researchers measured baseline psychotropic medication compliance, then provided patients with a free educational seminar on drug therapy, and then measured psychotropic medication compliance six months later. The one-day, 8-hour seminar included information on positive effects of psychotropic medication, side effects of psychotropic medication, psychotropic medication interactions with other substances such as alcohol and non-prescribed drugs, and information on accessing Medicare benefits. Compliance was measured by number of doses of prescribed psychotropic medication that the patients took in a week, over the course of 12 weeks, as compared to the number of doctor-recommended doses per week. Compliance was measured using a self-report questionnaire.

Results indicated that post-seminar, mentally ill patients from middle or upper class backgrounds (Upper and Middle SES) were significantly more compliant with their psychotropic medication regimens than prior to the seminar. However, no significant differences were found in patients at or below the poverty level (Lower SES). Table 1 displays psychotropic medication compliance by SES and disorder.

Disorder	SES	Pre-Seminar Compliance	Post-Seminar Compliance
Bipolar I	Upper	60%	73%
	Middle	57%	61%
	Lower	25%	27%
Schizophrenia	Upper	53%	65%
	Middle	51%	62%
	Lower	22%	26%

Table 1 Psychotropic Medication Compliance by Socioeconomic Status (SES) and Disorder

MAPPING A PASSAGE

"Mapping a passage" refers to the combination of skimming, on-screen highlighting, and noteboard notes that you take while working through a passage.

Reading the Passage

"Reading" in the sense that we commonly use the word is seldom the best way to read MCAT passages. A kind of "informed skimming" is usually the best strategy. A quick scan of the passage, including reading the first sentence, should be enough to tell you its topic and type, and it will help you decide whether to do it now or postpone it until you've tackled easier passages. Once you decide to do a passage, try not to get bogged down reading all the little details. Generally, you should read for location of information, without doing too much heavy analysis of data or experiments at this time. You can always come back and ponder them further if you are asked a question about them.

Highlighting

Resist the temptation to highlight everything! (Everyone has done this: you're reading a science textbook with a highlighter, and then look back and realize that the whole page is yellow!) Restrict your highlighting to a few things:

- the main theme of a paragraph
- an unusual or unfamiliar term that is defined specifically for that passage (e.g., something that is italicized)
- statements that either support the main theme or contradict the main theme
- list topics
- equations
- relationships (for example, one thing increases while another decreases)

The Noteboard Booklet

Keep your noteboard organized! Resist the temptation to write on any blank space.

1) Label your noteboard with the passage number, range of questions, and topic for that passage (for example, "P2, Q5–9, enzymes").
2) For each paragraph, note P1, P2, etc. on the noteboard and jot down a few notes about that paragraph.
3) Jot down any important conclusions you come to as you skim the passage and/or answer the questions.
4) For physics passages only: write down any given equations and leave some space to work with them. Also, redraw any simple diagrams and label any values given (note that some values might be found in the text around the diagram). In some cases, you may need to manipulate the figures to answer questions, and you can't do this with figures on the computer screen. For passages that don't include many diagrams or equations, write down any equations and basic ideas you recall about the passage topic. For example, in a passage about perfectly inelastic collisions, you might write down $p = m\mathbf{v}$, and "momentum conserved, KE not."
5) As you tackle the questions, label each question and its work (if needed) on the noteboard.

2.4 SCIENCE QUESTION TYPES

Questions in the science sections are generally one of three main types: Memory, Explicit, or Implicit.

Memory Questions

These questions can be answered directly from prior knowledge, with no need to reference the passage or question text. Memory questions represent approximately 25 percent of the science questions on the MCAT. Usually, Memory questions are found as FSQs, but they can also be tucked into a passage. Here's an example of a Memory question:

> Which of the following acetylating conditions will convert diethylamine into an amide at the fastest rate?
>
> A) Acetic acid / HCl
> B) Acetic anhydride
> C) Acetyl chloride
> D) Ethyl acetate

If you find that you are missing a fair number of Memory questions, it is a sure sign that you don't know the science content well enough. Go back and review.

Explicit Questions

Explicit questions can be answered primarily with information from the passage, along with prior knowledge. They may require data retrieval, graph analysis, or making a simple connection. Explicit questions make up approximately 35–40 percent of the science questions on the MCAT; here's an example (taken from the Information/Situation Presentation passage above):

> The sensor device D shown in Figure 1 performs its function by acting as:
>
> A) an ohmmeter.
> B) a voltmeter.
> C) a potentiometer.
> D) an ammeter.

If you find that you are missing Explicit questions, practice your passage mapping. Make sure you aren't missing the critical items in the passage that lead you to the right answer. Slow down a little; take an extra 15–30 seconds per passage to read or think about it more carefully.

Implicit Questions

These questions require you to take information from the passage, combine it with your prior knowledge, apply it to a new situation, and come to some logical conclusion. They typically require more complex connections than do Explicit questions, and they may also require data retrieval, graph analysis, etc. Implicit questions usually require a solid understanding of the passage information. They make up approximately 35–40 percent of the science questions on the MCAT; here's an example (taken from the Experiment/Research Presentation passage above):

If Experiment 2 were repeated, but this time exposing the cells first to Pesticide A and then to Pesticide B before exposing them to the green fluorescent-labeled estrogen and the red fluorescent probe, which of the following statements will most likely be true?

A) Pesticide A and Pesticide B bind to the same site on the estrogen receptor.
B) Estrogen effects would be observed.
C) Only green fluorescence would be observed.
D) Both green and red fluorescence would be observed.

Here's another example of an Implicit Question taken from the Psych/Soc passage above:

Suppose the experiment described in the passage were repeated, but instead of testing how drug education affects compliance, researchers measured how incentives affect compliance in low SES schizophrenics. The low SES schizophrenia group was broken into two groups. Group A received an incentive every time they took their medication for seven consecutive days, while Group B received an incentive every two weeks, regardless of compliance level. Based on operant conditioning principles, what results should the researchers see?

A) No difference in compliance levels from the first study.
B) Group A's compliance should be higher than Group B's compliance.
C) Group B's compliance should be higher than Group A's compliance.
D) Both groups should demonstrate increased compliance from the first study, but it is impossible to tell which group's compliance is expected to be higher.

If you find that you are missing a lot of Implicit questions, make sure first of all that you are using POE aggressively. Second, go back and review the explanations for the correct answers, and figure out where your logic went awry. Did you miss an important fact in the passage? Did you forget the relevant science content? Did you miss a connection to the data? Did you follow the logical train of thought to the right answer? Once you figure out where you made your mistake, you will know how to correct it.

Science Question Strategies

1) Remember that the potential content in the science sections is vast, so don't panic if something seems completely unfamiliar. Understand the basic content well, find the basics in the unfamiliar topic, and apply them to the question.

2) Process of Elimination is paramount! The Strikethrough button allows you to eliminate answer choices; this will improve your chances of guessing the correct answer if you are unable to narrow it down to one choice.

3) Answer the straightforward questions first (typically the memory questions). Leave questions that require analysis of experiments and graphs for later. Take the test in the order YOU want. Make sure to use your noteboard to indicate questions you have skipped.

4) Make sure that the answer you choose actually answers the question, and isn't just a true statement.

5) Try to avoid answer choices with extreme words such as "always," "never," etc. In the sciences, there is almost always an exception and answers are rarely black-and-white.

6) I-II-III questions: Whenever possible, start by evaluating the Roman numeral item that shows up in exactly two answer choices. This will allow you to quickly eliminate two wrong answer choices regardless of whether the item is true or false. Typically then, you will only have to assess one of the other Roman numeral items to determine the correct answer. Always work between the I-II-III statements and the answer choices. Once an item is found to be true (or false), strike out answer choices which do not contain (or do contain) that item number. Make sure to strike out the actual Roman numeral item as well, and highlight those items that are true.

7) LEAST/EXCEPT/NOT questions: Don't get tricked by these questions that ask you to pick the answer that doesn't fit (the incorrect or false statement). It's often good to use your noteboard and write a T or F next to answer choices A–D. The one that stands out as different is the correct answer!

8) 2 × 2 style questions: These questions require you to know two pieces of information to get the correct answer, and are easily identified by their answer choices, which commonly take the form A because X, B because X, A because Y, B because Y. Tackle one piece of information at a time, which should allow you to quickly eliminate two answer choices.

9) Ranking questions: When asked to rank items, look for an extreme—either the greatest or the smallest item—and eliminate answer choices that do not have that item shown at the correct end of the ranking. This is often enough to eliminate one to three answer choices. Based on the remaining choices, look for the other extreme at the other end of the ranking and use POE again.

10) If you read a question and do not know how to answer it, look to the passage for help. It is likely that the passage contains information pertinent to answering the question, either within the text or in the form of experimental data.

11) If a question requires a lengthy calculation, mark it and return to it later, particularly if you are slow with arithmetic or dimensional analysis.

12) Don't leave any question blank. There is no guessing penalty on the MCAT.

2.5 SUMMARY OF THE APPROACH TO SCIENCE PASSAGES AND QUESTIONS

How to Map the Passage and Use the Noteboard Booklet

1) The passage should not be read like textbook material, with the intent of learning something from every sentence (science majors especially will be tempted to read this way). Passages should be read to get a feel for the type of questions that will follow, and to get a general idea of the location of information within the passage.

2) Highlighting—Use this tool sparingly, or you will end up with a passage that is completely covered in yellow highlighter! Highlighting in a science passage should be used to draw attention to a few words that demonstrate one of the following:
   - the main theme of a paragraph
   - an unusual or unfamiliar term that is defined specifically for that passage (e.g., something that is italicized)
   - statements that either support the main theme or counteract the main theme
   - list topics (see below)

3) Pay brief attention to equations, figures, and experiments, noting only what information they deal with. Do not spend a lot of time analyzing at this point. For physics passages, jot down the equations in a row with room to work beneath them. Copy simple figures to which you can add force or kinematics vectors, simplified circuit diagrams, or other details that allow you to see directly what's happening. Physics generally involves the most noteboard work of all the sciences.

4) For each passage, start by noting the passage number, the general topic, and the range of questions on your noteboard. You can then work between your noteboard and the Review screen to easily get to the questions you want to.

5) For each paragraph, note "P1," "P2," etc. on the noteboard and jot down a few notes about that paragraph. Try to translate science jargon into your own words using everyday language. Especially note down simple relationships (for example, the relationship between two variables).

6) Lists—Whenever a list appears in paragraph form, jot down on the noteboard the paragraph and the general topic of the list. It will make returning to the passage more efficient and help to organize your thoughts.

7) The noteboard will only be useful if it is kept organized! Make sure that your notes for each passage are clearly delineated and marked with the passage number and question range. This will allow you to easily read your notes when you come back to a review a Flagged question. Resist the temptation to write in the first available blank space as this makes it much more difficult to refer back to your work.

Chapter 3
CARS Strategy

This chapter is designed to present you with an overview of the types of passages and questions that will appear in the Critical Analysis and Reasoning Skills (CARS) section of the MCAT, and to give you some general strategies for dealing with them. For more in-depth information on strategy for both the science and CARS sections, check out our comprehensive resource, *The Princeton Review MCAT*.

3.1 CRITICAL ANALYSIS AND REASONING SKILLS STRATEGY OVERVIEW

Critical Analysis and Reasoning Skills (CARS) is the second section of the test. It consists of nine passages, which typically average 500–700 words each. Each passage is followed by 5–7 questions (with four answer choices per question), for a total of 53 questions. Unlike the science sections, CARS has no freestanding questions.

Pacing

You will have 90 minutes to complete the section. However, you do not necessarily need to complete all 53 questions and all nine passages to get a competitive score. Many people will maximize their score by randomly guessing on at least one passage and focusing on getting a high percentage of the rest of the questions correct. Also, keep in mind that there is no guessing penalty. Never leave a question blank; always select a random guess for questions that you choose not to complete. You have a 25 percent chance of getting those questions right.

Content

The passages may be on any subject in the humanities and social sciences. This possible range of topics may seem overwhelming. However, unlike the science sections of the test, **CARS does not test your outside knowledge of the subject.** In fact, using your own factual knowledge or opinions of the subject can lead you to pick incorrect answers; the questions require you to use only the information provided in the question and in the passage. Clearly, you can't prepare for or approach the CARS section of the test in the same way as physics or chemistry!

Skill Development

There are many false beliefs regarding the CARS section, one of which is that your score depends on luck. That is, if you happen to get "good" passages, all is well, but if you don't, you are in trouble. However, this is entirely untrue. There are ways that you can improve your CARS score regardless of the passages you happen to get on your test. BUT...to achieve this improvement, many, if not most, of you will need to fundamentally change how you read the passages and go about answering the questions. You will need to develop new skills that have little to do with memorization and everything to do with reading efficiently and thinking critically. The good news is that these are skills that everyone can acquire and refine through practice and careful self-evaluation. These core skills fall into three basic categories.

Working the Passage

- Reading the passage efficiently: identifying the most important points made by the author while moving quickly through the details
- Following the logical structure of the author's argument: identifying such things as key shifts in direction, comparisons and contrasts, conclusions, and the author's tone
- Synthesizing the Bottom Line of the entire passage: identifying the author's Main Idea and Attitude

Attacking the Questions

- Correctly identifying and translating the questions: knowing what each question is asking you to do in order to choose the correct answer
- Using the passage (and only the passage) as a resource: quickly locating the relevant passage information for each question
- Answering in your own words: predicting what the correct answer will do before considering the answer choices
- Using Process of Elimination (POE): eliminating down to the "least wrong" choice rather than just picking an answer that "sounds good"

General Test Strategy

- Time management: getting what you need from the passage without getting bogged down in irrelevant facts or spending too much time on one question
- Pacing and accuracy: not going so fast that you miss a high percentage of the questions that you complete, or so slow that you overthink the questions or do not complete enough questions to reach your target score
- Stress management: thinking clearly and working efficiently under stressful conditions

Self-Evaluation

Every student has different strengths and weaknesses on the MCAT CARS section. To improve on your weaknesses, you must first recognize them. From now on, keep a chart or log of every passage that you do. After you complete a passage, go through each question. Pay particular attention to those questions that you got wrong. Don't just go over why the right answer is right and the wrong answers are wrong. It is even more important to diagnose what led you to your wrong answer. In order to increase your score, you'll need to assess and change the way that you read and think. You may not even realize that you're making the same mistake over and over again until you see it logged into your chart several times.

However, don't just think about the questions you got wrong—also analyze how you arrived at the credited response when your answers are correct. Did you avoid a common trap? Are there question types on which you are particularly strong? Did you successfully apply one of our techniques?

Look for patterns in your mistakes and successes; based on those patterns, define specific aspects of your approach that you can change in order to raise your score.

3.2 FUNDAMENTALS: THE SIX STEPS

Here are the six steps to follow when working the CARS section.

■ STEP 1: RANK AND ORDER THE PASSAGES

Ranking: Now, Later, or Killer

The passages are not necessarily, or even usually, presented in order of difficulty. There is no reason to waste time on the hardest passage or passages, only to skip or rush through an easy passage at the end of the section. Therefore, your first step as you hit each new passage is to decide if it is a Now (or easier) passage, a Later (or harder) passage, or a Killer passage (one that you will simply randomly guess on, or do last). To assign a rank, skim a few sentences of the passage and see if you can easily paraphrase it. If you can, it's most likely an easier passage. If not, it is likely to be a harder passage that you should either come back to later during your 90 minutes or just randomly guess on.

Ordering: The Two Pass System

Take two passes through the section, doing the easier passages first, and then coming back in a second pass for at least some of the harder passages. If a passage is a Now passage, go ahead and work it through, completing all of the questions. If it is a Later or Killer passage, first write "Skipped" on your noteboard under a heading with the passage number and range of questions. Then, as you move forward through the questions to the next passage, "Flag" each question and at the same time fill in a random guess (always guess the same letter). Once you have completed the Now passages in the section, come back through the section for your second pass, completing the Later passages.

■ STEP 2: PREVIEW THE QUESTIONS

Knowing what topics show up in the questions will help you work the passage more quickly and effectively. Before working the passage, read through the question stems from first to last (not the answer choices), identifying and highlighting any words or phrases that indicate important passage content. Do not worry at this stage about understanding the question or identifying the question type.

■ STEP 3: WORK THE PASSAGE

Stay on the screen for the last question and work the passage from there. As you read through the passage, use the highlighting function (sparingly) to annotate the most important references in the text. This includes things like question topics from the preview, topic sentences, shifts in direction or continuations, indications of the author's tone, different points of view, and conclusions. As you read, articulate the Main Point of each chunk of information (usually, each paragraph). Use your noteboard, especially on difficult passages, to jot down these main points. As you move through the passage, think about how these chunks relate to each other; that is, track the logical structure of the author's argument in the passage.

■ STEP 4: BOTTOM LINE

After you have read the entire passage, sum up the Bottom Line: the main idea and tone of the entire passage. For particularly difficult passages, write this down on your noteboard to make sure that you have a reasonably clear idea of the point and purpose of the passage as a whole.

■ STEP 5: ATTACK THE QUESTIONS

Answer the questions in reverse order, so that you don't need to click back to the first question for that passage. As you work through each question, follow these steps:

- Read the question word for word and identify the question type (see Section 3.3 for more on this).
- Translate the question task into your own words, thinking about what the question is asking you to do with or to the passage.
- When the question stem provides a specific reference to the passage, go back to the passage before reading the answer choices and find the relevant information (reading at least five lines above and below the reference).
- Paraphrase the passage information. Then, with the question type firmly in mind, think about what the correct answer needs to do.
- As you go through the choices, use POE actively. Look for reasons to strike out incorrect choices, and select the "least wrong" of the four.
- If you hit a particularly difficult question, skip over it for the moment and complete the other easier questions for that passage. Then move forward through the questions toward the next passage, completing any questions that you initially skipped.

■ STEP 6: INSPECT THE SECTION

At or before the 5-minute mark (ideally, before you begin your last passage), double-check to make sure that you haven't left any incomplete questions. You can use the Review Screen functions at this stage, if you like. Do NOT rethink questions you have already completed. Your goal in this step is simply to make sure that you have selected an answer for each question.

3.3 CARS QUESTION TYPES

In order to effectively attack a question, you must understand what that question is asking you to do. There are four categories of CARS questions, including ten different question types.

Specific Questions

1. Retrieval

Retrieval questions test your ability to locate information in the passage. They may also involve simple paraphrasing and summarizing, but they do not require any substantial analysis or interpretation. They will include some specific reference to passage information (a person's name, a theory, a time period, etc.). The correct answer will often be a paraphrase of something stated in the passage about that reference.

Retrieval questions may be phrased in the following ways:

- "According to the passage, the three components of Brown's theory are…"
- "The passage states that Brown's theory is rejected by…"

2. Inference

Inference questions are the most common question type in the CARS section. They require you to choose the answer that is best supported by the passage.

There is no such thing as being "too close" to the passage to qualify as a correct answer to an Inference question. An answer that directly paraphrases the passage may in fact be the credited response. On the other hand, the correct answer may seem debatable (that is, you could argue that it isn't literally deducible from the passage information), but it will still be better supported by the passage text than the other three choices.

There are a variety of ways in which Inference questions can be phrased. Here are some examples of how these questions can be worded:

- "It can be inferred from the passage that…"
- "An assumption underlying the author's discussion of Brown's theory is that…"
- "The author implies/suggests/indicates that Brown's theory is most closely linked to…"
- "By 'only dimly perceived,' the author most likely means:"
- "Based on information in the passage, it can be most reasonably concluded that…"
- "With which of the following statements would the author be most likely to agree?"
- "Which of the following statements is best supported by the passage?"

General Questions

3. Main Idea/Primary Purpose

These questions require you to summarize the various claims made in the text into a general statement of the central point or primary activity of the passage. Think of the passage as an argument. The Main Idea is the overall claim, supported by specific evidence in the various paragraphs, that the author wants to convince you to accept as true. The Primary Purpose is very closely related; it will express what the author does in order to convey the Main Idea.

Good active reading is the key to these questions. Connect the main points of the paragraphs as you read the passage. At the end of the passage, define a main theme or claim that links those main points to each other. Include the author's tone or attitude; an answer may have the correct content and scope, but if the tone or attitude doesn't match the passage, the choice is incorrect. Additionally, if an answer is too narrow (for example, only one of several points made by the author), it is also incorrect.

Main Idea questions are often phrased in the following ways:

- "The main idea of the passage is that…"
- "The central thesis of this passage is…"

Primary Purpose questions are often phrased as follows:

- "The author's primary purpose is to explain that…"

4. General Tone/Attitude

Tone and Attitude questions ask you to evaluate whether or not the author expresses an opinion regarding the material in the passage, and if so, to judge how strongly positive or negative that opinion is. Wrong answers may have the wrong tone overall (for example, the author is critical of an idea but the answer indicates the author is in favor of that idea) or they may be too extreme (for example, the author is moderately critical of an idea, and the wrong answer indicates that the author strongly condemns it).

Tone/Attitude questions are often phrase as follows:

- "In this passage, the author's tone is one of…"
- "The author's attitude can best be described as…"

Reasoning Questions

5. Structure

Structure questions ask you to describe how the author makes his or her argument. They differ from other questions in that they address the passage's construction or logical structure along with its content. Structure questions most often ask you for the purpose of a particular reference within the passage. Alternatively, a Structure question might cite a claim from the passage and ask you how that claim is supported by the author.

To answer these questions, it is crucial to identify the Main Point of the paragraph or chunk of information in which a reference cited in the question appears, and to separate the claims made by the author from the evidence (if any is given) supporting those claims. Look for words—like "for example" or "for instance"—that indicate that what comes next is the support or evidence, and conclusion words—like "therefore" or "thus"—that indicate that what comes next is the claim being supported.

Structure questions may be worded as follows:

- "The author most likely mentions the controversy surrounding Brown's ideas in order to…"
- "The author's claim that Brown's theory is unique is supported by:"

6. Evaluate

Evaluate questions are similar to Structure questions in that you need to identify the logical structure of the author's argument. Evaluate questions, however, go a step farther by asking **how well** an author supports his or her claims. That is, the question asks you to evaluate whether or not the author does a good job justifying his or her conclusions.

The answers for these questions often come in two parts. One part will be some version of "strongly" or "weakly" supported. The other part will be the explanation or justification for that evaluation (for example, that it is weakly supported because no examples are given, or, strongly supported because relevant examples are provided).

Alternatively, an Evaluate question may ask you whether or not the author's logic is valid or internally consistent, or how the author's argument is flawed. The answers to this form of the question may not include the words "strongly" or "weakly," but they will still evaluate the strength (or lack thereof) of the author's argument.

These questions may be phrased as follows:

- "The author asserts that Brown's theoretical model is 'dangerously incomplete.' The support offered for this conclusion is…"
- "Is Brown's analysis of the implications of Herrera's theoretical model well supported?"
- "The author's criticism of Brown's argument is flawed because it:"

Application Questions

7. Strengthen

A Strengthen question asks you to find the answer that most supports the passage. That is, the correct answer will make the author's argument more convincing than it already was.

Notice that Strengthen questions often use the phrase, "which of the following, if true…." Take those words "if true"—whether implied or explicitly stated—seriously. Do not try to find the answer choices in the passage. Instead, take each statement as a fact and find the one that does what it needs to do to the relevant part of the passage. These questions are quite different from Specific, General, and Reasoning questions in that they give you new information in the answer choices; the correct answer will change (for the better), not just describe or reflect, the passage. These questions are also distinct from other question types (except for Weaken questions) in that it is impossible for an answer to be "too extreme" to be correct.

Strengthen questions may be phrased as follows:

- "Which of the following, if valid, would provide the best support for the author's conclusion in the last paragraph?"
- "Which of the following, if true, would most strengthen the author's claim regarding Brown's theory?"

8. Weaken

A Weaken question requires you to find the answer choice that most undermines or calls into question the claim or claims made by the author. Notice that just like Strengthen questions, Weaken questions often use the phrase, "which of the following, if true…." Take those words "if true"—whether implied or explicitly stated—seriously. Do not try to find the answer choices in the passage. Take each statement as if it were true and find the one that is **most inconsistent** with the relevant part of the passage. These questions are quite different from Specific, General, and Reasoning questions in that they give you new information in the answer choices; the correct answer will change the passage by making the author's argument less convincing than it originally was. These questions are also distinct from other question types (except for Strengthen questions) in that it is impossible for an answer to be "too extreme" to be correct.

Weaken questions are often phrased as follows (the weakening words are always in italics):

- "Which of the following, if valid, would most *weaken* the author's main claim in the third paragraph?"
- "Which of the following, if true, would most *undermine* the author's claim regarding Brown's theory?"

9. New Information

All New Information questions have one thing in common: they provide new facts or scenarios in the question stem that are never mentioned in the passage. That said, the question may require you to do a variety of things with that new information. They may ask you what can be concluded based on the new information in the question in combination with passage information. Or, they might ask what effect the new information has on the passage, or what in the passage would be most weakened or strengthened by it. Regardless, the answer has to have a connection to the new information in the question stem, not just to the passage text.

New Information questions might be phrased as follows:

- "If China experienced an unusually rainy winter, what would also be true, based on the passage?"
- "Which of the following claims made in the passage would be most strengthened by data showing that industrialization has affected global weather patterns?"

10. Analogy

These questions ask you to take something described in the passage, abstract or generalize it, and then apply it to an entirely new situation. They differ from New Information questions in that the new information is in the answer choices, not in the question stem. They differ from Strengthen questions in that the new information in the correct choice will not make the original argument stronger than it already was. It will be similar to it in logic, but is likely to be on a different issue or subject matter. These questions can be tricky, as all the answers at first glance may seem to have nothing to do with the passage. However, you are matching the logic or purpose of the author's argument, not the informational content of the passage. Therefore, the correct answer can match the logic of the passage (or relevant part of the passage) while still bringing in entirely new content.

Analogy questions can be phrased as follows:

- Which of the following is most logically similar to the school reform policy described in the passage?
- The author's discussion of the historical importance of pasta is most comparable to which of the following?

Part 2

MCAT Biochemistry

Chapter 4
Enzymes and Inhibition

FREESTANDING QUESTIONS: ENZYMES AND INHIBITION

1. Assuming that temperature is consistent and not so high as to denature proteins, which of the following would indicate that a chemical reaction is NOT spontaneous?

A) A reaction with a large positive ΔH and a large positive ΔS
B) A reaction with a large positive ΔH and a large negative ΔS
C) A reaction with a small negative ΔH and a large positive ΔS
D) A reaction with a small positive ΔH and a large positive ΔS

2. Which of the following is a true statement?

A) Catalysts increase the energy of activation for a reaction, thus reducing ΔG.
B) Catalysts are always specific and reduce the energy of activation for a reaction.
C) ΔG is unaffected by a catalyst; however, the energy of activation is increased, thereby increasing the rate of the reaction.
D) ΔG remains unaffected by a catalyst, while the energy of activation is reduced.

3. In an oxidation-reduction reaction:

A) the molecule being oxidized loses electrons and the molecule being reduced is known as the oxidizing agent.
B) the molecule being oxidized gains electrons and the molecule being reduced is known as the oxidizing agent.
C) the molecule being reduced loses electrons and is known as the oxidizing agent.
D) the molecule being oxidized loses electrons and is known as the oxidizing agent.

4. Metoprolol, a competitive antagonist (inhibitor) of β-adrenergic receptors, is a commonly prescribed medication resulting in a decrease in heart rate and blood pressure. Which of the following is most likely true?

A) Metoprolol principally affects the parasympathetic division of the autonomic nervous system.
B) The quantity of norepinephrine in the synaptic cleft directly affects the degree of inhibition.
C) Metoprolol binds to an allosteric site on the receptor.
D) K_d (a measure of a receptor's affinity for its ligand) will be unaffected by metoprolol.

5. During the initiation of cytotoxic chemotherapy in select types of cancer, massive tumor lysis (leading to the spilling of cellular contents into circulation) can result in *tumor lysis syndrome*. This potentially life-threatening condition can cause elevated levels of uric acid leading to renal failure. One such contributing pathway results from conversion of xanthine to uric acid (seen below).

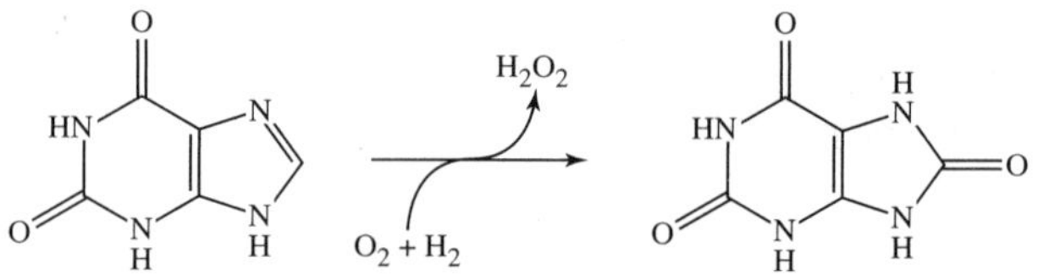

xanthine   uric acid

Which of the following best characterizes this reaction?

A) Carbon serves as an oxidizing agent.
B) Oxygen serves as a reducing agent.
C) There is an increase in the oxidation state of carbon.
D) There is a decrease in the oxidation state of carbon.

6. In a study of mRNA folding, researchers discovered that the fall in free energy due to folding was heavily impacted by nucleotide sequence. What is most likely to be true regarding mRNA folding?

A) mRNA folding results in an increase in ΔS of the transcript.
B) Folded mRNA exists in greater quantities than the unfolded transcript at equilibrium.
C) Folded mRNA exhibits a greater degree of rotational freedom.
D) The intra-molecular nucleotide interactions alone dictate the energetics of mRNA folding.

7. Patients requiring anticoagulation via warfarin are carefully monitored to ensure the medication remains in the therapeutic range. In patients with supratherapeutic (very high) levels of warfarin, elimination of the drug displays zero-order kinetics. Which of the following would be true regarding these patients?

A) The patients would have a decreased risk of bleeding relative to patients in the therapeutic range.
B) Patients would show increased elimination of warfarin with higher serum concentrations of the drug.
C) Elimination rates would be increased by concurrent treatment with injections of vitamin K.
D) The half-life of drug elimination would be dependent on the initial medication concentration.

ENZYMES AND INHIBITION PRACTICE PASSAGE 1

The rough endoplasmic reticulum (ER) is known to be the site of secreted and membrane-bound protein translation, with the proteins being inserted into the lumen of the ER cotranslationally. Animal cells infected with enveloped viruses also use the ER to synthesize and modify viral proteins prior to their insertion in the cell membrane or their assembly into mature virus. The ER is the site of protein folding and disulfide bond formation, which plays a significant role in the final folded structure of many proteins. Disulfide bond formation can occur within a single polypeptide, or between two or more different polypeptides.

Vaccinia virus is a complex virus belonging to the poxvirus family. It is an enveloped virus with a dsDNA genome that encodes approximately 250 genes. It is closely related to the cowpox virus and variola virus (the cause of smallpox), and can be used as a vaccine to prevent smallpox infection. Some of the proteins encoded by the genome are listed in Table 1 below.

Protein Name	Molecular mass (kDa)	Gene Name	Location in Virus
4a	65	A10L	C
p16	14–16	A14L	M
p21	23–25	A17L	M
p25	25	L4R	C
p35	35	H3L	M
p39	40–45	A4L	C

Table 1 Some vaccinia virus proteins; C = core, M = membrane

The formation of intracellular mature virus (IMV) is highly dependent on disulfide bonding. p16 and p21 form dimers in mature virus (more than 50% of these proteins were found in dimer form), while p35 also dimerizes, but to a lesser extent (approximately 30% of p35 was found as a dimer).

To track the dimer formation of p16, HeLa cells were infected with vaccinia virus and pulse-labeled with ^{35}S-methionine at 6 hours after infection, then chased for 4 hours. Pulse-labeling is a technique where a small amount of radioactivity is introduced for a short time period, then tracked for several hours afterwards. Cell lysates were prepared at different time periods and p16 was immunoprecipitated from them, then separated by gel electrophoresis in both reducing and nonreducing conditions. Dithiothreitol (DTT) was used as a reducing agent. Visualization was via autoradiography; the results are shown in Figure 1.

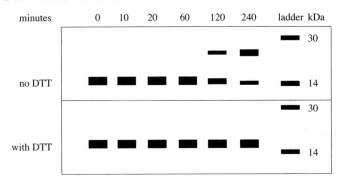

Figure 1 Results of pulse-chase experiment on p16 dimerization

Adapted from Locker, J.K. and Griffiths, G, *An Unconventional Role for Cytoplasmic Disulfide Bonds in Vaccinia Virus Proteins*, J Cell Biol, 1999.

1. Given that most disulfide bond formation occurs in the lumen of the ER and not in the cytoplasm, which of the following statements is true?

   A) Both the ER lumen and the cytoplasm are reducing environments.
   B) Both the ER lumen and the cytoplasm are oxidizing environments.
   C) The ER lumen is an oxidizing environment, while the cytoplasm is a reducing environment.
   D) The ER lumen is a reducing environment, while the cytoplasm is an oxidizing environment.

2. The results shown in Figure 1 indicate that:

   A) p16 dimerization was prevented by DTT because it prevents the formation of, or breaks, disulfide bonds.
   B) the additional band at 240 minutes in the absence of DTT must be due to dimerization with a different protein.
   C) the absence of reducing conditions prevented the dimerization of p16.
   D) because the band indicating dimerization is less than 30 kDa, no conclusion can be made about the effect of DTT on dimerization.

3. A researcher identified protein disulfide isomerase (PDI) as the enzyme responsible for catalyzing the formation of disulfide bonds in the ER. She combines viral p16 monomers with PDI *in vitro* and detects the formation of p16 dimers. Which of the following is true once the solution has reached equilibrium?

A) The rate of p16 dimer formation is the same the rate of p16 dimer dissociation.
B) Removal of PDI from solution will decrease the amount of p16 dimers in solution.
C) Addition of more PDI will increase the amount of p16 dimers in solution.
D) p16 monomers have ceased to associate together to form p16 dimers.

4. Which of the following is most likely true if the formation of the p21 dimer in the ER is an exothermic process?

A) The formation of a p21 dimer is spontaneous at all temperatures.
B) The formation of a p21 dimer is nonspontaneous at all temperatures.
C) The formation of a p21 dimer is spontaneous only at low temperatures.
D) The formation of a p21 dimer is spontaneous only at high temperatures.

ENZYMES AND INHIBITION PRACTICE PASSAGE 2

Hexokinase, an enzyme facilitating the phosphorylation of glucose, catalyzes the first step in glycolysis. Multiple isoforms of the enzyme have been identified, with several displaying differing tissue-specific expression patterns in humans. While hexokinase I/A is detectable across many tissues and cell-types, hexokinase IV/D, also known as *glucokinase*, is preferentially expressed in the liver and pancreatic β-cells. Glucokinase is nearly half the size of other isoforms and is composed of a single subunit. In the liver, it plays a critical role in glucose uptake, while in β-cells it serves as part of the glucose sensing-machinery.

In addition to structural differences, hexokinase I and glucokinase display differing enzymatic properties. Hexokinase I exhibits a low K_m, a measure of substrate concentration required to reach half maximal velocity, while glucokinase displays a high K_m. These differences allow the enzymes to function in differing physiological states.

In a series of experiments evaluating the impact of the amino acid sequence of human glucokinase on enzymatic function, a group of researchers created missense mutations in glucokinase to assess for changes in both K_m and V_{max} (maximal reaction velocity). The results are shown in Table 1.

Mutation	V_{max}, units/mg	K_m (glucose), mM	K_m (ATP), mM
Native liver enzyme	98 ± 9	6.8 ± 1.3	0.23 ± 0.19
Native β-cell enzyme	100 ± 8	8 ± 2	0.15 ± 0.18
Mutant 1 (G175R)	51 ± 5	39 ± 12	0.10 ± 0.03
Mutant 2 (T228M)	0.4 ± 0.03	10 ± 2	0.20 ± 0.17
Mutant 3 (E279Q)	55 ± 6	41 ± 1	0.20 ± 0.2
Mutant 4 (E300Q)	100 ± 3	20 ± 1.2	0.19 ± 0.04

Table 1 Enzymatic properties of native and mutant forms of human β-cell glucokinase. Error values represent standard errors of the mean.

Adapted from Gidh-Jain, M., et al. "Glucokinase mutations associated with non-insulin-dependent (type 2) diabetes mellitus have decreased enzymatic activity: implications for structure/function relationships." *Proceedings of the National Academy of Sciences* 90.5 (1993): 1932-1936.

1. Which of the following best characterizes the differences between hexokinase I/A and glucokinase?

A) Hexokinase I/A has a greater affinity for glucose and can function at lower substrate concentrations than glucokinase.

B) Hexokinase I/A has a greater affinity for glucose and requires higher substrate concentrations than glucokinase.

C) Glucokinase has a greater affinity for glucose and can function at lower substrate concentrations than hexokinase I/A.

D) Glucokinase has a greater affinity for glucose and requires higher substrate concentrations than hexokinase I/A.

2. Researchers investigating the structure of glucokinase determine that the binding sites of glucose and ATP are significantly further from one another in the active site than had been anticipated, given the size of glucose-6-phosphate. Which of the following best explains this observation?

A) Binding of the substrates results in a change in the tertiary structure of the enzyme.

B) A shift in the quaternary structure of the peptide brings the two groups in apposition to one another.

C) Hydrogen bonding between the peptide and substrate stabilize the transition state.

D) ATP is serving as an allosteric inhibitor and not a substrate.

3. Glucose-6-phosphate serves as an allosteric inhibitor for hexokinase I/A but not for glucokinase. The most likely reason for this difference is to:

A) decrease competition for the active site in glucokinase.

B) allow for continued glycogen production in hepatocytes at high substrate concentrations.

C) increase carbohydrate storage in β-cells.

D) shunt glucose through the Krebs cycle by inhibition of hexokinase I/A.

4. Glucokinase works in conjunction with GLUT2 (a glucose transporter facilitating glucose uptake from the blood) serving as a glucose sensor in pancreatic β-cells. What would be the most likely abnormality noted in a patient with a loss-of-function mutation in the GLUT2 gene?

A) Increase in apparent K_m of glucokinase
B) Decrease in apparent K_m of glucokinase
C) Hyperglycemia (elevated blood sugar)
D) Hypoglycemia (low blood sugar)

5. Of the mutants evaluated by the researchers, which is most likely to demonstrate activity most similar to endogenous glucokinase?

A) Mutant 1
B) Mutant 2
C) Mutant 3
D) Mutant 4

SOLUTIONS TO FREESTANDING QUESTIONS: ENZYMES AND INHIBITION

1. **B** Recall the equation for Gibbs Free Energy: $\Delta G = \Delta H - T\Delta S$. Reactions with a negative ΔG are spontaneous, and with a positive ΔG are not spontaneous. A large negative ΔS multiplied by T gives a large negative number. In choice B, a large positive ΔH minus a large negative number gives a large positive number as a result, and a positive ΔG means that the reaction is not spontaneous. Another way to look at it is that a negative ΔS means that entropy is decreasing, and things are becoming more ordered; this is rarely spontaneous. All other answer choices have a large positive ΔS multiplied by T; this gives a large positive number. Subtracting a large positive number from a large positive number (such as in choice A) might give a negative number, or might give a positive number, so this *might* be a spontaneous reaction (choice B is better than choice A). Subtracting a large positive number from a small negative number (such as in choice C) gives a large negative number; this would indicate a spontaneous reaction (choice C is wrong), and subtracting a large positive number from a small positive number would also give a negative number as a result and indicate a spontaneous reaction (choice D is wrong).

2. **D** Catalysts reduce the energy of activation for a reaction (choices A and C can be eliminated), thus making it easier to get to the transition state (TS). This increases the rate of the reaction. ΔG is not affected by the addition of a catalyst; catalysts only affect the kinetics of a reaction, not the thermodynamics. Catalysts are not always specific. Heat and sparks are good general catalysts, but are not specific for particular reactions (choice B is wrong, and choice D is correct).

3. **A** In an oxidation-reduction reaction, the molecule being oxidized loses electrons (choice B can be eliminated) and the molecule being reduced gains electrons (choice C is wrong). The molecule being reduced is accepting those electrons and thus "allowing" the oxidation of the other molecule to occur; the molecule being reduced is therefore known as the oxidizing agent (choice A is correct, and choice D is wrong).

4. **B** The question stem describes metoprolol as a competitive inhibitor impacting β-adrenergic receptors, the predominant postsynaptic receptors of the sympathetic nervous system (choice A is wrong). Competitive antagonists bind to the same site on the receptor as the ligand and, unlike non-competitive or other allosteric inhibitors, can be displaced with sufficient quantities of ligand (choice B is correct, and choice C is wrong). K_d for receptors and their ligands is analogous to K_m in enzyme-substrate interactions. It is the concentration of ligand at which half the receptors are occupied, and it will increase in the presence of a competitive antagonist (higher concentrations of ligand are required to reach the same saturation point (choice D is wrong).

5. **C** During the reaction, carbon gains two bonds to oxygen (and loses a bond to hydrogen) indicating that an oxidation reaction occurred and therefore the oxidation state must have increased (choice D is wrong, and C is correct). If carbon had served as an oxidizing agent, it would have been reduced in the process (choice A is wrong). If oxygen had served as a reducing agent, it would have been oxidized in the process. Since the products of this reaction are uric acid and H_2O_2, oxygen is gaining bonds to hydrogen, indicating that it is reduced (choice B is wrong). Note that it is not necessary to assign oxidation states to answer the question.

6. **B** By definition, products are favored over reactants in an exergonic process (choice B is correct). The predominant contributor to net free energy depends both on enthalpic and entropic factors involving both the transcript and solvent. The stem of the question does not provide adequate information to conclude that intra-molecular nucleotide interactions are the principal factor driving the reaction (choice D is wrong). Folding decreases entropy (ΔS, choice A is wrong), and transcript folding (as with protein folding), results in a decrease in degree of rotational freedom as the macromolecule forms new interactions (choice C is wrong).

7. **D** Zero-order processes exhibit rates that are independent of substrate concentration. In the case of drug elimination, zero order kinetics means that the drug is eliminated at a constant rate regardless of drug concentration (choice B is wrong). Given a constant rate of elimination, the half-life will depend upon the initial concentration of the medication (choice D is correct). With supratherapeutic levels of an anticoagulant, patients would be at an increased, not decreased, risk of bleeding (choice A is wrong). Vitamin K treatment would increase coagulation, but would not impact the elimination rate of the warfarin (choice C is wrong).

SOLUTIONS TO ENZYMES AND INHIBITION PRACTICE PASSAGE 1

1. **C** The formation of disulfide bonds requires an oxidation; thus the ER lumen must be an oxidizing environment (choices A and D can be eliminated). Since disulfide bond formation generally does not occur in the cytoplasm, it must be a reducing environment (choice B can be eliminated, and choice C is correct).

2. **A** DTT (dithiothreitol) is a reducing agent, thus it would break, or prevent the formation of, disulfide bonds. Figure 1 supports this, showing that in the absence of DTT, dimerization of p16 occurs beginning at 120 minutes (the presence of a second, larger band). This band is absent in the presence of DTT (choice A is correct, and choice C is wrong). Since only p16 was immunoprecipitated, no other proteins should be present, plus the band at 14 kDa in the absence of DTT gets smaller at 120 and 240 minutes, indicating that the amount of that protein decreases. The band at about 28 kDa gets bigger, indicating that the amount of that protein increases; this must be due to loss of the individual p16 polypeptides as they dimerize (choice B is wrong). Just because the band indicating dimerization is less than 30 kDa doesn't mean you can't form conclusions. p16 was described as being 14-16 kDa; thus a dimer would have a size in the range of 28–32 kDa. The band in no DTT at 120 and 240 minutes is about that size (choice D is wrong).

3. **A** At equilibrium, the rate of the forward reaction is equal to that of the reverse reaction (choice A is correct). It's not that p16 dimers are not forming (choice D is wrong), but rather that p16 dimers are forming just as fast as p16 dimers are breaking down. As a result, the net amount of p16 dimers is not changing. Enzymes decrease the amount of time it takes for a reaction to reach equilibrium. However, once a reaction has reached equilibrium, the addition or removal of the enzyme will have no affect (choices B and C are wrong).

4. **C** The formation of a dimer is associated with a decrease in entropy ($\Delta S < 0$). The question stem states the formation of a protein dimer is an exothermic process ($\Delta H < 0$). A reaction is spontaneous if $\Delta G < 0$. Based on ΔS and ΔH values and the equation $\Delta G = \Delta H - T\Delta S$, ΔG for the formation of the p21 dimer will be less than 0 only at low temperatures.

SOLUTIONS TO ENZYMES AND INHIBITION PRACTICE PASSAGE 2

1. **A** The answer choices are presented in a 2 × 2 format, meaning that if either portion of the answer choice can be disproven, two answers can be eliminated. The passage states that hexokinase has a low K_m, while glucokinase has a high K_m; this indicates that hexokinase has a greater affinity for glucose than glucokinase (choices C and D can be eliminated). An enzyme with a high affinity for a substrate would not require a high concentration of that substrate in order to function (choice A is correct, and choice B is wrong).

2. **A** The change in peptide structure associated with substrate bonding often results in changing interactions between the enzyme and substrate, including bringing substrates closer to one another (choice A is correct). In this instance, the passage states that glucokinase has only a single subunit and therefore has no quaternary structure (choice B is wrong). While it is likely true that hydrogen bonding helps stabilize the transition state, this does not answer the question (choice C is wrong). The stem of the question states that ATP binds to the active site, which would not be expected for an allosteric inhibitor (choice D is wrong).

3. **B** After eating, serum glucose concentrations are high and both hexokinase I/A and glucokinase generate glucose-6-phosphate. In hepatocytes (not β cells, choice C is wrong), some of this glucose-6-P is stored as glycogen for later consumption. Allowing glucokinase to continue to function even when there are high levels of glucose-6-P ensures that there will be plenty of glucose-6-P to store as glycogen (choice B is correct). The stem notes that glucose-6-P serves as an allosteric inhibitor and therefore would not be in competition for the active site (choice A is wrong). While it is true that glucose-6-P inhibits the function of hexokinase I/A, glucose does not directly serve as a reagent in the Krebs cycle, thus excess glucose cannot be shunted through that pathway (choice D is wrong).

4. **C** An impaired ability to detect serum glucose would likely impede the ability of β-cells to appropriately release insulin, thus leading to hyperglycemia (choice C is correct, and choice D is wrong). K_m reflects the relative affinity of the enzyme (glucokinase) for its substrate (glucose) and would not be affected by a change in GLUT2 (choices A and B are wrong).

5.   **D**   In order to maintain enzymatic activity, find the mutant with those enzyme kinetic constants most similar to wild type. While Mutant 2 (T228M) mutation results in a K_m indistinguishable from the endogenous enzyme, its maximal velocity falls to nearly zero indicating it cannot form significant quantities of product (choice B is wrong). Of the remaining three answer choices, Mutant 4 results in no change in maximal velocity with only a mild fall in affinity as noted by a rise in K_m (choice D is correct). The remaining two choices demonstrate both lower V_{max} as well as lower affinity (higher K_m) and would be less likely to demonstrate similar activity to the wild type enzyme (choices A and C are wrong).

Chapter 5
Amino Acids and Proteins

FREESTANDING QUESTIONS: AMINO ACIDS AND PROTEINS

1. What best characterizes the active site of an enzyme designed to catalyze a reaction with a positively charged transition state?

A) Hydrophobic amino acids to stabilize the transition state with weak interactions
B) Acidic amino acids to stabilize the transition state with electrostatic interactions
C) Basic amino acids to stabilize the transition state with electrostatic interactions
D) Large variability in the active site within a species

2. All of the following are true of uncompetitive inhibition EXCEPT:

A) increasing inhibitor concentration decreases V_{max}.
B) decreasing inhibitor concentration increases K_m.
C) the inhibitor binds to the active site.
D) inhibition results in an increase in apparent affinity of the enzyme for the substrate.

3. Posttranslational modification includes a broad set of processes by which translated proteins are converted into mature protein products through folding, cleavage, addition of functional groups, and other processes. Which of the following examples of posttranslational modification generally requires the consumption of ATP?

A) Folding by chaperone proteins
B) Cleavage by a protease
C) Formation of disulfide bridges
D) Phosphorylation

4. Proopiomelanocortin (POMC) is 241 amino acids long and is synthesized from pre-POMC, which is 285 amino acids long. POMC is cleaved to give rise to multiple peptide hormones, such as melanocyte-stimulating hormone, adrenocorticotropic hormone, and β-endorphin. This means that POMC:

A) is generated via proteolytic cleavage of a precursor molecule and contains 240 peptide bonds.
B) is hydrophilic in nature and must start with a sulfur-containing amino acid.
C) costs the cell approximately 950 high-energy bonds to synthesize.
D) is a protein with at least quaternary structure.

5. A scientist isolated a protein from a cell. A portion of the primary sequence from the transmembrane region is Leu-Leu-Ile-Val-Leu-Asp-Leu. Which amino acid, if deleted, would likely cause the biggest change to the functionality of the protein?

A) L
B) I
C) V
D) D

6. An experiment is conducted to measure enzyme kinetics with an inhibitor. The baseline measurements as well as those of the inhibitor are plotted on a Lineweaver-Burk graph and the inhibitor's results share only an x-intercept with the baseline results. What conclusion can be drawn about the apparent affinity of the enzyme for its substrate when this inhibitor is present?

A) The apparent affinity has decreased along with an increase in V_{max}.
B) The apparent affinity remains unchanged in the presence of the inhibitor.
C) The apparent affinity has decreased based on the change in K_m.
D) The apparent affinity could increase or decrease, based on the concentration of the enzyme.

7. During glycolysis, the production of fructose-1,6-bisphosphate can lead to an increase in pyruvate production via pyruvate kinase. This type of enzymatic regulation would be an example of:

A) feedback stimulation.
B) cooperativity.
C) feedback inhibition.
D) feedforward stimulation.

8. Which of the following amino acids would be LEAST helpful in the formation of an α-helix?

A) G
B) P
C) V
D) W

Questions 9 and 10 relate to the following experiment:

Thymidylate synthetase functions in nucleotide biosynthesis metabolism and catalyzes the conversion of deoxyuridine monophosphate (dUMP) to deoxythymidine monophosphate (dTMP). A biochemist is collecting enzyme kinetic data for this enzyme and runs three experiments: one using only substrate, one adding a compound called DHV52 and one adding a compound called HKA10. The following data are obtained:

[Substrate] (nmol)	Reaction Rate (pmol/min)	Reaction Rate with DHV52 (pmol/min)	Reaction Rate with HKA10 (pmol/min)
0	0	0	0
5	12	9	16
10	24	18	24
15	33	23	28
20	39	27	30
25	42	30	31
30	44	32	32
35	44	32	32

9. Which of the following is true?

A) Both DHV52 and HKA10 have a similar mechanism of inhibition and both bind an allosteric site on the thymidylate synthetase peptide chain.
B) DHV52 binds an allosteric site of the enzyme, effectively decreasing the maximum reaction rate; in contrast, HKA10 binds the enzyme-substrate complex, decreasing enzymatic activity, maximum reaction rate and apparent K_m.
C) DHV52 is an uncompetitive inhibitor that binds the enzyme and enzyme-substrate complex with similar affinity, while HKA10 is a noncompetitive inhibitor.
D) HKA10 is likely a noncompetitive inhibitor that binds the active site, while DHV52 is either an uncompetitive or mixed inhibitor.

10. Which of the following graphs represents the Lineweaver-Burk plot for DHV52?

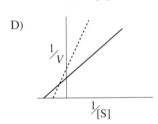

A)

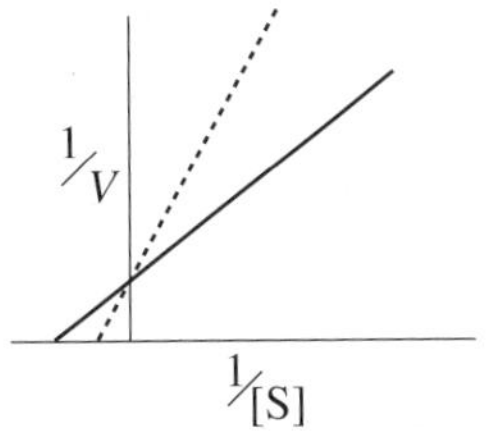

B)

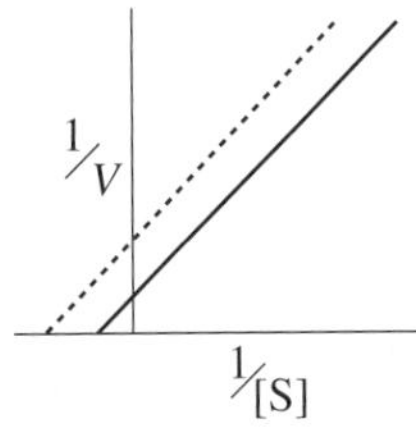

C)

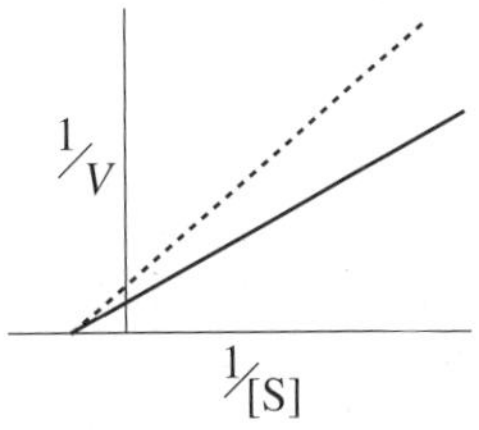

D)

11. Tissue plasminogen activator, or tPA, is a serine protease used clinically to facilitate thrombolysis (the destruction of blood clots). A variant of the enzyme was found with a missense mutation at position 117 in the active protease domain, however, in spite of the mutation, enzymatic activity was maintained. Which of the following was the most likely substitution?

A) N117D
B) N117I
C) N117G
D) N117Q

AMINO ACIDS AND PROTEINS PRACTICE PASSAGE 1

"Growth factor" is a general term encompassing a number of different compounds that can have a variety of effects on cellular activity, including cell migration, proliferation, and adhesion. Responses to growth factors involve a complex web of interacting proteins, including receptor dimerization and various kinases.

Integrin-linked kinase (ILK) is a 59 kDa protein that functions in cell migration, cell proliferation, cell-adhesion, and signal transduction. In resting cells, ILK has low basal kinase activity. However, in response to transient stimulation by a subset of growth factors, ILK can function as a serine/threonine kinase in the cell. Recent publications have shown ILK can modify protein kinase B (PKB) on amino acid S473 and myosin light chain (MLC) on T19 in certain, but not all, cell types.

In order to investigate cooperation between ILK and a novel potential substrate (glycogen synthase kinase 3 or GSK3) in renal cells, a Western blot was performed. To do this, three different kidney proximal tubule epithelial cell lines were used. The first (JV32) is known to express ILK. One sample of these cells was left untreated and the other was exposed to a growth factor known to activate ILK. NA13 cells were also used; these cells do not express ILK but were subjected to the same treatment as JV32. Finally, DK5 cells were used and these cells express a dominant negative isoform of ILK, which has no kinase activity. Each plate of adherent cells was treated with trypsin to release cells and then collected by centrifugation. The cell pellet was resuspended in cell lysis buffer that included protease inhibitors. The remaining lysate was cleared and lysates were separated by electrophoresis on a polyacrylamide gel. Six different Western blots were generated, using different primary antibodies for phospho-GSK3, phospho-PKB, phospho-MLC, and total amounts of PKB, MLC and β-actin (see Figure 1). Western blot results are often quantified and normalized with respect to a housekeeper protein, but this normalization was not necessary for the experimental results obtained.

Based on this data, researchers hypothesized that ILK phosphorylates GSK3. A collaborating lab has data indicating this is the case in sympathetic neurons, and that in these cells, this results in decreased GSK3 activity, thus promoting dendrite initiation and growth.

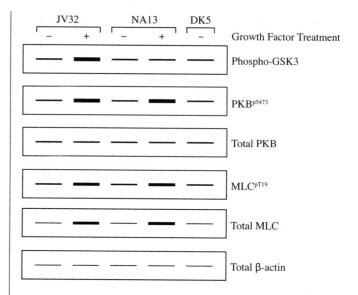

Figure 1 Western blot analysis of renal epithelial cell lines with and without growth factor treatment

1. Is the hypothesis reached by the ILK research team supported by the data in Figure 1?

A) Yes: in both JV32 and NA13, phospho-GSK3 levels increased with growth factor treatment, while DK5 cells had low phospho-GSK3.

B) No: if ILK is the only protein phosphorylating GSK3, phospho-GSK3 levels should increase in JV32 cells when treated with growth factor, but should not increase in NA13 cells.

C) No: There is no way to determine the effect of ILK on GSK3 phosphorylation, since the researchers did not show if the total amount of GSK3 changed with growth factor treatment.

D) No: The researchers cannot determine the effect of ILK on GSK3 without knowing how phospho-GSK3 changes in DK5 cells after growth factor treatment.

2. Which of the following could support the conclusions drawn by the collaborating neurobiology lab mentioned in the passage?

   I. Pharmacologically inhibiting ILK activity in cultured sympathetic neurons reduces dendrite formation.
   II. Expressing a dominant negative GSK3 allele causes robust dendrite initiation.
   III. Inhibition of GSK3 by genetic knockdown promotes dendrite initiation even when ILK is simultaneously inhibited.

A) I only
B) I and II
C) II and III
D) I, II, and III

3. Which of the following is true regarding the housekeeper protein used in Figure 1?

A) β-actin was not a good control to use, since it is found predominantly in intermediate filaments and expression of these cytoskeleton components varies with the cell cycle.
B) β-actin was a good housekeeper protein to use because it is expressed in most cells and is a major component of microfilaments.
C) β-actin was a good housekeeper protein to use because it is commonly expressed in many cell types; it was used to make sure lysate separation occurred during gel electrophoresis.
D) Since there was no housekeeper protein used in this experiment, the researchers should have quantified Western blot signals and compared each phospho-protein to the total amount of that protein.

4. Phosphomimetics are amino acid substitutions that mimic a phosphorylated protein in structure and charge, and often, biological activity. Which of the following is most likely a true statement?

A) A point mutation at residue 473 of PKB (S to D) would be phosphomimetic.
B) A nonsense mutation at residue T19 of MLC or S473 of PKB will closely match the outcome of a phosphomimetic at the same site.
C) Changing residue 19 of MLC to amino acid A instead of T will have the same effect as a phosphomimetic.
D) None of the above statements is likely true.

5. Which of the following represents substrate residue structures in MLC and PKB, respectively, after the ILK-mediated reaction?

A)

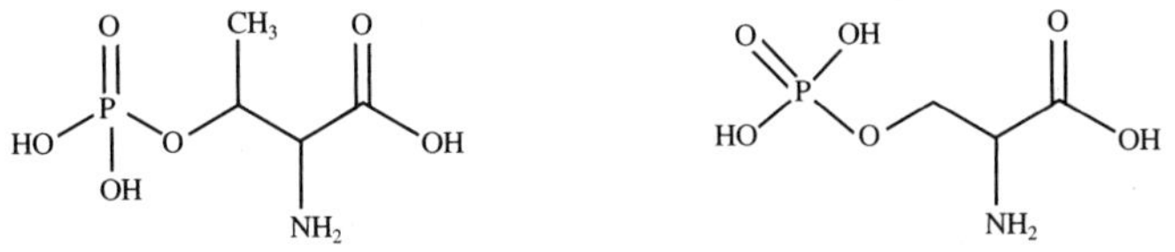

B)

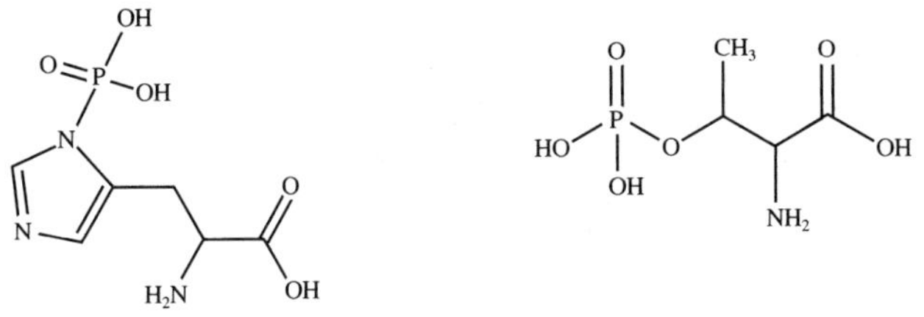

C)

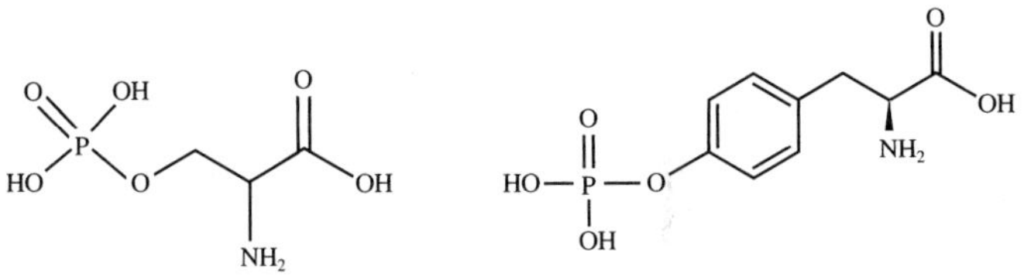

D)

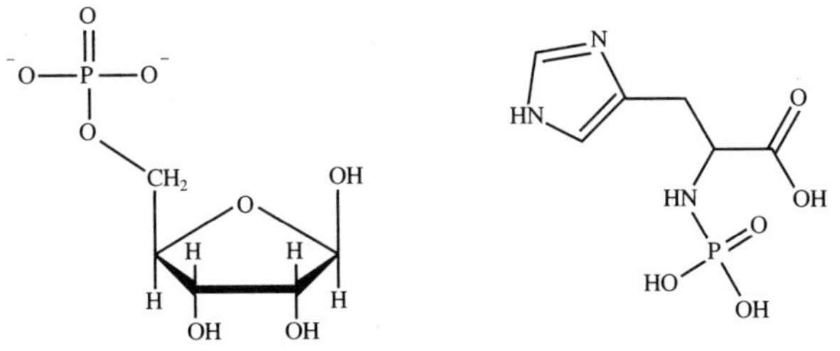

6. Based on the data in Figure 1, which of the following is true?

A) ILK phosphorylates T19 of MLC in kidney proximal tubule epithelial cells.
B) S473 is phosphorylated solely by ILK in kidney proximal tubule epithelial cells.
C) Each lane of the Western blot contained the same amount of β-actin, indicating equal amounts of each lysate were used, and eliminating the need for normalization.
D) The variation in the total MLC Western blot could be due to protein degradation of some lysate samples but not others.

AMINO ACIDS AND PROTEINS PRACTICE PASSAGE 2

The mucosa of the small intestine plays an essential role in the absorption of nutrients. Uptake of amino acids and glucose across the brush border is accomplished by distinct transporter proteins, the majority of which require ion cotransport. Enterocytes (intestinal cells) collected from patient biopsies can form vesicles after isolation and treatment, and these vesicles can be used to study transport processes within the intestine. Hepatocytes (liver cells) also transport amino acids, and do so using similar transport systems. These cells can also be induced to form vesicle structures in a tube.

Both enterocytes and hepatocytes express a Na⁺/H⁺-antiporter, an ion-dependent glucose transporter, and many different types of amino acid transporters. The transport of glutamine and alanine are mediated by System B amino acid transporter complexes. Leucine, arginine, and glycine are transported by Systems L, Y and B3, respectively. Many of the neutral amino acids are transported by amino acid transport A system, and this transport can be inhibited by the small molecule α-(Methylamino)isobutyric acid (MeAIB, see Figure 1).

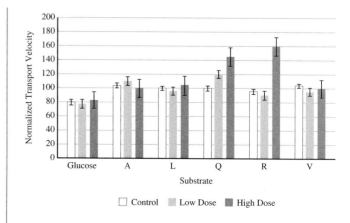

Figure 2A Nutrient transport in BBMVs, measured in a sodium-rich buffer

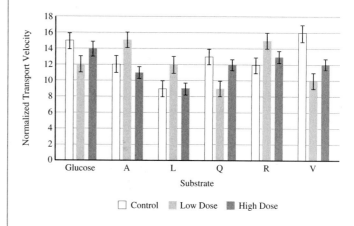

Figure 2B Nutrient transport in BBMVs, measured in a potassium-rich buffer

Figure 1 α-(Methylamino)isobutyric acid

In order to study how amino acid transport may be controlled by the endocrine system, patients undergoing abdominal surgery were randomized into one of three groups: placebo, low dose, or high dose. The experimental groups were treated with a synthetic adenohypophysic peptide hormone 191 residues in length for three days prior to surgery. Tissue biopsy samples were collected from patients undergoing surgery and used to generate hepatic plasma membrane vesicles (HPMVs) or brush border membrane vesicles (BBMVs). Nutrient uptake was measured by adding radiolabeled substrate to the vesicles and using a rapid mixing and filtration technique. Results from this experiment are presented in Figures 2A–C.

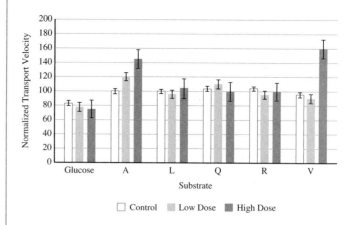

Figure 2C Nutrient transport in HPMVs, measured in a sodium-rich buffer

1. The effects of MeAIB can be overcome when local amino acid concentrations are high. Which of the following is most likely true?

A) MeAIB competitively inhibits the intestinal import of

B) MeAIB noncompetitively inhibits the intestinal import of

C) MeAIB competitively inhibits the intestinal import of

D) MeAIB noncompetitively inhibits the intestinal import of

2. The results in Figure 2 support which of the following conclusions?

A) Insulin at a high dose increases intestinal absorption of glutamine and arginine.
B) Growth hormone at a high dose enhances the activity of intestinal absorption of system B amino acid transporter complexes.
C) Insulin at a high dose enhances the activity of intestinal absorption of system B and system Y amino acid transporter complexes.
D) Growth hormone at a high dose increases intestinal absorption of glutamine and arginine.

3. Which of the following is true of both enterocyte and hepatocyte amino acid transporter complexes?

A) High dose groups show elevated transport of nonpolar neutral amino acids.
B) Amino acid transport is coupled to sodium ion transport.
C) System Y amino acid transporters are sensitive to hormone treatment.
D) Glucose transport is high in the presence of sodium but not potassium.

4. Which of the following observations matches the data from high dose patients in Figure 2?

A) ^{3}[H]-Glutamine is found in HPMV lumens.
B) ^{3}[H]-Lysine is found in HPMV lumens.
C) ^{3}[H]-Arginine is found in BBMV lumens.
D) ^{3}[H]-Glutamic acid is found in BBMV lumens.

5. Which of the following is true?

A) MeAIB is a chiral molecule.
B) All amino acid system complexes transport chiral amino acids.
C) System B complexes transport chiral amino acids.
D) System B3 complexes transport chiral amino acids.

SOLUTIONS TO FREESTANDING QUESTIONS: AMINO ACIDS AND PROTEINS

1. **B** Enzymes decrease the activation energy of a reaction by stabilizing the transition state. Given that the transition state for the reaction in question is positively charged, the active site will likely possess acidic amino acids that have a negative charge at physiological pH. This would stabilize the positive charge of the transition state due to electrostatic interactions (choice B is correct). Basic amino acids have a positive charge at physiological pH and would destabilize a positively charged species (choice C is wrong). Hydrophobic amino acids are important for dictating overall enzymatic structure, but they would not significantly stabilize charge on the substrate (choice A is wrong). The active site is incredibly important for enzymatic function and minimal variability will be seen within a given species (choice D is wrong).

2. **C** Uncompetitive inhibition occurs when an inhibitor binds to the enzyme-substrate complex. This decreases the maximal rate of enzyme activity (choice A is a true statement and is not the correct answer) and increases the apparent affinity of the enzyme for the substrate (choice D is a true statement and is not the correct answer). Decreasing the quantity of inhibitor would therefore result in a decrease in apparent affinity (an increase in K_m; choice B is a true statement and is not the correct answer). As the inhibitor must bind to the enzyme-substrate complex, it is unlikely that the inhibitor could bind to the active site after the substrate had already bound (choice C is a false statement and is the correct answer).

3. **D** The source of the phosphate group required for phosphorylation is often ATP (choice D is correct). Chaperone proteins generally serve as "containers" in which newly produced proteins will reach a certain conformation prior to release without consuming any ATP (choice A is wrong). Proteases generally do not require ATP to cleave peptide bonds (choice B is wrong). Reactions in which disulfide bridges are formed are oxidation-reduction reactions; they are typically catalyzed by enzymes that do not consume ATP (choice C is wrong).

4. **A** Pre-POMC has 285 amino acids and POMC has only 241 amino acids (with 240 peptide bonds connecting them). This means pre-POMC must be cleaved by a protease to form POMC (choice A is correct). Most proteins are hydrophilic, especially peptide hormones, but there is no guarantee POMC starts with methionine, a sulfur-containing amino acid. The N-terminus is cleaved from many proteins, including those that go through the secretory pathway (as does POMC), so not all peptide chains start with a methionine residue (choice B can be eliminated). The cell that makes pre-POMC must synthesize a 285 amino acid peptide chain, and thus must spend (4)(285) = 1140 high-energy bonds to do so (eliminate choice C). Proteins in general have three levels of structure (tertiary structure); only proteins that contain more than one peptide chain have quaternary structure. There is no information on whether POMC contains more than one peptide chain, so choice D is not supported.

5. **D** Amino acids in the transmembrane region of proteins are typically hydrophobic due to the hydrophobicity of the cell membrane. Leucine, isoleucine, and valine are all hydrophobic, and one of them could likely be deleted without too much consequence, as there are six of these hydrophobic amino acids in this short sequence. However, aspartic acid is charged (acidic); the presence of a charged amino acid, especially in an otherwise hydrophobic region, almost always indicates functional significance. A deletion of this Asp residue would most likely effect the functionality of the protein (choice D is correct). Note also that you could use the "one of these things is not like the other" technique here.

6.   **B**   The experimental scenario in the question describes an inhibitor with a plot line that runs through the same x-intercept as the uninhibited measurements; this is indicative of a noncompetitive inhibitor. The x-intercept represents $-1/K_m$; if both the uninhibited and inhibited reactions share the same K_m, then the affinity of the enzyme for its substrate has not changed (choice B is correct, and choices A and C are wrong). Changing the concentration of the enzyme will change V_{max}, not K_m; affinity is not affected by enzyme concentration (choice D is wrong).

7.   **D**   Pyruvate kinase is the last enzyme in the glycolytic pathway, and it is being stimulated by an earlier intermediate, fructose-1,6-bisphosphate. This describes an example of feed-forward stimulation (choice D is correct). In feedback stimulation, an intermediate from later in the pathway would need to trigger the enzyme (choice A is incorrect). Cooperativity is not related to this type of pathway regulation (choice B is irrelevant and incorrect). In feedback inhibition, an intermediate or end product decreases, rather than increases, production by acting on an enzyme used in an earlier step (choice C is incorrect).

8.   **B**   Because of its unique ring structure, when proline (P) forms a peptide bond with another amino acid as part of the primary structure of a protein, its only hydrogen is displaced. Thus, there is not another one available for the hydrogen bonds that characterize a protein's secondary structures (as would be necessary in α-helices, choice B is least helpful and is the correct answer choice). Glycine (G), valine (V), and tryptophan (W) all have the hydrogen atoms needed to be involved in creating secondary levels of structure (choices A, C, and D are incorrect).

9.   **B**   The V_{max} of the control reaction is 44 pmol/min. K_m is the substrate concentration required to reach $\frac{1}{2}V_{max}$ (22 pmol/min). Based on data in the chart, this will be a little below 10 nmol for the control reaction. DHV52 decreases the V_{max} to 32 pmol/min; so for this reaction $\frac{1}{2}V_{max}$ is 16 pmol/min. This corresponds to a substrate concentration a little below 10 nmol. In other words, the control experiment and the DHV52 have the same K_m value. This means DHV52 must be a noncompetitive inhibitor that binds an allosteric site or a mixed inhibitor with a similar affinity for the enzyme and the enzyme-substrate complex (choice C can be eliminated). HKA10 also decreases V_{max} to 32 pmol/min. $\frac{1}{2}V_{max}$ for this reaction is 16 pmol/min, and this corresponds to a substrate concentration of 5 nmol. Because the K_m for the HKA10 reaction is different than the control, HKA10 is not a noncompetitive inhibitor (choice D can be eliminated), and must have a different mechanism of inhibition than DHV52 (choice A is wrong). This means HKA10 is likely an uncompetitive inhibitor, or a mixed inhibitor that preferentially binds the enzyme-substrate complex (choice B is correct).

10.   **C**   By analyzing the data, you can see that DHV52 is a noncompetitive inhibitor (see solution to question 9 above). Noncompetitive inhibitors have the same K_m as the uninhibited reaction, but have a lower V_{max}. On the Lineweaver-Burk plot, the x-intercept represents $-1/K_m$ and the y-intercept represents $1/V_{max}$. Choice C, with an unchanged x-intercept and a greater y-intercept (representing a smaller V_{max}, or a bigger $1/V_{max}$), is the correct plot. Choice A, showing the same V_{max} but a greater K_m (a smaller $-1/K_m$), represents competitive inhibition; choice B, with a smaller K_m (a bigger $-1/K_m$) and a smaller V_{max} (a bigger $1/V_{max}$), represents uncompetitive inhibition; and choice D represents mixed inhibition.

11. **D** Enzymatic activity relies on the association of the enzyme and substrate at the active site, which is a function of both electrostatic interaction and amino acid size. If enzymatic activity is to be maintained following a point mutation, there cannot be significant deviations in these attributes. Glutamine, a polar amino acid, differs from asparagine by a single $-CH_2-$. It is therefore most similar to the endogenous enzyme and most likely to maintain activity (choice D is correct). Neither glycine nor isoleucine possess a polar R group (choices B and C are wrong), and aspartate has a full negative charge at physiological pH (choice A is wrong).

SOLUTIONS TO AMINO ACIDS AND PROTEINS PRACTICE PASSAGE 1

1. **C** The passage states that growth factors can have a number of different effects on cells (including proliferation), mediated by a number of different proteins (including, but not limited to, various kinases). The results in the Western blot for phospho-GSK3 show an increase in phospho-GSK3 on treatment with a growth factor in both JV32 cells (that express ILK) and in NA13 cells (that do not express ILK); this suggests first that ILK is not the only protein involved in phosphorylating GSK3 (choices A and B are wrong). However, the researchers do not show a Western blot that gives information on the total amount of GSK3, and if it is also changing on treatment with growth factors. Without this information, researchers cannot claim that phospho-GSK3 levels are changing only due to ILK effects; it may be, for example, that total cell counts (and thus total cell protein) is increased on treatment with growth factors, and that alone contributes to the increase in phospho-GSK3. Consider the results in Figure 1 for phospho-PKB (PKB^{pS473}). These results match the idea that ILK phosphorylates PKB on amino acid S473; phospho-PKB increases in JV32 cells after growth factor treatment, and the total amount of PKB does not change across the samples. This suggests that the increase in phospho-PKB is due to the activity of ILK and not due to increased cell numbers (and thus cell protein levels). Note also that this response is more robust than what happens in NA13 cells (which have no ILK), further supporting the idea that ILK is not the only protein phosphorylating GSK3. DK5 cells express a dominant-negative isoform of ILK, meaning that ILK will be nonfunctional in these cells. Knowing how these cells respond to growth factors would strengthen the experiment but is not strictly necessary in order to conclude how ILK is affecting GSK3 (eliminate choice D).

2. **D** Since Item III appears in only two of the answer choices, start by analyzing Item III. This will turn the question in to a 50:50 elimination. Item III is true: the collaborating lab has shown that a decrease in GSK3 activity promotes dendrite initiation and growth. If the inhibition of GSK3 by genetic knockdown (i.e., there is not GSK3, and thus no GSK3 activity) produces the same effect, this supports their conclusion, regardless of the activation or inhibition of ILK (choices A and B can be eliminated). Both remaining choices include Item II, so it must be true; take a look at Item I. Item I is true: the collaborating neurobiology lab has data indicating that ILK phosphorylates GSK3 in sympathetic neurons, and that in these cells, this results in decreased GSK3 activity to promote dendrite initiation and growth. In other words, they believe that ILK negatively regulates GSK3, thereby positively regulating dendrite initiation and growth. If ILK were inhibited, it would no longer

be able to negatively regulate GSK3, and there would be a reduction in dendrite formation. Item I supports their conclusion (choice C can be eliminated, and choice D is correct). Note that Item II is in fact true: a "dominant negative" GSK3 allele means that either GSK3 will not be expressed, or if it is expressed it will be non-functional. This is consistent with the idea of inhibiting GSK3 and seeing dendrite growth.

3. **B**   Since most cells express β-actin, it is a good housekeeper protein to use in Western blot analysis (choice D is wrong). The purpose of checking housekeeper protein (β-actin) levels across the different samples is to ensure each lane of the Western blot contains the same amount of total lysate. This is important if lanes are going to be compared to each other. As the passage explains, if β-actin levels were not the same across the different lanes, Western blot signals would be quantified and normalized with respect to β-actin (or total lysate) amounts. Since the β-actin levels were the same, it was not necessary to do this; β-actin was a good housekeeper protein. Actin is the major component of microfilaments, not intermediate filaments (choice A is wrong). Intermediate filaments are made of proteins such as keratin, vimentin, lamin, and desmin. The purpose of a housekeeper protein is not to make sure separation occurred during gel electrophoresis. This could be checked by looking at how the molecular weight ladder separated on the gel, or by staining the gel to look at how the lysate samples have separated after electrophoresis (choice C is wrong).

4. **A**   Phosphate groups are deprotonated at physiological pH and thus have negative charge. The same is true of R-groups on the two acidic amino acids (aspartic acid or D, and glutamic acid or E). These two amino acids can be used to mimic phosphorylated amino acids (choice A is correct, and choice D is wrong). A nonsense mutation will result in an early stop codon and a truncated protein. This will not have the same effect as a phosphomimetic (choice B is wrong). Alanine (A) is a small and hydrophobic amino acid that cannot be phosphorylated. If T19 of MLC were mutated to alanine, it could not be phosphorylated and this would not have the effect of a phosphomimetic (choice C is wrong).

5. **A**   The passage says that ILK phosphorylates T (threonine) 19 of MLC and S (serine) 473 of PKB. Choice A shows these two amino acids in their phosphorylated forms (choice A is correct). Choice B shows one type of phospho-histidine and phospho-threonine (eliminate choice B), Choice C shows phospho-serine and phospho-tyrosine (eliminate choice C), and choice D shows ribose 5-phosphate and a different type of phospho-histidine (eliminate choice D). Note that you did not have to know absolutely the structures of the amino acids; simply knowing that threonine and serine do not contain any ring structures allows the elimination of choices B, C, and D.

6. **C**   Figure 1 shows that phospho-MLC increased in both JV32 and NA13 cells when growth factor was added. This change was similar in the two cells types in spite of the fact that NA13 cells do not express ILK. Also notice that total MLC protein levels change in a similar way for both cell types. This suggests growth factor treatment is causing an increase in total MLC in kidney proximal tubule epithelial cells, and that this effect is independent of ILK expression. While the passage says that ILK phosphorylates MLC on T19, this must occur in other cell types and not the cells used here (choice A can be eliminated). ILK is causing phosphorylation of PKB in JV32 cells, but since phospho-PKB levels also increase slightly in NA13 cells, there must be other proteins contributing to PKB phosphorylation in these cells (choice B can be eliminated). β-actin is the housekeeper protein used in this

experiment to determine how much lysate is present in each lane. Since each lane has a similar amount of β-actin, it also likely contains the same amount of overall lysate (choice C is correct). The passage says that protease inhibitors were added to the lysis buffer. It is therefore unlikely for protein degradation to occur in some samples but not others (choice D is wrong).

SOLUTIONS TO AMINO ACIDS AND PROTEINS PRACTICE PASSAGE 2

1. **A** The question stem tells you that the inhibitory effects of MeAIB can be overcome if amino acid concentrations are high. This is characteristic of a competitive inhibitor (choices B and D can be eliminated). The effects of noncompetitive inhibitors cannot be overcome at high substrate concentrations. Paragraph 2 of the passage says that MeAIB inhibits the amino acid transport A system, which functions in the absorption of many neutral amino acids. The amino acid in choice A is valine (a neutral amino acid; choice A is correct), while the amino acid in choice C is histidine (normally charged at physiological pH; choice C is wrong).

2. **D** Paragraph 3 says that the hormone being used is a peptide hormone from the adenohypophysis, another name for the anterior pituitary. Since insulin comes from the pancreas, choices A and C can be eliminated. Paragraph 2 says that the System B amino acid transporter complexes transport glutamine (Q) and alanine (A). Intestinal vesicles from the high dose group (Figure 2A) show higher glutamine (Q) and arginine (R) absorption (choice D is correct), but no change in alanine (A) transport (choice B is wrong).

3. **B** Figure 2A shows intestinal (enterocyte) transport in a sodium buffer. Figure 2B shows intestinal (enterocyte) transport in a potassium buffer. Figure 2C shows liver (hepatocyte) transport in a sodium buffer. Figure 2A shows elevated glutamine (Q) and arginine (R) transport in high dose patients (both of these amino acids are polar), and no increase in the transport of alanine (A), leucine (L), or valine (V); in fact, valine transport decreases (choice A is a false statement). Figure 2C shows elevated alanine (A) and valine (V) transport in high dose patients. Both of these are nonpolar and neutral amino acids. Overall then, it cannot be said that both enterocytes and hepatocytes show elevated transport of nonpolar neutral amino acids. Now consider the y-axes of the graphs. Figure 2A and 2C have high numbers, thus showing high amounts of transport. The y-axis numbers in Figure 2B are quite a bit lower. This supports the fact that transport events are coupled to the presence of sodium and not potassium (choice B is correct). Paragraph 2 says that system Y amino acid transporters move arginine. Based on Figure 2, these complexes respond to hormone treatment in intestinal cells, but not in liver cells (choice C is wrong). Finally, choice D is a completely true statement, but has nothing to do with the question stem, which asks about amino acid transporters, not glucose transporters (choice D is wrong).

4. **C** First, data on neither lysine nor glutamic acid is found in Figure 2 (choices B and D can be eliminated). The passage says that hepatic plasma membrane vesicles (HPMVs) and brush border membrane vesicles (BBMVs) are generated from patient biopsy samples and are used to study transport processes in the liver and intestine, respectively. Vesicles have a lumen on the inside, and the passage says that radiolabeled substrates were used to track transport events. It therefore makes sense that the presence of a radiolabeled substrate on the inside of the vesicle (or in the lumen) would indicate a transport event had occurred. HPMVs are shown in Figure 2C; glutamine transport is unchanged in all groups (error bars overlap, choice A can be eliminated, and choice C is correct). Note that choice C is supported by the data in Figure 2A; the high dose patients showed elevated transport of arginine (R).

5. **C** There are no chiral centers in the structure of MeAIB in Figure 1 (choice A is wrong). Remember, a chiral center is a carbon or nitrogen atom with sp^3 hybridization and bound to four different groups. The passage contains information on some but not all amino acid system complexes, so the statement in choice B is too strong and not supported (choice B can be eliminated). Paragraph 2 says that System B amino acid transporter complexes transport glutamine and alanine. Both these amino acids have a chiral center and are chiral molecules (choice C is correct). Finally, paragraph 2 says that glycine is transported by System B3. Because the side chain of glycine is a hydrogen atom, glycine is an achiral molecule (choice D is wrong).

Chapter 6
Carbohydrates

FREESTANDING QUESTIONS: CARBOHYDRATES

1. What is the most likely value for the equilibrium constant for the combustion of glucose?

A) $K_{eq} > 1$
B) $K_{eq} \approx 1$
C) $K_{eq} < 1$
D) Unable to determine from the information provided

2. Given the information below, which of the following reactions results in the largest liberation of free energy?

Glucose-6-phosphate → Glucose + Inorganic Phosphate	$\Delta G° = -13.9$ kJ/mol
ADP + Inorganic Phosphate → ATP	$\Delta G° = 30.5$ kJ/mol

A) Glucose + ATP → Glucose-6-phosphate
B) Glucose + 2 Inorganic Phosphate + ADP → Glucose-6-phosphate
C) Glucose-6-phosphate + ATP → Glucose + 2 Inorganic Phosphate + ADP
D) Glucose-6-phosphate + ADP → Glucose + ATP

3. If a yeast culture is treated with 2-deoxyglucose (an inhibitor of glycolysis), which of the following is the most likely result?

A) Increased anaerobic fermentation
B) Increased production of ethanol
C) Decreased production of pyruvate
D) Decreased fatty acid catabolism

4. A patient presents to the emergency room complaining of shortness of breath and a headache. She is shortly diagnosed with acute carbon monoxide poisoning. What best describes glucose metabolism in this patient's cells?

A) Increased production of lactic acid
B) Increased activity of the electron transport chain
C) Increased citrate production
D) Increased ATP production

5. During the Krebs cycle, one mole of glucose will result in the generation of how many ATP equivalents via substrate-level phosphorylation?

A) 2 moles
B) 6 moles
C) 10 moles
D) 20 moles

6. In a newly discovered fungus, an unknown protein is isolated that has a localization sequence directing it to the inner mitochondrial membrane. When this gene is knocked out, the cell appears to be capable of metabolizing $FADH_2$, however, products of fermentation rapidly begin to accumulate. What is the most likely identity of this protein?

A) Hexokinase
B) Pyruvate decarboxylase
C) Citrate synthase
D) NADH dehydrogenase

7. Glucagon has what impact on glucose metabolism?

A) Increased glycogen synthesis
B) Decreased glycogen synthesis
C) Increased glucose uptake from the bloodstream
D) Decreased gluconeogenesis activity

8. In an experiment, hexokinase is exposed to an inhibitor such that feedback inhibition on the enzyme no longer occurs. Which reaction is most likely to be favored in this situation?

A) Conversion of glucose-6-phosphate to glucose-1-phosphate by phosphoglucomutase
B) Conversion of glucose-6-phosphate to glucose by hexokinase
C) Conversion of pyruvate to oxaloacetate by pyruvate carboxylase
D) Conversion of glycogen to glucose-1-phosphate by glycogen phosphorylase

9. What cellular need provides the most consistent reason to stimulate the pentose phosphate pathway?

A) Production of nucleotides to be used in mismatch repair
B) Increased demand for glycolytic intermediates during times of stress
C) Exposure to reactive oxygen species as part of cellular respiration
D) Ongoing β-oxidation of fatty acids

10. A side effect of an investigational medication causes fatty acid β-oxidation to be favored in cells exposed to the drug. What aspect of metabolism is most likely to be directly impacted in treated cells?

A) Stimulation of phosphofructokinase, inhibition of PEP carboxykinase
B) Stimulation of glycogen phosphorylase, inhibition of phosphoglucomutase
C) Stimulation of ATP synthase, inhibition of hexokinase
D) Stimulation of fructose-1,6-bisphosphatase, inhibition of phosphofructokinase

CARBOHYDRATES PRACTICE PASSAGE

Obesity and adult-onset diabetes mellitus present problems of epidemic proportions in much of the developed Western world. The ubiquity of high fructose corn syrup, as well as other metabolized sugars in processed food has been consistently cited as the chief culprit in the widespread nature of these chronic conditions. Although the first artificial sweeteners were discovered centuries ago, over the past few decades they have been increasingly used as sugar substitutes in a wide range of mass-produced food products. The proposed benefits of utilizing such sweeteners are multiple: increasing potential for weight loss, minimizing tooth decay, and mitigating development of type 2 diabetes mellitus. Though it might seem reasonable to assume that non-metabolized artificial sweeteners would help individuals reduce the risk of developing a chronic metabolic condition like obesity or type 2 diabetes, recent research has drawn into question their utility in maintaining a person's health.

One such study focused on a comparative assessment of caloric intake versus post-prandial (after a meal) glucose and insulin levels. The study was conducted in both normal and obese individuals in a laboratory setting. All subjects consumed the same breakfast, and the researchers provided a lunch and dinner preload meal to each participant. Preload meals were supplemented with either aspartame, stevia, or sucrose. The participants were allowed to eat to satiety for the lunch and dinner meals. Total caloric consumption for each meal is shown in Figure 1.

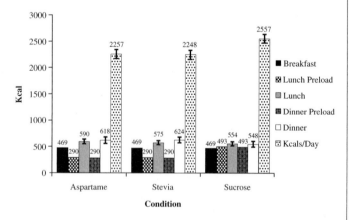

Figure 1   Total caloric consumption by meal and preloads across the entire study group including both normal weight and obese participants

Plasma glucose and insulin levels were monitored for each subject for two hours following each meal. Data for post-lunch measurements are shown in Figures 2 and 3. * indicates significant difference between stevia and sucrose, ** indicates significant difference between stevia and aspartame, and *** indicates significant difference between sucrose and aspartame.

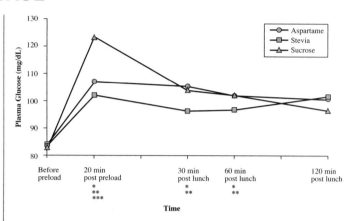

Figure 2   Post-prandial plasma glucose levels across the entire study group including both normal weight and obese participants

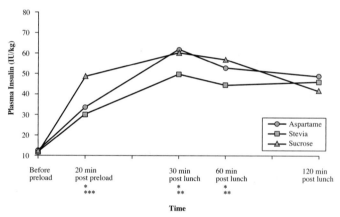

Figure 3   Post-prandial plasma insulin levels across the entire group including both normal weight and obese participants

An important metric utilized in the authors' analysis is the *insulinogenic index* which is described in Equation 1. The purpose of this ratio is to assess the effect of any given treatment (in this case, stevia vs. aspartame vs. sucrose) on insulin release per unit of blood glucose. Higher ratios indicate a relatively large change in insulin levels with respect to glucose, whereas lower ratios indicate relatively smaller changes in insulin level with respect to glucose over some specified time interval.

$$\frac{\Delta\ insulin}{\Delta\ glucose}\ \text{at 30–60 minutes post-load}$$

Equation 1   Formula for calculating the insulinogenic index

All figures and information adapted from Anton SD, et al. *Effects of stevia, aspartame, and sucrose on food intake, satiety, and postprandial glucose and insulin levels.* Appetite. 2010 Aug; 55(1): 37–43.

1. Which of the following conclusions about the insulinogenic index between 30 and 60 minutes after lunch is the most likely?

A) Aspartame has a higher insulinogenic index than sucrose.
B) Stevia has a lower insulinogenic index than sucrose.
C) Aspartame has a lower insulinogenic index than sucrose.
D) Stevia has a higher insulinogenic index than sucrose.

2. The authors were able to confirm that there was no difference in post-prandial satiety and satisfaction across the three conditions. Assuming that the authors' other results can be externally validated in the context of participants' dietary routines at home, which of the following outcomes would be most likely over the long term?

A) Supplementation with aspartame would decrease incidence of type 2 diabetes mellitus.
B) Supplementation with stevia would decrease incidence of type 2 diabetes mellitus.
C) Supplementation with stevia would increase incidence of obesity.
D) Supplementation with aspartame would increase incidence of obesity.

3. Which of the following statements best describes the mechanism by which insulin decreases blood glucose levels?

A) Insulin binds directly to individual molecules of glucose in the bloodstream, facilitating uptake.
B) Insulin passes easily through the lipophilic cell membrane and travels to the nucleus where it upregulates the synthesis of glucose transporter proteins.
C) Insulin binds to the extracellular portion of the insulin receptor, triggering an intracellular cascade resulting in increased expression of glucose transporters on the cell surface.
D) Insulin binds to a receptor in the brain, leading to increase autonomic nervous system activity and, thus, cellular respiration.

4. The rate of which of the following biochemical processes would increase with increasing insulin secretion?

A) Lipolysis
B) Proteolysis
C) Gluconeogenesis
D) Glycogen synthesis

5. Which of the following cofactors is NOT produced during glycolysis?

A) ADP
B) ATP
C) NAD^+
D) NADH

SOLUTIONS TO FREESTANDING QUESTIONS: CARBOHYDRATES

1. **A** The combustion of glucose is an exergonic process ($\Delta G < 0$) that is carried out during cellular respiration in order to generate ATP. The equilibrium constant (K_{eq}) is the ratio of products to reactants at equilibrium; a spontaneous reaction will favor products resulting in an equilibrium constant greater than 1 (choice A is correct). Alternatively, you can use the equation $\Delta G° = -RT \ln K_{eq}$ to calculate that a large negative $\Delta G°$ indicates a large K_{eq}.

2. **C** The Gibbs free energy values for reactions are additive when the reactions are coupled. This allows nonspontaneous reactions to proceed when coupled to a spontaneous reaction with a large negative ΔG. In this case, the question asks for the reaction liberating the greatest amount of free energy (the most negative $\Delta G°$). By reversing the second reaction, you could obtain a coupled reaction where $\Delta G° = -44.4$ (choice C is correct).

3. **C** Glycolysis results in the cleavage of glucose into two molecules of pyruvate. Blocking the glycolytic pathway with an inhibitor will decrease the quantity of products generated by the pathway (choice C is correct). Fermentation is essentially glycolysis in the absence of oxygen; if glycolysis is inhibited, fermentation cannot occur either (choice A is wrong). In yeast, fermentation results in the formation of ethanol (choice B is effectively the same as choice A and is wrong). If glycolysis is no longer functional, the cell must obtain energy via an alternative pathway. One such option would be fatty acid catabolism, so this is likely to increase, not decrease (choice D is wrong).

4. **A** Carbon monoxide poisoning prevents the delivery of oxygen throughout the body by increasing hemoglobin's affinity for oxygen. Oxygen normally serves as the terminal electron acceptor in the electron transport chain (ETC). When a cell lacks oxygen, the ETC cannot run and the cell turns to fermentation in order to meet its metabolic demands (choice B is wrong). In humans, this results in the production of lactic acid from pyruvate (choice A is correct). Citrate formation occurs in the first step of the citric acid cycle which cannot operate under anaerobic conditions (choice C is wrong), and there is no reason to suppose that fermentation will result in a net increase in ATP production; ATP levels will likely fall since fermentation produces only 2 net ATP as opposed to 30 from aerobic respiration (choice D is wrong).

5. **A** Each turn of the Krebs cycle produces one GTP, one $FADH_2$, and three NADH. One mole of glucose produces two moles of pyruvate during glycolysis, each of which would be fed into the Krebs cycle. This would generate a total of two moles of ATP equivalents (GTP is the energy equivalent of ATP; choice A is correct). Note that substrate-level phosphorylation occurs only during glycolysis and the Krebs cycle during cellular respiration. The generation of ATP in the electron transport chain occurs via oxidative phosphorylation.

6. **D** Since the protein of interest is localized to the inner mitochondrial membrane, and since knockout of the gene (and thus elimination of the protein) still allows glycolysis to occur, the protein is likely not hexokinase, which catalyzes the first step in glycolysis and is located in the cytosol (choice A can be eliminated). The protein must be involved in a reaction occurring within the mitochondrion, and given that the products of fermentation rapidly accumulate, this appears to indicate a defect in the electron transport chain. Since $FADH_2$ is still able to

deliver its electrons to the chain, the defect must occur upstream of this process. NADH, the other commonly used electron carrier, unloads its high-energy electrons in the first step of the electron transport chain, at NADH dehydrogenase. If this protein were rendered nonfunctional, NADH would no longer be able to make this delivery but $FADH_2$ would remain able to do so. As the cell begins to deplete its store of NAD^+, it would begin to undergo fermentation in order to regenerate NAD^+ (choice D is correct). Knockout of pyruvate decarboxylase or citrate synthase would effectively shut down the Krebs cycle but would not account for the difference in NADH versus $FADH_2$ metabolism (choices B and C are wrong).

7. **B**   Glucagon, a hormone released when blood glucose levels fall, serves to increase blood glucose by increasing the breakdown of glycogen and reciprocally decreasing its rate of synthesis (choice A is wrong, and choice B is correct). Glucagon also increases gluconeogenesis (choice D is wrong). Insulin serves to drive the absorption of glucose from the bloodstream, not glucagon (choice C is wrong).

8. **A**   Hexokinase phosphorylates glucose (glucose → glucose-6-P), and it typically receives negative feedback from rising levels of glucose-6-phosphate. If this regulatory step is no longer possible, glucose-6-phosphate is likely to accumulate and will need to be moved into pathways other than glycolysis. This would favor its conversion into glucose-1-phosphate by PGM (phosphoglucomutase), so choice A is correct. Glucose-6-phosphate is converted to glucose by glucose-6-phosphatase (choice B is incorrect). The conversion of pyruvate to oxaloacetate would promote gluconeogenesis; this could lead to further increases in the levels of glucose-6-phosphate further up the pathway and thus would not be favored (choice C is incorrect). Similarly, producing more glucose-1-phosphate could lead to more glucose-6-phosphate, which would not be favored (choice D is incorrect).

9. **C**   The pentose phosphate pathway (PPP) produces NADPH, which is used to neutralize the ROS (reactive oxygen species) to which a cell is constantly exposed as part of engaging in ATP production through cellular respiration (choice C is correct). While PPP does produce ribose-5-phosphate for use in nucleotide synthesis, mismatch repair occurs during replication and is not as consistent a need as the need to neutralize ROS (choice A is incorrect). Other pathways besides PPP are the primary producers of glycolytic intermediates (choice B is incorrect). NADPH is used to synthesize fatty acids, not to break them down (choice D is incorrect).

10. **D**   High levels of β-oxidation would lead to increases in acetyl-CoA levels and Krebs cycle activity. This would contribute to electron transport chain ATP production. Both citrate and ATP levels would rise in the cell, causing the inhibition of phosphofructokinase and glycolysis (there is no point in running glycolysis if the Krebs cycle is overwhelmed). The rise in citrate and ATP would also lead to the stimulation of fructose-1,6-bisphosphatase and gluconeogenesis; although the increase in gluconeogenesis would be less due to the lack of glucose and more due to the side effect of the drug (choice D is correct, and choice A is wrong). The other enzymes listed could be impacted (for example, hexokinase might be impacted by changing glucose levels), but these would not be as direct as the stimulation and inhibition by citrate and ATP (choices B and C are wrong).

SOLUTIONS TO CARBOHYDRATES PRACTICE PASSAGE

1. **A**   Equation 1 shows that the insulinogenic index is a ratio of the change in insulin to the change in glucose over a specified time interval. Looking at Figure 2, the change in glucose levels is relatively similar for all three sweeteners 30 to 60 minutes after lunch; however, looking at Figure 3, the greatest change in insulin levels during that same time period is for those consuming aspartame. Thus, the insulinogenic index for aspartame should be higher than for the other two sweeteners (choice A is correct). With little change in glucose levels between 30 and 60 minutes, the similar changes in insulin level for both stevia and sucrose consumption, as shown in Figure 3, would yield similar insulinogenic indices for these two conditions (choices B and D can be eliminated). The larger change in insulin level with aspartame consumption in the presence of similar glucose levels indicates that aspartame would have a higher, not lower, insulinogenic index as described above (choice C can be eliminated).

2. **B**   Type 2 diabetes mellitus (adult-onset) is thought to be caused by persistently elevated levels of post-prandial glucose which lead to persistently elevated insulin levels and eventual insulin resistance; because the stevia was found to have consistently lowered post-prandial blood glucose and insulin levels, it can be predicted that supplementation of one's diet with stevia-sweetened food would produce similar levels of satisfaction with a decreased risk of type 2 diabetes over the long term (choice B is correct). The aspartame condition was found to significantly decrease levels of blood glucose and insulin 20 minutes after the preload, but there was no difference after the meal; these results are not as strong as those for stevia which had decreased levels both post pre-load and post-meal (choice A can be eliminated). Figure 1 in combination with the information in the question stem show that the consumption of artificial sweeteners resulted in lower caloric intake for the same level of satisfaction and satiety; thus, it would be expected that decreased caloric intake would lead to more normal weight over the long term (choices C and D can be eliminated).

3. **C**   Insulin is a peptide hormone which will bind to a receptor on the extracellular surface of the cell membrane to induce an intracellular biochemical cascade for the desired effect, in this case, increasing expression of glucose (GLUT4) channels on the cell membrane surface. These channels then allow for increased influx of glucose from the blood into the intracellular space (choice C is correct). Insulin does not bind directly to glucose in the blood (choice A is wrong). Insulin is not a steroid hormone and does not pass easily through lipophilic membranes (choice B is wrong). While insulin actually does bind to receptors in the brain to induce increased autonomic system activity, this is not known to be a major contributor to glucose metabolism (choice D is wrong).

4. **D**   Insulin release and elevated blood insulin levels are typically associated with an anabolic state in which fats, proteins, and complex carbohydrates are synthesized by the body; thus, it is reasonable to expect that glycogen (a complex, branching carbohydrate) will be synthesized during these times (choice D is correct). Lipolysis and proteolysis will primarily take place during catabolic states, times when the body needs to break down stored fats and proteins for energy in a fasting state (choices A and B are wrong). Gluconeogenesis produces glucose which can be released into the blood in a fasting state (choice C is wrong).

5.   **C**   In the conversion of glyceraldehyde-3-phosphate to 1,3-bisphosphoglycerate, both NAD^+ and inorganic phosphate (P_i) are consumed and NADH is produced; thus, NAD^+ is not generated in glycolysis (choice D can be eliminated, and choice C is correct). ADP is produced twice (choice A can be eliminated), first in the step in which glucose is converted to glucose-6-phosphate and second when fructose-6-phosphate is converted to fructose-1,6-bisphosphate. In both of these steps, ATP provides the P_i to the carbohydrate undergoing metabolism. In addition to generating pyruvate for the Krebs cycle, the primary purpose of glycolysis is to generate ATP (choice B can be eliminated).

Chapter 7
Lipids

FREESTANDING QUESTIONS: LIPIDS

1. Fatty acid catabolism will cause which of the following:

A) increased glycolytic activity.
B) decreased phosphofructokinase activity.
C) increased utilization of the malate-aspartate shuttle.
D) decreased electron transport chain activity.

2. Taxadiene is a diterpene, and a precursor to taxol, a common drug used to treat breast, lung, pancreatic, and ovarian cancers. How many isoprene units would be found in taxadiene?

A) 1
B) 2
C) 3
D) 4

3. All of the following statements about cholesterol are true EXCEPT that it:

A) is the precursor for testosterone, estrogen, and progesterone.
B) is used by the liver to produce bile.
C) is the precursor for the fat-soluble vitamins A and D.
D) helps to maintain optimal membrane fluidity.

4. Which of the following correctly pairs a metabolic pathway with its cellular location?

　　I.　Beta-oxidation—mitochondria only
　　II.　Fatty acid synthesis—mitochondria only
　　III.　Gluconeogenesis—cytoplasm only

A) I only
B) II only
C) I and III
D) II and III

5. In humans, leucine and lysine are exclusively ketogenic. This means their α-keto acid carbon skeleton is degraded into acetyl-CoA or acetoacetate, an acetyl-CoA precursor. These amino acids can be:

A) catabolized for energy in the Krebs cycle, converted to ketone bodies, or used for fatty acid synthesis.
B) converted to acetone, acetoacetate, or β-hydroxybutyrate via ketogenesis, or enter gluconeogenesis to generate new glucose in the liver or kidney.
C) catabolized for energy in the Krebs cycle or via β-oxidation, but cannot be converted into glucose.
D) converted to pyruvate to enter gluconeogenesis.

6. mTORC1 is a protein complex that coordinates cell growth with the availability of nutrients and energy. Inhibition of mTORC1 is required for fasting-induced activation of ketogenesis. Two proteins, TSC1 (tuberous sclerosis 1) and raptor act on mTORC1. TSC1 inhibits mTORC1, and raptor is an essential for normal mTORC1 function. Loss of TSC1, or loss of raptor, would lead to which of the following, respectively?

A) Defect in ketone body production; decreased amounts of acetone, acetoacetate, and β-hydroxybutyrate
B) Defect in ketone body production; increased amounts of acetone, acetoacetate, and β-hydroxybutyrate
C) Decreased acetyl-CoA levels in the plasma; decreased ketone body production in hepatocyte mitochondria
D) Decreased acetyl-CoA levels in the plasma; increased ketone body production in hepatocyte mitochondria

7. After a meal rich in carbohydrates and fats:

A) fatty acids and triglycerides are synthesized to generate reduced energy-storage molecules.
B) β-oxidation levels increase to convert dietary fats to acetyl-CoA for entry into the Krebs cycle.
C) glucagon and epinephrine activate signaling cascades that result in activation of hormone-sensitive lipase.
D) Glycogenesis will be favored over glycolysis if ADP:ATP and NAD$^+$:NADH ratios are high.

8. A patient presents with musculoskeletal issues and laboratory tests confirm low levels of Vitamin D in the person's blood. A supplement is recommended, but despite daily consumption, the patient's Vitamin D levels do not show an increase in subsequent testing. What is the most likely cause of this outcome?

A) The patient is consuming too little dietary fiber with the supplement.
B) The patient is not consuming dietary fats along with the supplement.
C) The patient is also taking oral contraceptives.
D) The patient is spending more time outdoors.

9. Unsaturated fats produce less energy during β-oxidation than saturated fats with an equal number of carbons. What is the primary difference leading to this lower level of production?

A) The need to create a double bond within a saturated fat also generates $FADH_2$.
B) The $FADH_2$ generated by saturated fats stores more energy than those generated by processing unsaturated fats.
C) The number of NADH molecules produced by saturated fats is greater than for unsaturated fats.
D) NADH is produced earlier when processing saturated fats and can be sent more directly into the electron transport chain.

10. What is the best description for lipids that are being stored in the body as a potential source of energy?

A) Glycerol backbone, three fatty acid chains, required to have equivalent R groups
B) Glycerol backbone, two fatty acid chains, four isoprene units
C) Glycerol backbone, three fatty acids chains, possibly equivalent R groups
D) Glycerol backbone, two fatty acid chains, one phosphate group

LIPIDS PRACTICE PASSAGE 1

Sphingolipids are a class of lipids that contain a sphingosine (2-amino-4-octadecene-1,3-diol) moiety. Sphingomyelin, a type of sphingolipid, is found in animal cell membranes and is especially prevalent in the myelin sheath of neurons. In addition to a sphingosine moiety, sphingomyelin also consists of a fatty acid residue and a phosphocholine head group, as depicted below, where R represents another fatty acid:

Figure 1   Sphingomyelin

Sphingomyelin also plays an indirect role in cellular metabolism. During the synthesis of sphingomyelin by the enzyme sphingomyelin synthase, diacylglycerol is produced as a metabolic side-product. Diglyceride acyltransferase can convert diacylglycerol into triacylglycerol that can then be degraded by lipases to provide cellular energy.

Acid sphingomyelinase (ASM) is an enzyme involved in the breakdown of sphingomyelin. When the encoding gene for ASM—the *SMPD1* gene—is mutated, toxic amounts of sphingomyelin build up within cells, potentially leading to several metabolic disorders within humans. The group of metabolic disorders caused by mutations in the *SMPD1* gene is referred to as *Niemann-Pick disease*, and is inherited in an autosomal recessive fashion.

An experiment was performed to identify the role of two candidate *SMPD1* missense mutations in Niemann-Pick disease. ASM activity was assessed after transfection of HeLa cells with two variant cDNA constructs formed by site-directed mutagenesis of wild-type cDNA. The results of these experiments are summarized below (Table 1):

cDNA construct	ASM activity (pmol/mg/h)	% of Wild-type ASM activity
C1460T	24,579	100
C973G	737	3

Table 1   ASM activities of transiently expressed ASM variants in HeLa cells

Adapted from: Rhein C., Naumann J., Mühle C., Zill P., Adli M., Hegerl U., Hiemke C., Mergl R., Moller H.J., Reichel M., et al. *The acid sphingomyelinase sequence variant p.A487V is not associated with decreased levels of enzymatic activity.* JIMD Rep. 2013;8:1–6.

1. When sphingomyelin is broken down by sphingomyelinases, it is degraded into two components: phosphocholine and ceramide. One of these components diffuses through the cell membrane and participates in the apoptotic signaling pathway. The component that most likely participates in the apoptotic signaling pathway is:

A) phosphocholine, because its size relative to ceramide allows it to diffuse through the cell membrane more easily.
B) phosphocholine, because its polarity relative to ceramide allows it to diffuse through the cell membrane more easily.
C) ceramide, because its size relative to phosphocholine allows it to diffuse through the cell membrane more easily.
D) ceramide, because its polarity relative to phosphocholine allows it to diffuse through the cell membrane more easily.

2. Subject A and Subject B each have siblings with Niemann-Pick disease but are themselves unaffected. The parents of both subjects are also unaffected. If Subject A and a separate individual have a child with Niemann-Pick disease, what is the chance that a child from Subject A and Subject B will also have Niemann-Pick disease?

A) 0
B) 4/9
C) 1/6
D) 1/4

3. Which of the following will result from an increase in levels of acid sphingomyelinase on neuronal communication?

    I. Increased length of time for voltage-gated Na^+ channel inactivation
    II. Increased leakage of Na^+ into the extracellular fluid following an action potential
    III. Decrease in maximum membrane potential during depolarization

A) I only
B) II only
C) III only
D) II and III only

4. In the experiment performed in the passage, suppose that instead of cDNA constructs being mutated, wild-type DNA constructs were mutated at the same physical site as that of the cDNA constructs. How would the ASM activity of both constructs be affected?

A) No change in ASM activity of both
B) Increase in ASM activity of both
C) Decrease in ASM activity of both
D) Increase in ASM activity in one of the constructs only

5. From the results of the experiment, what is the most reasonable conclusion that can be made from the data?

A) Only the mutation represented by construct C1460T could be responsible for symptoms of Niemann-Pick disease.
B) Only the mutation represented by construct C973G could be responsible for symptoms of Niemann-Pick disease.
C) Both mutations represented by the two constructs could be responsible for symptoms of Niemann-Pick disease.
D) Neither of the mutations represented by the two constructs could be responsible for symptoms of Niemann-Pick disease.

6. The reaction catalyzed by diglyceride acyltransferase involves the formation of:

A) an ester bond.
B) a peptide bond.
C) a disulfide bond.
D) a glycosidic bond.

LIPIDS PRACTICE PASSAGE 2

Phospholipids are the main structural component of biological membranes. In order to build a phospholipid, a cell must generate large amounts phosphatidic acid (or 1,2-diacyl-sn-glycerol 3-phosphate) from glycerol. Phosphatidic acid can be derived from glycerol by phosphorylating it to glycerol-3-phosphate; this reaction is catalyzed by glycerol kinase. Reduction of DHAP (dihydroxyacetone phosphate), a glycolytic intermediate, is another source of glycerol-3-phosphate, and this reaction is catalyzed by glycerol-3-P dehydrogenase. Glycerol-3-phosphate is then twice esterified using acyl-CoA precursors as fatty acid donors to form phosphatidic acid. The first acylation to 1-acyl-sn-glycerol 3-phosphate is catalyzed by glycerol-3-phosphate O-acyltransferase and the second fatty acylation is catalyzed by 1-acylglycerol-3-phosphate O-acyltransferase. The final step in phospholipid synthesis is to esterify an alcohol, such as choline or inositol, to the phosphate group.

The first acylation of glycerol-3-phosphate takes place at either the endoplasmic reticulum membrane or the mitochondrial membrane. The latter reaction is significant in the liver, an organ with large numbers of mitochondria. The product of this acylation is lysophosphatidic acid, which is itself a membrane component. Indeed, all metabolic intermediates from this stage onwards are themselves components of biological membranes. Adipocytes have a higher mass ratio of phospholipids than all other cells, and so must anabolize large amounts of phospholipids. Generally, phospholipids are categorized into one of five types: phosphatidylserine, phosphatidylcholine, phosphatidylethanolamine, phosphatidylinositol, and phosphatidyl sphingomyelin.

Cerebral ischemia is a condition in which there is insufficient blood flow to the brain, resulting in brain tissue death. Depending on its severity and location, there are several categories and effects of ischemic injury. Specifically, phospholipases can be activated, thus changing membrane phospholipid composition. To determine the effect of ischemia on phospholipid composition, tissue from the cerebrum was collected from normal rats and those that had undergone an ischemic episode. Phospholipids were isolated and analyzed via matrix assisted laser desorption/ionization-imaging mass spectrometry (MALDI-IMS). Some results from this study are shown in Figure 1.

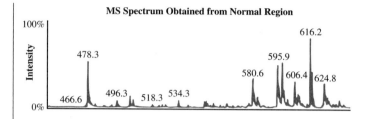

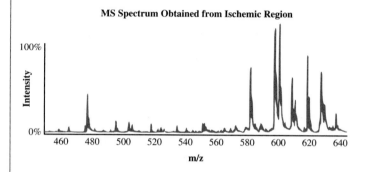

Figure 1 MALDI-IMS data from normal and ischemic *Rattus norvegicus* cerebral core tissue

1. Which of the following describes how neuronal cell membranes change in response to ischemia?

A) Cells express a different set of phospholipids.
B) Cells express the same phospholipids at the same relative proportions.
C) Cells express the same phospholipids but in different relative proportions.
D) Cells express phospholipids along the length of the long axon process.

2. Which of the following is LEAST likely to be an effect of ischemic injury?

A) Altered production of second messengers
B) Elevated levels of apoptosis
C) Upregulation of citrate synthase and isocitrate dehydrogenase
D) Altered activity of glucose 6-phosphate dehydrogenase

3. Enzymes involved in phospholipid synthesis pathways can be mutated, thus altering their activity. Which of the following would be the effect of a hyper-activating mutation in glycerol-3-P dehydrogenase and an inactivating mutation in glycerol-3-phosphate O-acyltransferase, respectively?

A) Elevated levels of glycerol-3-phosphate and decreased levels of lysophosphatidic acid

B) Elevated levels of DHAP and elevated levels of phosphatidic acid

C) Elevated levels of glycerol-3-phosphate and elevated levels of phosphatidic acid

D) Elevated levels of DHAP and lysophosphatidic acid

4. In order to collect brain samples from experimental rats, which of the following steps would NOT be required?

A) Penetrate three membranes of connective tissue (dura mater, arachnoid mater, pia mater)

B) Isolation of the cerebellum, which is located posterior to the pons

C) Removal of cortex tissue, which is composed of soma and dendrites

D) Mechanical disruption of the flat bones of the skull

5. Which of the following statements is supported by information in the passage?

A) The experimental samples contained at least two cell types.

B) Neurons have the highest concentration of phospholipids.

C) The activities of glycerol kinase and 1-acylglycerol-3-phosphate O-acyltransferase require ATP.

D) There are no first order connections between carbohydrate and lipid metabolic pathways.

SOLUTIONS TO FREESTANDING QUESTIONS: LIPIDS

1. **B** Fatty acid catabolism, also known as beta oxidation, results in the cleavage of two-carbon units from fatty acids to generate multiple acetyl-CoA molecules. Elevated levels of acetyl-CoA result in a decrease in glycolytic activity, including phosphofructokinase, which serves as the rate-limiting enzyme in glycolysis (choice A is wrong, and choice B is correct). Fatty acid catabolism occurs in the mitochondria so the malate-aspartate shuttle, which normally serves to deliver the electrons from cytoplasmic NADH into the electron transport chain, would not be required (choice C is wrong). Given the large quantity of NADH and $FADH_2$ generated during beta oxidation, it is unlikely that there would be a significant deficit in electron transport chain activity (choice D is wrong).

2. **D** A terpene is made up of two isoprene units. If taxadiene is a diterpene, then it has two terpenes, and thus four isoprene units.

3. **C** Cholesterol is the precursor to all of the steroid hormones (choice A is a true statement about cholesterol and can be eliminated), and it is used by the liver to make bile (choice B is a true statement about cholesterol and can be eliminated). It is an important component of cell lipid bilayers; its presence helps maintain the correct level of membrane fluidity (choice D is a true statement about cholesterol and can be eliminated). However, while cholesterol is an important precursor for vitamin D (a steroid-like vitamin), it is not the precursor for vitamin A (choice C is not true of cholesterol and is the correct answer choice).

4. **A** Item I is correct: beta-oxidation begins once an activated fatty acid is transported into the mitochondrial matrix (choices B and D can be eliminated). Note that neither of the remaining choices includes Item II, so it must be incorrect; jump straight to Item III. Item III is incorrect: gluconeogenesis is one of three biochemical pathways that occur in both the cytoplasm and mitochondria (the other two are heme synthesis and the urea cycle). Gluconeogenesis begins in the matrix and finishes in the cytosol (choice C can be eliminated, and choice A is correct). Note that Item II is in fact incorrect: unlike fatty acid breakdown, fatty acid synthesis occurs in the cytoplasm.

5. **A** Acetyl-CoA can enter the Krebs cycle to generate ATP, can be converted into ketone bodies (such as acetone, acetoacetate, or β-hydroxybutyrate), or can be used to build fatty acids. Acetyl-CoA cannot be converted to glucose (choices B and D are wrong). β-oxidation is the breakdown of fatty acids and generates acetyl-CoA; it does not use acetyl-CoA (choice C is wrong).

6. **B** The question stem describes a complex signaling system, where the inhibition of mTORC1 stimulates ketogenesis. This means mTORC1 must normally inhibit ketogenesis. TSC1 normally inhibits mTORC1, so TSC1 would stimulate ketogenesis, and the loss of TSC1 will have the opposite effect (inhibit ketogenesis, so choices C and D can be eliminated; note that TSC1 and mTORC1 do not affect acetyl-CoA production). Raptor is an essential component of mTORC1, so the loss of raptor will lead to loss of mTORC1 function. This means mTORC1 will not be able to inhibit ketogenesis, and the formation of the ketone bodies (acetone, acetoacetate, and β-hydroxybutyrate) will increase (choice A is wrong, and choice B is correct).

7. **A** After a meal rich in carbohydrates and fats, dietary nutrients will be extracted from food then put into storage molecules. Fats are more reduced than carbohydrates and proteins, which is why they store more energy per carbon; this means that fatty acids and triglycerides will be synthesized, not broken down (choice B is wrong). Glucagon and epinephrine levels increase during times of low blood glucose, not after a meal (choice C is wrong). If the ADP/ATP and NAD^+:NADH ratios are high, this indicates an energy deficit, which would favor glycolysis over glycogenesis. Glycogenesis is favored when ADP:ATP and NAD^+:NADH ratios are low (or, conversely, when the ATP/ADP and NADH:NAD^+ ratios are high; choice D is wrong).

8. **B** Vitamin D is a fat-soluble vitamin and is best absorbed along with some dietary fat; a lack of that consumption could explain this clinical result (choice B is correct). Consuming too little fiber would not have this impact on Vitamin D (choice A is incorrect), nor would taking oral contraceptives, which contain steroid hormones (choice C is incorrect). If the patient were spending more time outdoors, this would increase blood levels of Vitamin D rather than keeping them low (choice D is incorrect).

9. **A** Saturated fats lack double bonds between their carbons; the initial step in their β-oxidation pathway creates a double bond (an oxidation) while also producing an $FADH_2$ (a reduction). Since this step does not necessarily need to happen in an unsaturated fat, fewer high energy electron carriers are produced and thus the overall energy yield is lower (choice A is correct). $FADH_2$ molecules are equivalent no matter how they are produced (choice B is incorrect), and both versions of β-oxidation produce the same amount of NADH at the same point in the pathway (choices C and D are incorrect).

10. **C** Dietary fats are stored as triglycerides which have a glycerol backbone and three fatty acid chains which may or may not be the same (choice C is correct, and choice A is wrong). The inclusion of isoprene units is not relevant to dietary fats (choice B is wrong), and the inclusion of a phosphate group creates a phospholipid used in constructing membranes (choice D is wrong).

SOLUTIONS TO LIPIDS PRACTICE PASSAGE 1

1. **D** This is a 2 × 2 type of question. As stated in the question stub, the products of sphingomyelin degradation are phosphocholine (Figure 1) and ceramide (everything in sphingomyelin except for phosphocholine). The cell membrane is comprised of a lipid bilayer, with an interior hydrophobic core. Because of this hydrophobic core, charged, polar molecules such as phosphocholine will not be permeable (choices A and B are wrong). Smaller molecules in general diffuse through the membrane faster than larger molecules. However, ceramide is a larger molecule than phosphocholine, so size is not a reasonable explanation as to why ceramide can diffuse through the membrane (choice C is wrong; choice D is correct). Because of its long hydrocarbon chains, the hydrophobic ceramide can diffuse through the also hydrophobic membrane interior and participate in the apoptotic signaling pathway.

2. **C** Niemann-Pick disease is inherited in an autosomal recessive fashion, so only homozygous recessive individuals will be affected. If two carriers (heterozygous individuals) mate, there will be a 1/4 chance of the child having the disease. Since Subject A had a child with the disease, she must be a carrier. Subject B could either be homozygous dominant or a carrier. Because you know Subject B does not have the disease (is not homozygous recessive) and both Subject B's parents are carriers (since Subject B has siblings with the disease), there is a 2/3 chance that Subject B is heterozygous. The likelihood that Subject B is a carrier and that Subject B and Subject A have a child with the disease is therefore 2/3 × 1/4 = 1/6 (choice C is correct; choices A, B, and D are wrong).

3. **B** Since Items II and III both appear in the answer choices twice, it is best to start by analyzing one of these items first. Identification as either true or false will eliminate half the answer choices. Item II is true: acid sphingomyelinase (ASM) is involved in the breakdown of sphingomyelin. Sphingomyelin is a key component in neuronal myelin sheaths. Consequently, if ASM levels are increased, we would expect a decrease in the integrity of the myelin sheath. This will allow increased leakage of sodium ions out of the axon into the extracellular fluid and consequently decrease conduction velocity. This is because the myelin sheath serves as an insulator of sodium ions (choices A and C can be eliminated). Since Item I does not appear in either remaining choice, it must be false; look at Item III. Item III is false: action potentials are an "all-or-none" response; a decrease in myelin will not change the maximum depolarization potential during an action potential. The magnitudes of depolarization for action potentials in neurons are equivalent as long as threshold potential is reached, regardless of the strength of the stimulus (choice D can be eliminated, and choice B is correct). Note that Item I is false: decreasing the amount of myelin will not increase the length of time it takes for opened sodium channels to inactivate. Once voltage gated sodium channels reach threshold potential, the amount of time it takes for inactivation is a constant.

4. **A** In wild-type DNA, after transcription of the SMPD1 gene, the hnRNA is modified and introns are spliced out. The resulting mRNA is then translated into acid sphingomyelinase (ASM). The cDNA constructs in the experiment are created by reverse transcription of the mRNA post-splicing, followed by site-directed mutation. However, when these constructs are transfected into cell lines and then transcribed into mRNA, no further splicing occurs; the introns were already spliced out to make the cDNA in the first place. Thus, whether using wild-type DNA or using constructed cDNA, the ASM that is produced is a result of translation of already-spliced mRNA. Because of this, mutating wild-type DNA in the same location as the cDNA constructs will have no effect on the amount of ASM activity (choice A is correct; choices B, C, and D can be eliminated).

5. **B** This is a data-interpretation type of question. From the data table, the mutation represented by cDNA construct C1460T resulted in no change in ASM activity from the non-mutated wild-type DNA; the construct produces ASM with 100% of wild-type ASM activity (choices A and C are wrong). In contrast, the mutation represented by cDNA construct C973G has a large decrease in ASM activity, having only 3% of wild-type activity. Niemann-pick disease results in a build-up of sphingomyelin due to decreased ASM activity; thus, the mutation in this second construct is more likely to be responsible for symptoms of Niemann-Pick disease (choice B is correct, and choice D is wrong).

6. **A** The passage states that diglyceride acyltransferase converts a diglyceride into a triglyceride. Diglycerides are made up of a glycerol molecule with two fatty acids attached; conversion into a triglyceride means that another fatty acid would be attached (hence the name acyltransferase). The connection of a fatty acid to a glycerol molecule involves the formation of an ester bond (choice A is correct). Peptide bonds are found between amino acids in a protein (choice B is wrong), disulfide bonds are covalent bonds between sulfur atoms in tertiary or quaternary protein structure (choice C is wrong), and glycosidic bonds join monosaccharides in di- and poly-saccharide structures (choice D is wrong).

SOLUTIONS TO LIPIDS PRACTICE PASSAGE 2

1. **C** Paragraph 2 says that in response to cerebral ischemia, phospholipases can be activated, thus changing membrane phospholipid composition. This means it is unlikely that cells will express the same phospholipids at the same relative proportions (choice B is wrong, and choice C is correct). Figure 1 shows mass spectrometry (MS) data for phospholipids isolated from normal and ischemic brains. Both spectra (top and bottom) have a similar peak pattern, suggesting the two brain samples express the same phospholipids (choice A is wrong). Note also that the y-axis of a mass spectrometry graph is intensity or abundance. Because the peaks in the top and bottom of Figure 1 are different heights, it is logical that cells are expressing different relative proportions of the same phospholipids (additional support for choice C). Finally, note that choice D is a true statement, but is not relevant to the question stem.

2. **C** Paragraph 2 says that cerebral ischemia is a condition in which there is insufficient blood flow to the brain. If brain cells are experiencing limited blood flow, they are not going to receive sufficient oxygen. Citrate synthase and isocitrate dehydrogenase are Krebs cycle enzymes, and Krebs is part of aerobic respiration. There is no reason for low oxygen conditions to upregulate the Krebs cycle (choice C is least likely to be an effect of ischemia and is the correct answer choice). The passage states that ischemia can cause changes in membrane phospholipid composition, and since phospholipids are involved in cell signaling, ischemia may alter second messenger production (choice A could be an effect of ischemic injury and can be eliminated). Remember that some G-protein-linked receptors activate phospholipase C; this enzyme generates DAG (diacylglycerol) and IP_3 (inositol triphosphate) second messenger molecules by breaking down phosphatidylinositol-4,5-bisphosphate (or PIP_2, a phospholipid). Paragraph 2 also says that cerebral ischemia can lead to brain tissue death, which is likely due to apoptosis (choice B could be an effect of ischemic injury and can be eliminated). Finally, glucose 6-phosphate dehydrogenase (or G6PDH) is an enzyme in the pentose phosphate pathway. It reduces $NADP^+$ to NADPH and oxidizes glucose 6-phosphate at the same time. NADPH is a reducing agent with important roles in anabolism (fatty acid synthesis), and it also helps the cell neutralize reactive oxygen species. There are two reasons why this enzyme may have altered activity in response to ischemia. First, the passage says that phospholipid composition is altered, which may require fatty acid metabolism. Second, in low oxygen conditions, reactive oxygen species are not likely a major concern for the cell. There is no way to predict exactly what will happen to G6PDH activity in ischemia, but the point is that it is likely or possible that activity of this enzyme will change (choice D can be eliminated).

3. **A** Because of the "respectively" in the question stem, the first result in the answer choices goes with "a hyper-activating mutation in glycerol-3-P dehydrogenase," and the second result pairs with "an inactivating mutation in glycerol-3-phosphate O-acyltransferase." According to paragraph one, glycerol-3-P dehydrogenase reduces DHAP to form glycerol-3-phosphate. A hyper-activating mutation in this enzyme would increase its activity, resulting in a decrease in DHAP levels (the substrate) and an increase in glycerol-3-phosphate (the product, choices B and D can be eliminated). According to paragraphs 1 and 2, glycerol-3-phosphate O-acyltransferase adds an acyl group to glycerol-3-phosphate, forming 1-acyl-sn-glycerol 3-phosphate. Paragraph 2 says that this molecule can also be called lysophosphatidic acid. An inactivating mutation in glycerol-3-phosphate O-acyltransferase would cause reduced enzyme activity and thus more substrate (glycerol-3-phosphate) and less product (lysophosphatidic acid, choice A, is correct; choice C is wrong).

4. **B** The last paragraph of the passage says that cerebral tissue samples were used in the experiment. To access the cerebrum, researchers would have to remove skull bones (choice D would be required and can be eliminated) and the meninges (choice A would be required and can be eliminated). The cerebral cortex would certainly have been included in a cerebral tissue sample, and is made of gray matter, or dendrites and cell bodies (choice C is required and can be eliminated). However, there is no reason that the cerebellum would have to be isolated in this experiment (choice B would not be required and is the correct answer choice).

5. **A** The last paragraph of the passage says that tissue samples from the cerebrum were used in the experiment. The outer region of the cerebrum (the cortex) is made of gray matter (somas and dendrites), and the inner region is made of white matter (myelinated axons). This means that the samples likely contained both neuron tissue (the axons) and oligodendrocytes (myelin-producing cells of the central nervous system). Overall, choice A is supported and the correct answer. Note however that you did not have to realize this to get the right answer, as none of the other choices are supported and can therefore be eliminated. Paragraph 2 says that adipocytes have a higher mass ratio of phospholipids than all other cells (choice B is not supported). Glycerol kinase activity will require ATP because this enzyme is a kinase; however, there is no information in the passage that 1-acylglycerol-3-phosphate O-acyltransferase also requires ATP (choice C is not supported). Paragraph 1 says that DHAP (an intermediate of glycolysis) can be used to synthesize phospholipid precursor molecules (choice D is not supported).

Chapter 8
Nucleic Acids

FREESTANDING QUESTIONS: NUCLEIC ACIDS

1. All of the following types of bonds are involved in synthesizing double-stranded DNA EXCEPT:

A) β-N-glycosidic linkages.
B) disulfide bridges.
C) phosphodiester bonds.
D) hydrogen bonds.

2. Biological aging, or senescence, is the process by which molecular changes that disrupt metabolism accumulate in cells with time. All of the following would contribute to cellular senescence EXCEPT:

A) mitotic debris divided unevenly among daughter cells.
B) persistence of mutations from errors in DNA synthesis during mitosis.
C) activation of the apoptotic pathway following a metabolic insult.
D) shortening of chromosomal telomeres with increasing divisions of the cell.

3. The primary difference between euchromatin and heterochromatin is their accessibility for the purpose of transcription. Euchromatin is generally considered the "accessible" form in which DNA is ready for transcription while heterochromatin is the less accessible form in which DNA is stored. Which of the following is the protein around which DNA is wrapped during storage?

A) Nucleosome
B) Endosome
C) Histone
D) Centrosome

4. NADH (see below) plays important roles in cell metabolism. It is a:

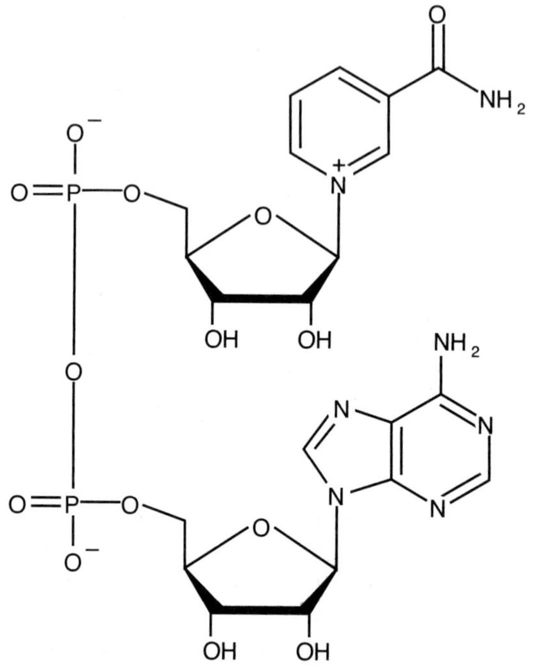

A) dideoxynucleotide with a pyrimidine base and nicotinamide group.
B) dinucleotide with a pyrimidine base and nicotinamide group.
C) dideoxynucleotide with a purine base and nicotinamide group.
D) dinucleotide with a purine base and nicotinamide group.

5. A substantial part of the information in the human genome does not lead to translation of functional proteins. The initial RNA transcript is hnRNA, which includes both introns (non-coding regions) and exons (protein coding regions). Small nuclear ribonucleic particles (snRNPs) facilitate splicing, which involves removal of the introns and ligation of the exons. Which of the following is NOT a process by which splicing of introns and exons leads to unique mRNAs?

A) Alternative splicing
B) Interruption
C) Exon shuffling
D) Nesting of genes

6. Ribose 5-phosphate is converted into phosphoribosyl pyrophosphate (PRPP) by the enzyme ribose-phosphate diphosphokinase, and PRPP can react with nitrogenous bases to generate purines. Which of the following is a true statement?

A) Both ribose 5-phosphate and PRPP are hexose phosphates.
B) Ribose 5-phosphate contains one covalent phosphoester bond, while phosphoribosyl pyrophosphate contains two.
C) Adenosine monophosphate and cytidine monophosphate biosynthesis require PRPP.
D) The pentose phosphate pathway supports nucleotide biosynthesis primarily through generating NADPH, but secondarily by producing ribose 5-phosphate.

7. A graduate researcher is performing an experiment in the lab and requires genomic DNA samples from animal tissue. She collects the tissue and then accidentally leaves it out at room temperature overnight. The next day she isolates DNA and determines it is of relatively high quality. Another graduate researcher makes a similar mistake the next week when she is trying to isolate RNA from the same animal tissue. Unfortunately, her sample has very low quality RNA at an extremely low concentration. The difference in these two scenarios is most likely due to the fact that:

A) RNA is more stable than DNA because it contains uracil and is single stranded.
B) DNA is more stable than RNA because DNA is double-stranded and its 2′ OH group allows increased hydrogen bonding with the second strand.
C) RNA is less stable than DNA because it is single stranded and has a nucleophilic OH group on carbon 2 of ribose.
D) DNA is easier to handle and isolate than RNA.

8. When designing a protocol to perform polymerase chain reactions (PCR), temperatures for each stage of the cycle need to be optimized based on available information concerning the sequences involved in the process. What would allow for the lowest melting temperatures in the cycle?

A) Template sequences with a high level of guanine
B) Primers with a high level of cytosine
C) Primers with a high level of thymine
D) Template sequences with a high percentage of adenine

9. A strain of *Streptococcus* is found to have a premature stop codon in the sequence for its DNA gyrase. What is the most likely effect this will have on the strain?

A) The bacteria will not be able to remove primers.
B) The bacteria will not be able to compress its chromosome.
C) The bacteria will not be able to initiate replication.
D) The bacteria will not engage in DNA repair.

10. The diameter of the DNA helix measures 20 Å and is a constant throughout the genome. What allows this measurement to remain the same?

A) Pyrimidines consist of one ring while purines consist of two rings.
B) The phosphodiester bonds in the backbone compress the aromatic bases.
C) Hydrogen bonding determines the diameter and the bonds are always the same length.
D) Pyrimidine dimers control the diameter of the DNA molecule.

NUCLEIC ACIDS PRACTICE PASSAGE

A zinc finger (Znf) domain is a protein motif comprised of approximately 30 amino acids which fold to form an elongated loop held together and by a Zn^{2+} cation. Within the zinc finger domain, two cysteine and two histidine residues coordinate the zinc cation, stabilizing the fold (Figure 1). A unique characteristic of each zinc finger domain is its ability to bind to a specific sequence in DNA and it was first discovered as a DNA-binding motif in a transcription factor from the frog *Xenopus laevis.*

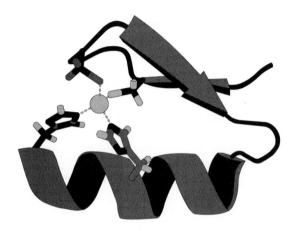

Figure 1   A zinc finger motif

Scientists have recently utilized zinc finger domains as a tool to experimentally facilitate genomic modifications. By tethering a specific zinc finger domain to an endonuclease, these enzymes can be targeted to specific regions in the genome. A construct of one or more zinc finger domains combined with an endonuclease is known as a zinc-finger nuclease (ZFN). If the DNA sequence of interest is palindromic, one ZFN will attach to one strand of DNA, while another ZFN attaches to the other strand, ultimately causing a double stranded break (Figure 2). Thus, either new mutations can be formed or foreign DNA can be added to the genome by various DNA repair mechanisms. If the DNA sequence is not palindromic, two different ZFNs must be constructed in order to get specific targeting of the DNA.

Nuclease Domains

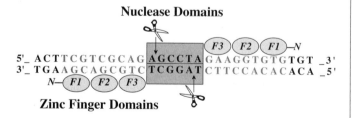

Zinc Finger Domains

Figure 2   Illustration of two zinc finger nucleases primed to make a double-stranded break

The human immunodeficiency virus (HIV) relies on a virally coded reverse transcriptase in order to propagate its genome. The nucleocapsid protein of HIV has two zinc finger motifs. Studies suggest that the zinc finger motifs are needed by the virus in order to facilitate viral infection. In order to combat HIV, scientists have employed azodicarbonamide, a small molecule which undergoes an electrophilic attack on the HIV zinc finger domain, ultimately disrupting the domain's folding.

1. Of the following sources, which can damage DNA in a similar manner to that of zinc finger nucleases?

    I.   UV radiation
    II.   X-ray radiation
    III. Benzene

A) I only
B) II only
C) I and II only
D) III only

2. How will adding more zinc finger domains to a zinc finger nuclease complex likely impact the quantity of resulting fragments when mixed with DNA?

A) Increase number of fragments
B) Decrease number of fragments
C) No effect on number of fragments
D) Increase number of fragments only if DNA is palindromic

3. Since the drug azodicarbonamide is electrophilic, it will most likely be reactive at the molecular level with which of the following components of the zinc finger domain?

A) Zinc cation
B) Valine side-chains within the zinc finger
C) Cysteine residues coordinating the zinc cation
D) Nitrogen lone-pairs within the peptide bonds of the peptide backbone

4. Which of the following is the most likely repair method for DNA damage caused by zinc finger nucleases?

A) Nucleotide excision repair
B) Direct reversal
C) Mismatch repair pathway
D) Non-homologous end joining

5. An experiment is performed in which four strains of a lysogenic (+)-ss RNA virus are reverse transcribed to ultimately form dsDNA. Each DNA sample is then heated to separate the strands. Which initial viral sequence results in a dsDNA molecule with the most negative change in enthalpy during separation?

A) 5′-GAUAAUAAA-3′
B) 5′-AAAGGAUUU-3′
C) 5′-ACACACACA-3′
D) 5′-CCAAUUUCC-3′

SOLUTIONS TO FREESTANDING QUESTIONS: NUCLEIC ACIDS

1. **B** Disulfide bridges are formed as part of post-translational protein modification and are not one of the bonds involved in double-stranded DNA (choice B is wrong and therefore the correct answer). β-N-glycosidic linkages connect the ribose in a nucleotide (or nucleoside) to its aromatic base (choice A is correct and can be eliminated), phosphodiester bonds connect nucleotides (choice C is correct and can be eliminated), and hydrogen bonds connect the aromatic bases to create the double-stranded property of the DNA molecule (choice D is correct and can be eliminated).

2. **C** Uneven division of mitotic intracellular debris would lead to increased accumulation of debris in certain cells; this may have an inhibitory effect on the metabolism of those cells, leading to senescence (choice A could contribute to senescence and can be eliminated). Persistence of mutations from errors in DNA synthesis could result in mounting abnormal genetic material. In turn, this would lead to the production of potentially dysfunctional or harmful proteins, increasing senescence (choice B could contribute to senescence and can be eliminated). Telomeres are short sequence repeats found on the ends of linear chromosomes and are typically degraded and shortened during cell division. Initially, because the telomeres are long, this does not present a problem; however, with ongoing rounds of cell division, the telomeres become increasingly shorter and are eventually lost altogether. The loss of the telomere means that with subsequent cell divisions, as the chromosome continues to shorten, there may be losses of important protein coding regions. This could lead to problems with the cell and cellular senescence (choice D can contribute to senescence and can be eliminated). However, the activation of the apoptotic pathway would result in cell death shortly thereafter; once the cell ceases to exist, molecular changes will no longer accumulate in the cell and, thus, it ceases to age (choice C would not contribute to cellular senescence and is the correct answer choice). (Note that telomerase is an enzyme that can lengthen telomeres; cells expressing telomerase are often immortal cells and are able to divide an infinite number of times, further emphasizing the importance of the telomeres in preventing senescence.)

3. **C** Histones are the proteins around which DNA is wrapped (choice C is correct). Nucleosomes are formed when multiple DNA-wrapped histones are bundled together (choice A is wrong). The endosome is a membrane-bound compartment of the eukaryotic cell responsible for transport of materials from the plasma membrane to the lysosome (choice B is wrong). The centrosome is an organelle that is responsible for organizing microtubules during cell division (choice D is wrong).

4. **D** This is a 2 × 2 question. NADH contains two nucleotides, each with a phosphate, a ribose and a nitrogenous base. The riboses in the middle of each have OH groups on both carbons 2 and 3; this means they are not dideoxynucleotides, which are missing both of these OH groups (eliminate choices A and C). The nitrogenous bases are attached to carbon 1; and the base at the top is not one you have likely seen before, but all the answer choices call this a nicotinamide group. The bottom nucleotide contains a nitrogenous base with two rings, and so must be a purine (choice B can be eliminated and choice D is correct).

5. **B** Alternative splicing is the process by which different exons are included in or excluded from the final mRNA (choice A directly leads to unique mRNAs and variable proteins and can be eliminated). Exon shuffling connects exons from different genes and occurs via recombination or transposons (choice C can lead to variable mRNAs and proteins and can be eliminated). Nesting of genes occurs when the exons of one gene lie entirely within an intron of a separate gene. The spliced out intron has the proper start and stop signal for translation, but of course translates a different protein (choice D can lead to variable mRNAs and proteins and can be eliminated). However, interruption is the phenomenon by which introns separate exons on the mRNA strand; this is the typical situation, and it is not implicated directly in the generation of variable protein products (choice B is not a variability process and is the correct answer choice).

6. **B** Ribose-5-phosphate contains a ribose sugar and a phosphate group:

Ribose 5-phosphate

A covalent phosphoester bond connects the CH_2O of ribose with the phosphate group. A pyrophosphate (PP_i) contains two orthophosphates, so PRPP must also contain a second phosphoester bond (choice B is a true statement and the correct answer choice):

Phosphoribosyl pyrophosphate (PRPP)

Ribose-5-phosphate and PRPP are pentose phosphates (not hexose phosphates), because the carbohydrate ribose contains five carbons (choice A is wrong). Based on information in the question stem, ribose-5-phosphate and PRPP help in purine synthesis. The purines are adenine and guanine, not cytosine (choice C is wrong). The pentose phosphate pathway supports nucleotide biosynthesis primarily through generating ribose-5-phosphate. NADPH is used in fatty acid biosynthesis, not nucleotide synthesis (choice D is wrong).

7. **C** RNA is less stable than DNA as is indicated by the fact that the overnight sample had low quality RNA at a low concentration (choice A is wrong). DNA is more stable, but it lacks the 2′ OH group (choice B is wrong). While it is true that DNA is easier to handle and isolate, this statement does not explain the discrepancy described in the question stem (choice D is wrong). The correct answer is choice C; it is both a true statement and answers the question.

8. **D** Melting temperature (T_m) is the temperature at which half of the hydrogen bonds holding together two strands of DNA can be broken. Since G-C base pairs contain three hydrogen bonds (compared to two hydrogen bonds in an A-T base pair), the greater the G-C content of a DNA sequence, the higher the melting temperature (choices A and B can be eliminated). Having greater amounts of adenine and thus thymine would bring down the T_m (choice D is correct). While primers do need to dissociate from the template sequence, this does not involve nearly as many hydrogen bonds as the overall sequence to be amplified (choice D is better than choice C).

9. **B** DNA gyrase folds and twists the single circular chromosome present in prokaryotic cells. If this enzyme were not functional, the genome could not be properly packed (choice B is correct). DNA polymerase I removes primers in bacteria (choice A is incorrect), helicase initiates replication (choice C is incorrect), and multiple enzymes can perform DNA repair, but gyrase is not one of them (choice D is incorrect).

10. **A** Pyrimidines are hydrogen bonded to purines as part of DNA sequence pairing, and pyrimidines are composed of one ring while purines have two. The diameter of DNA is determined by the presence of three rings at each base pairing (choice A is correct). Phosphodiester bonds do create the backbone of DNA, but do not determine its diameter (choice B is incorrect). Hydrogen bonds do link base pairs, but similarly do not determine the diameter (choice C is incorrect). Pyrimidine dimers form when the hydrogen bonds between base pairs are broken and pyrimidines on one strand bond to one another; this is a form of mutation and not part of typical DNA structure (choice D is incorrect).

SOLUTIONS TO NUCLEIC ACIDS PRACTICE PASSAGE

1. **B** Item I is a good place to start because it appears twice in the answer choices; determining whether to keep or eliminate it turns the question into a 2 × 2 elimination. Item I is false: as stated in Paragraph 2, zinc finger nucleases cause double stranded breaks within DNA. UV radiation damages DNA by causing pyrimidine dimers to form (choices A and C can be eliminated). Both remaining choices include Item II, so it must be true; consider Item III. Item III is false: benzene, an aromatic compound, results in intercalation of DNA bases rather than causing double-stranded breaks (choice D can be eliminated, and choice B is correct). Note that Item II is true: X-ray radiation, like zinc finger nucleases, can cause double stranded breaks.

2. **B** As described in Paragraph 2, one or more zinc finger domains can be tethered to an endonuclease to make the zinc finger nuclease complex. The effect of adding additional zinc finger domains will be a higher specificity of the zinc finger nuclease for the strands of DNA. This is because the DNA strand complementary to the combined zinc finger domains will need to be longer in order to bind. Thus, there will be fewer locations on the DNA where the zinc finger nuclease can bind. If there are fewer binding locations, there will be fewer cuts along the DNA, and thus the number of resulting fragments will decrease (choice B is correct; choices A, C, and D are wrong).

3. **C** Azodicarbonamide is an electrophilic molecule that reacts with the zinc finger domain to inhibit the nucleocapsid formation within HIV. The component most reactive with the electrophilic drug will be one that is nucleophilic. Nucleophiles are electron-rich and have a lone pair to donate. Cysteine residues are nucleophilic, and if cysteine attacks the azodicarbonamide drug, its coordination with the zinc cation of the HIV zinc finger will be disrupted, making it a reasonable mechanism of drug action (choice C is correct). The zinc cation is a positively charged divalent ion and as a result is not electron-rich (choice A is wrong). Valine side chains cannot act as nucleophiles because they do not have free lone pairs to attack electrophiles (choice B is wrong). While the nitrogen atoms in the peptide bonds do have free lone pairs, they are not as nucleophilic, as the lone pairs are delocalized through resonance with the carbonyl oxygen in the peptide backbone (choice D is wrong).

4. **D** Zinc finger nucleases cause double stranded breaks within DNA, so this is the damage that needs to be addressed by the repair mechanism. Nucleotide excision repair and the mismatch repair pathway tend to occur when only one of the two strands has a defect, as the other strand is used as a template to repair the damaged strand (choices A and C can be eliminated). Direct reversal is a repair mechanism that occurs when there is no breakage of the phosphodiester backbone, such as the formation of dimers (choice B can be eliminated). Non-homologous end joining is a repair mechanism that frequently occurs to repair a double stranded break (choice D is correct).

5.   **A**   The change in enthalpy necessary to separate the dsDNA represents the energy required to break the hydrogen bonds of the base pairs. The more hydrogen bonds there are, the more energy will be required to break them. However, the question asks for the DNA with the most negative change in enthalpy, so the correct answer will be the viral strand yielding the DNA strand with the fewest hydrogen bonds formed. GC base pairs are held together by three hydrogen bonds, while AT base pairs are held together by two, thus the fewer GC base pairs a strand has, the easier it will be to separate. Out of the four candidate sequences, the first will form only one GC base pair, and hence will have the fewest hydrogen bonds in the DNA (choice A is correct). Choice B would generate two GC base pairs, while choices C and D would generate four each.

Part 3

MCAT Biology

Chapter 9
Molecular Biology

FREESTANDING QUESTIONS: MOLECULAR BIOLOGY

1. Which of the following is used to regulate prokaryotic transcription?

    I.   Pribnow box
    II. Promoters
    III. TATA box

    A) I and II only
    B) I and III only
    C) II and III only
    D) I, II, and III

2. Which of the following statements regarding methylation of bases in DNA is FALSE?

    A) Plays an important role in X chromosome inactivation
    B) Protects bacterial genomes from digestion by restriction enzymes
    C) Increases the rate of DNA mutation
    D) Marks a section of DNA for activation by transcription factors

3. The goal of a particular experimental procedure is to stop genome replication in tissue culture as early as possible. The researchers thus look for a chemical that can achieve this effect. Which of the following enzymes would be the best target for that chemical?

    A) Helicase
    B) Primase
    C) DNA polymerase
    D) Ligase

4. Growth of a bacterial culture appeared to stop unexpectedly. Upon sequencing the genomes of the colonies with the stalled growth, it was found that RNA sequence was mixed into the DNA genome. Which enzyme has likely become disabled in these cells?

    A) DNA polymerase I
    B) DNA polymerase II
    C) DNA polymerase III
    D) DNA polymerase IV

5. In a certain experimental cell line, the tRNA with an anticodon sequence of UAC experiences a folding error that makes it nonfunctional 10% of the time. What impact would this have on translation?

    A) Translation would proceed as normal because other tRNAs would take over the work of the nonfunctional copies.
    B) The initiation of translation would be facilitated by an increased association with sigma factors.
    C) Translation rates would be reduced because the transport of methionine to the ribosomes would be curtailed.
    D) The completion of translation would be impaired by a lack of the ability to recognize stop codons.

6. An autosomal recessive disease presents in a child who has one homozygous dominant parent and one heterozygous parent. What type of mutation would make this expression possible?

    A) Inversion
    B) Loss of heterozygosity
    C) Point mutation
    D) Translocation

7. What type of DNA is LEAST likely to contain repeated sequences such as single nucleotide polymorphisms and tandem repeats?

    A) Heterochromatin
    B) Telomeres
    C) Centromeres
    D) Euchromatin

8. What is the nature of the relationship between RNA transcript and the amino acids that are determined by its codons?

    A) The relationship is ambiguous and bidirectional.
    B) The relationship is ambiguous and degenerate.
    C) The relationship is unambiguous and degenerate.
    D) The relationship is unambiguous and bidirectional.

9. Under what circumstances would a cell be likely to trigger cap-independent translation?

    I.   Dysregulated cell growth
    II. Sustained anaerobic respiration
    III. Viral infection

    A) I only
    B) I and II only
    C) III only
    D) I, II, and III

MOLECULAR BIOLOGY PRACTICE PASSAGE

Adipose tissue is found in two forms: white fat cells, which store energy in the form of triglycerides, and brown fat cells, which oxidize fuels and dissipate energy in the form of heat. When activated, brown fat cells take up fatty acids and glucose from the circulation, as shown in Figure 1. Brown adipose tissue has abundant mitochondria, which, via uncoupling oxidative phosphorylation, release chemical energy in the form of heat. Uncoupling protein 1 (UCP1) causes the inner membrane of the mitochondria to become "leaky"; this dissipates the hydrogen ion gradient by allowing H^+ to re-enter the matrix without going through the ATP synthase. UCP1 is regulated by triiodothyronine (T3), which is generated when type 2 5′ deiodinase (D2) removes an iodine from the prohormone thyroxine (T4). A specific adrenergic receptor, known as a β_3-adrenergic receptor, stimulates this process. The β_3-adrenergic receptor is a G-protein coupled receptor (GPCR) and is activated by catecholamines, including epinephrine and norepinephrine. Brown adipose tissue is also rapidly activated by exposure to cold temperatures, and the activity of brown adipose tissue in adults is inversely correlated to age, body mass index (BMI), and fasting plasma glucose levels.

While brown fat cells are important for thermoregulation in small mammals and newborn humans, the vast majority of brown fat cells are replaced by white fat cells in adult humans. However, positron emission tomography (PET) with the tracer ^{18}F-fluorodeoxyglucose (^{18}F-FDG), has revealed that there are commonly multiple depots of brown adipose tissue in the cervical region of adults. This has been seen as a nuisance for ^{18}F-FDG PET scanning, since this technique is used to visualize the increased uptake of radiolabeled glucose by metabolically active cancers. Metabolically active brown fat has substantial uptake of the radiolabeled glucose, thus leading to false positive results.

Recently, a genetic "master switch" for brown adipose tissue differentiation has been discovered. PRDM16 (PRD1-BF1-RIZ1 homologous domain containing 16) was shown to be selectively expressed in brown fat cells versus white fat cells and stimulates nearly all of the characteristics of brown fat cells. A large majority of genes that are selectively expressed in brown adipocytes are positively regulated by PRDM16. Conversely, PRDM16 expression suppresses the mRNA levels of several genes, such as *resistin* and *serpin3ak*, which are selectively enriched in white fat. It has been further discovered that bone morphogenetic protein 7 (BMP7) activates the formation of brown fat including induction of PRDM16 and PGC-1α [peroxisome proliferator-activated receptor-γ (PPAR-γ) coactivator-1α], as well as increased expression of brown-fat-defining marker UCP1.

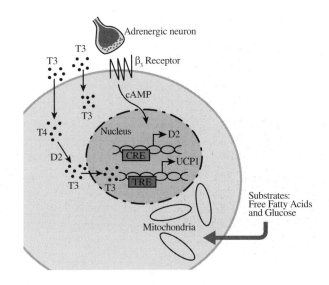

Figure 1   A brown fat cell. CRE = cAMP Response Element; TRE = Thyroid hormone response element; D2 = Type 2 5′ Deiodinase; UCP1 = Uncoupling Protein 1

Adapted from Celi FS. *Brown adipose tissue—when it pays to be inefficient.* N Engl J Med 2009;360:1553-6 and Seale P, Kajimura S, Yang W, et al. *Transcriptional control of brown fat determination by PRDM16.* Cell Metab 2007; 6:38-54.

1. A patient with a pheochromocytoma, a tumor of the adrenal gland that leads to hypersecretion of epinephrine, would be expected to have which of the following?

A) Decreased brown adipose tissue intracellular levels of T3
B) Decreased brown adipose tissue Krebs cycle activity
C) Increased brown adipose tissue levels of D2 mRNA
D) Increased fat cell activation, which would lead to increased weight gain

2. Which of the following treatments would help decrease the false positive rate of diagnostic ^{18}F-FDG PET scans for cancers?

    I.   Warming the room occupied by the study subject
    II. Administering beta-blockers (medications that block the β-adrenergic receptors)
    III. Administering a synthetic version of T4

A) I only
B) I and II
C) III only
D) I, II, and III

3. Based on the passage, which of the following may be inferred?

A) The regulation of brown fat cells appears to be a potential important therapeutic target for obesity.
B) Activation of brown fat cells leads to what may be considered a "local hypothyroid state."
C) A patient with diabetes who has frequent hyperglycemia would be likely to have a high state of brown adipose tissue metabolic activity.
D) The PRDM16 gene is selectively present in brown fat cell genomes.

4. Which of the following would be expected in a BMP7-knockout mouse embryo compared to a normal mouse embryo?

A) An increased amount of PRDM16 mRNA
B) A marked paucity of brown fat and almost a complete absence of UCP1 protein
C) An increase in PGC-1α activity
D) A decrease in the expression of the genes *resistin* and *serpin3ak*

5. In one experiment, an adenovirus vector was used to increase BMP7 expression in mice. Which of the following would be LEAST likely to occur?

A) A reduction in weight gain
B) An increase in brown fat mass
C) An increase in energy expenditure
D) An increase in fasting plasma glucose levels

6. Based on Figure 1, thyroid hormone (a peptide hormone) exerts its effect on brown fat cells via a mechanism of action that is most analogous to the mechanism of action of which of the following?

A) Adrenocorticotropic hormone (ACTH)
B) Cortisol
C) Antidiuretic hormone (ADH)
D) Insulin

SOLUTIONS TO FREESTANDING QUESTIONS: MOLECULAR BIOLOGY

1. **A** Item I is true: the Pribnow box is 10 nucleotides upstream of the start site in prokaryotes and is part of the promoter sequence required for the binding of RNA polymerase (choice C can be eliminated). Item II is true: promoters are involved in transcriptional regulation for both eukaryotes and prokaryotes (choice B can be eliminated). Item III is false: the TATA box has the same function as the Pribnow box, but it is found 25 nucleotides upstream of the start site in eukaryotes and is not involved in prokaryotic transcription (choice D can be eliminated, and choice A is correct). Remember, on Roman numeral questions, make POE do double work by eliminating answer choices based on whether individual statements are correct or not.

2. **D** The expression of genes is influenced by how the DNA is packaged in chromosomes and base modifications, such as methylation, can be involved in packaging. Regions that have low or no gene expression usually contain high levels of methylated cytosine bases; for example, cytosine methylation is important in X chromosome inactivation (choice A is true and can be eliminated). Bacteria methylate their genomes at the sequences recognized by restriction enzymes. This prevents binding of the bacterial genome to the active site of the enzyme, preventing digestion (choice B is true and can be eliminated). Methylation can lead to deamination, leaving behind a thymine base where there used to be a cytosine; methylated cytosines are therefore particularly prone to mutations (choice C is true and can be eliminated). However, methylation of bases interferes with the ability of the DNA to interact with transcription factors; this decreases the rate of transcription in methylated regions (choice D is false and is the correct answer choice).

3. **A** Helicase finds the origin on a DNA molecule and unwinds the helix at that point. Of the enzymes listed, it acts earliest in the process and thus would be the most appropriate target (choice A is correct). Primase is the RNA polymerase that creates primers and is involved in replication, but it acts after helicase (choice B can be eliminated). DNA polymerase adds nucleotides after the primers are in place and ligase connects the synthesized strands created by discontinuous replication; like primase, both are involved in replication, but act after helicase (choices C and D can be eliminated).

4. **A** DNA polymerase I is responsible for 5′ to 3′ exonuclease activity in prokaryotes (among other functions); thus, it removes the primers, which are composed of RNA. If this enzyme became non-functional, the bacterial genome would contain both RNA and DNA (choice A is correct). DNA polymerase II engages in both 5′ to 3′ polymerization and 3′ to 5′ exonuclease activity, but not in 5′ to 3′ exonuclease activity, so this would not explain the result (choice B is wrong). DNA polymerase III has the same functions as DNA polymerase II, but it is even more efficient and is in fact the primary enzyme for these tasks (choice C is wrong); DNA polymerase IV is primarily involved in slowing down the work of other polymerases when mistakes have been detected and need to be corrected (choice D is wrong).

5. **C** The anticodon UAC is complementary to the codon AUG which codes for methionine, the first amino acid used in translation (choice C is correct). Since methionine is always the first amino acid and has only one codon, other tRNAs could not pick up the slack (choice A is

wrong). While sigma factors are involved in the initiation of transcription, they do not play a role in translation (choice B is wrong). There are no tRNAs that recognize the stop codons (UAA, UGA, and UAG); thus, their recognition would not be impacted by this change (choice D is wrong).

6. **B** When heterozygosity is not present, a recessive trait can be expressed with only one copy of the allele present; this would explain the disease occurring in this child (choice B is correct). An inversion occurs when a piece of a chromosome gets turned in place, a point mutation would lead to a codon change (but possibly not even an amino acid change), and a translocation means recombination has occurred between non-homologous chromosomes. None of these would account for the expression of this recessive disease (choices A, C, and D can be eliminated).

7. **D** Euchromatin represents the least tightly packed DNA and thus contains sequences that are most likely to be transcribed to produce needed cellular products. Given their state of "information readiness," these sequences are least likely to contain confounding or unstable repetitious elements (choice D is correct). Heterochromatin represents the most tightly packed DNA; these sequences are least likely to be transcribed, so repeated sequences are more common (choice A is wrong). Telomeres represent the protective yet repetitious sequences on the ends of linear chromosomes. They make replication of the ends of the chromosomes possible (via a special enzyme called telomerase) without losing valuable DNA sequence; by definition, they contain repeats (choice B is wrong). Since centromeres are made of heterochromatin, choice C is also wrong.

8. **C** Each codon on mRNA specifies only a single amino acid; thus, the genetic code is unambiguous. Each piece of mRNA can only be read in one way (choices A and B can be eliminated). However, some (many!) amino acids can be specified by more than one codon, and so the process is also degenerate (choice D can be eliminated, and choice C is correct). Note that a one-to-one (bidirectional) relationship does not exist between all amino acids and codons.

9. **D** Always start Roman numeral questions by determining which of the three items appears in exactly two of the answer choices. Analyze this item first, since whether it is true or false, it will immediately eliminate half the answer choices. In this question, Items II and III both appear in exactly two answer choices, but Item III is short, so start analyzing that. Item III is true: cap-independent translation is used when the cell encounters circumstances that could require apoptosis. Viral infection can be a reason to trigger apoptosis (choices A and B can be eliminated). Note that either Item I or II can be used to determine the final answer. Item I is true: dysregulated cell growth, a precancerous state, would qualify for this intervention (choice C can be eliminated, and choice D is correct). Note that Item II is in fact true: long periods of anaerobic respiration would stress the cell, another trigger for this type of translation.

SOLUTIONS TO MOLECULAR BIOLOGY PRACTICE PASSAGE

1. **C**   As described in the first paragraph and the figure, increased epinephrine would lead to activation of the β_3 receptor, a GPCR, which triggers the production of D2 (choice C is correct). The increased D2 would convert more T4 to T3 (choice A is wrong). This would lead to increased metabolic activity, including the Krebs cycle (choice B is wrong). This increased metabolic activity, which would ultimately be in the form of uncoupled oxidative respiration, would be expected to lead to weight loss rather than weight gain (choice D is wrong).

2. **B**   The passage states that the increased metabolic activity and uptake of substrates, including glucose, by activated brown fat cells leads to "false positives" on ^{18}F-FDG PET scans for cancers. Therefore, in order to decrease the uptake of radiolabeled glucose at the brown fat cells, the intervention should decrease brown fat cell metabolic activity. Item I is true: the passage states that exposure to cold temperatures rapidly activates brown fat cells; thus, warming the room would lead to decreased brown fat activity (choice C can be eliminated). Item II is true: since activity of the β_3 receptor leads to increased brown fat cell metabolic activity, the administration of beta-blockers should lead to decreased activity (choice A can be eliminated). Item III is false: the passage and figure support that increased thyroid hormone (T4) levels lead to increased brown fat cell metabolic activity. Thus, the administration of a synthetic T4 would lead to increased metabolic activity and be counterproductive (choice D can be eliminated, and choice B is correct).

3. **A**   The regulation of brown fat cells as a potential therapeutic target for obesity is supported in the passage by various statements, including the fact that brown fat cell activity increases metabolism and dissipates energy, and also because it is inversely correlated with body-mass index (BMI). Therefore, choice A is correct. The increased levels of D2 in the brown fat cells leads to increased levels of active T3 hormone; therefore, it is considered to be a "local *hyper*thyroid state" (choice B is wrong). The passage directly states that the level of brown adipose tissue activity is inversely correlated with the serum glucose levels (choice C is wrong). While the PRDM16 gene is selectively *expressed* in brown fat cells, the gene is present in the genome of all cells (choice D is wrong). Remember that all of an individual's genes are present in their genome, and that specific genes are expressed (i.e., transcribed and translated) in specific tissue types.

4. **B**   As the passage states, BMP7 activates the formation of brown fat, including induction of PRDM16 and PGC-1α. Therefore, a mouse that lacked BMP7 would be expected *not* to express the PRDM16 gene, which would lead to decreased levels of PRDM16 mRNA (choice A is wrong). Since PRDM16 is the "master switch" for brown adipose tissue differentiation (as stated in the passage), the mouse would lack brown adipose tissue and would not express UCP1 (choice B is correct). Since BMP7 also leads to the expression of PGC-1α, it follows that lack of BMP7 would lead to decreased PGC-1α activity (choice C is wrong). Also, the passage states that PRDM16 inhibits the expression of the genes *resistin* and *serpin3ak*. Thus, a lack of BMP7, which leads to a lack of PRDM16, would result in an increased expression of *resistin* and *serpin3ak* (choice D is wrong).

5. **D** Since BMP7 induces brown fat cell metabolism, an increase in BMP7 would likely lead to weight loss due to increased metabolism and uncoupled cellular respiration (choice A is likely and can be eliminated). This would result in increased energy expenditure (choice C is likely and can be eliminated). BMP7 also induces many genes, including PRDM16, which would lead to brown fat cell differentiation; thus, the total brown fat cell mass would increase (choice B is likely and can be eliminated). However, the passage states that brown fat cell activity is inversely related to fasting plasma glucose; therefore, an increase in brown fat cell activity would lead to a decrease in fasting plasma glucose levels (choice D is not likely and is the correct answer choice).

6. **B** Despite the fact that thyroid hormone is a peptide hormone, Figure 1 supports the fact that this hormone works intracellularly to exert its effect on the cell at the level of gene expression. This is the mechanism of action primarily used by steroid hormones, such as cortisol (choice B is correct), aldosterone, testosterone, estrogen, and progesterone. Peptide hormones, including ACTH (choice A), ADH (choice C), insulin (choice D), and several others, exert their effect by binding to cell surface receptors and modifying intracellular enzyme activity.

Chapter 10
Microbiology

FREESTANDING QUESTIONS: MICROBIOLOGY

1. All functional viruses contain the following structure(s):

    I.   protein-based capsid.
    II. genomic DNA or RNA.
    III. phospholipid envelope.

    A) I only
    B) I and II only
    C) II and III only
    D) I, II, and III

2. The lysogenic act of an obligate, intracellular parasite excising portions of host DNA and transferring it to the next host is called:

    A) conjugation.
    B) transfection.
    C) transduction.
    D) transformation.

3. Which of the following nitrogenous bases would you NOT expect to find in the genome of a retrovirus?

    A) Adenine
    B) Uracil
    C) Thymine
    D) Guanine

4. Human immunodeficiency virus (HIV) is a lysogenic, (+) RNA retrovirus that carries a copy of reverse transcriptase in its capsid. What would happen to the virulence of its progeny that neglected to package reverse transcriptase within the capsid?

    A) The virulence will be unaffected; reverse transcriptase is not necessary for successful viral propagation.
    B) The virulence will be reduced, because reverse transcriptase will need to be translated by the host cell machinery before the virus can propagate.
    C) The virus will be rendered ineffective, because reverse transcriptase is necessary to copy the RNA genome into DNA for insertion into the host genome.
    D) The virus will be rendered ineffective, because reverse transcriptase is necessary for the virus to enter the host cell.

5. Which of the following is true regarding the productive cycle of viruses?

    A) The last stage of the cycle involves breaking open the host cell wall to release progeny viruses.
    B) The virus inserts its genome into the host cell genome and "hides" within the host cell.
    C) Imperfect excision can result in transduction of host cell genes to other host cells.
    D) The virus acquires an envelope from the host cell plasma membrane.

6. An auxotroph is a bacterium that has lost the ability to synthesize a compound. If the following auxotrophs were plated onto a growth medium containing arginine, lactose, and ampicillin, which would survive?

    A) Arg^-, lac^+, amp^r
    B) Arg^+, lac^-, amp^r
    C) Arg^-, lac^+, amp^s
    D) Arg^-, lac^-, amp^s

7. Which of the following structures is present in prokaryotes?

    A) Nucleus
    B) Mitochondria
    C) Ribosomes
    D) Golgi

8. Which of the following is true regarding prions?

    A) They are transmissible viruses that primarily attack neuromuscular junctions.
    B) They manifest themselves in the digestive tract of animals after ingestion of other animals within the same species.
    C) They are non-living, acellular structures only transmissible via ingestion and not inheritance.
    D) They are transmissible misfolded proteins responsible for several encephalopathies.

9. Hydrothermal vents on the sea floor emit geothermally heated water rich in minerals. They support thriving biological communities, including bacteria that oxidize sulfur compounds to generate energy. The energy is then used to produce organic material. How would these bacteria be classified?

A) Psychrophilic chemoautotrophs
B) Thermophilic chemoautotrophs
C) Psychrophilic chemoheterotrophs
D) Thermophilic chemoheterotrophs

10. Which of the following organisms would be forced to undergo fermentation in the presence of a toxin that blocks oxidative phosphorylation in mitochondria?

A) *Escherichia coli*, a facultative anaerobic bacterium
B) *Saccharomyces cerevisiae*, a facultative anaerobic yeast
C) *Propionibacterium acnes*, an obligate anaerobic bacterium
D) *Mycobacterium tuberculosis*, an obligate aerobic bacterium

MICROBIOLOGY PRACTICE PASSAGE

Bacillus anthracis is a gram-positive sporulating rod-shaped bacterium found extensively in the soil, and it causes the group of diseases collectively known as anthrax. Sporulation allows the bacterium to survive harsh conditions. Depending on the location of the bacteria in the body, an infection with *B. anthracis* can manifest as anthrax (either cutaneous, pulmonary, or gastrointestinal) or meningitis. The bacterium possess two virulence plasmids (pXO1 and pXO2), which code for exotoxins and a poly-D-glutamic acid capsule, respectively. When diagnosing a patient with anthrax, the outcome of the disease is highly dependent upon the speed of diagnosis due to the significant difference in mortality observed with the administration of antibiotics.

When identifying *B. anthracis* as the causative agent, physicians first attempt to culture and identify the living bacteria. Samples of blood, sputum, feces, or cerebrospinal fluid are cultured on blood agar at 37°C, and if gram-positive chains of rods are observed, further confirmatory tests are performed. These tests include phenotypic typing, gamma phage lysis, real-time PCR assays, direct fluorescent assays, and time-resolved fluorescent assays. Commercially available immunochromatographic tests have recently been developed and are now available.

While cultures of the bacteria are ideal for diagnosis, they are not always possible to obtain and often indirect methods of identification must be used. A recently developed PCR assay targets three loci on the bacterial chromosome and one on each of the virulence plasmids; this allows detection of an infection of as few as 167 total cells. PCR-amplified DNA fragments are identified through gel electrophoresis, in which fragments are separated by size and can be compared to a standard to confirm their respective lengths. Another method detects the antibodies produced by the body against the anthrax toxin protein (PA). This Enzyme-Linked Immunosorbent Assay (ELISA) is commercially available to quantify the level of human anti-PA IgG rapidly; this allows for more directed treatment.

1. A physician collects two blood samples and sends them to the lab for culture and an ELISA. The culture comes back negative but the ELISA is positive for human anti-PA IgG. What is a possible reason for this result?

A) The patient is infected with a virus producing similar symptoms.
B) The patient does not have an active infection.
C) The ELISA results are not conclusive because the test is nonspecific.
D) *B. anthracis* do not grow in culture.

2. According to the passage, which of the following samples is LEAST likely to result in an anthrax diagnosis?

A) Blood
B) Sputum
C) Feces
D) Cerebrospinal fluid

3. A new blood sample arrives at a lab and grows a gram-positive bacterium later identified as *B. anthracis*; however, the ELISA registers a negative result. Is this patient infected with *B. anthracis* and what most likely accounted for this result?

A) No; the laboratory sample was contaminated.
B) No; the cultured bacteria were part of the natural flora of the body.
C) Yes; the tested blood sample would register a positive ELISA in approximately seven days.
D) Yes; the infection was recently acquired.

4. In the PCR detection of the bacterium, a laboratory technician obtains a positive result. How many bands should the technician detect on the gel?

A) 2
B) 3
C) 4
D) 5

5. A culture from a sputum sample develops into colonies of round bacterial cells. Which of the following could be the pathogen causing infection in this patient?

A) *Streptococcus sp.* (streptococcal pharyngitis; "strep throat")
B) *Mycobacterium tuberculosis* (tuberculosis, TB, tubercle bacillus)
C) *Bacillus anthracis* (anthrax)
D) *Spirillum minus* (rat-bite fever)

6. One of the potential complications of inhalation or pulmonary anthrax is the development of hypotension. Which of the following would NOT cause hypotension in a healthy patient?

A) SA node depression
B) Destruction of the posterior pituitary
C) ACTH secreting lung tumor
D) Hemorrhage

SOLUTIONS TO FREESTANDING QUESTIONS: MICROBIOLOGY

1. **B** Since Item III appears in exactly two of the answer choices, start by analyzing this item. Whether it is true or false, you can eliminate half the answer choices. Item III is false: only animal viruses can have lipid-based envelopes, derived from the plasma membrane of their host cell (choices C and D can be eliminated). Both remaining answer choices include Item I, so it must be true, and you can now analyze Item II. Item II is true: the genome can contain either DNA or RNA (choice A can be eliminated, and choice B is correct). Note that Item I is in fact true: in order to function, all viruses have a protein coat (called a capsid) that surrounds and protects their genome.

2. **C** In the lysogenic cycle of bacteriophages, the genomic DNA of one bacterium can be transferred to another bacterium through a viral vector in a process called transduction (choice C is correct). Conjugation is the transfer of genomic material between bacteria via a physical bridge (choice A is wrong). Transfection and transformation are the process of incorporating DNA from the external environment in eukaryotes and prokaryotes, respectively (choices B and D are wrong).

3. **C** A retrovirus is a lysogenic virus with an RNA genome that uses reverse transcriptase to make DNA for insertion into the host genome. Because the innate genome of retroviruses is RNA, it does not carry thymine, which is only found in DNA (choice C is correct). Adenine and guanine can be found in both DNA and RNA (choices A and D are wrong), and uracil is found only in RNA (choice B is wrong).

4. **B** A (+) RNA virus contains a genome made of RNA that is ready to be translated into viral proteins. Because the genome can be immediately translated by the host cell machinery, it is not absolutely necessary for the virus to carry reverse transcriptase within the capsid; it only needs to code for it. However, this will take time and there is a risk that the (+) RNA would be degraded; virulence may be reduced, but the virus would not be rendered ineffective altogether (choice B is correct, and choice C is wrong). Reverse transcriptase is a required enzyme (choice A is wrong), needed to copy the RNA genome into DNA; it is not involved in the initial infection of the cell (choice D is wrong).

5. **D** The productive cycle refers to the life cycle of an animal virus. It is similar to the lytic cycle of bacteriophages, but the last stage involves budding rather than lysis (choice A is wrong), during which the virus acquires an envelope from the host membrane (choice D is correct). Insertion of the viral genome into the host genome is characteristic of the lysogenic cycle (choice B is wrong). Imperfect excision from the host genome during the lysogenic cycle can result in transduction (choice C is wrong).

6. **A** An arg$^-$ auxotroph is unable to synthesize the amino acid arginine, and needs arginine added to the medium in order to survive. Because arginine has been added to the medium, both the arg+ (able to synthesize arginine) and arg$^-$ (unable to synthesize arginine) bacteria can survive. A lac$^-$ auxotroph is unable to synthesize β-galactosidase, the enzyme that allows the bacteria to break down lactose. Thus, lac$^-$ auxotrophs cannot survive on a lactose-based medium (choices B and D can be eliminated). Only amp^r (ampicillin resistant) bacteria can survive in the presence of the antibiotic ampicillin (choice C is wrong; choice A is correct).

7. **C** The primary difference between prokaryotes and eukaryotes is that prokaryotes have no membrane-bound organelles, which means all cellular processes occur in the cytosol. Ribosomes are organelles, but they are not membrane-bound and are thus present in prokaryotes (choice C is correct). The nucleus, mitochondria, and Golgi apparatus are all membrane-bound organelles, which are only present in eukaryotes (choices A, B, and D are wrong).

8. **D** Prions are acellular, non-living proteins that are misfolded and can be transmissible through several modalities; they primarily attack the central nervous system, and cause encephalopathies such as Creutzfeldt-Jakob disease and bovine spongiform encephalopathy (choice D is correct). Prions lack a genome and are considered sub-viral particles, not viruses (choice A is wrong). Although the media popularized "mad cow disease" as a disease transmitted from cows to other cows, it was primarily transmitted through feed containing infected sheep meat (choice B is wrong). Prions can be transmitted through ingested material, blood, and soil; additionally, some prions can be inherited through mutations that code for misfolded proteins (choice C is wrong).

9. **B** This is a 2 × 2 question. Organisms that thrive in extreme cold are called psychrophiles, whereas organisms that thrive in extreme heat are called thermophiles (choices A and C are wrong). Organisms that generate energy by oxidizing organic or inorganic compounds are chemotrophs, and if these organisms can produce their own carbon compounds, they are autotrophs (choice B is correct, and choice D is wrong).

10. **B** Facultative anaerobes are capable of both aerobic and anaerobic respiration. However, only eukaryotic cells have mitochondria, so a toxin that targets mitochondria should have no effect on prokaryotes (choices A, C, and D are wrong). Yeast are eukaryotic, and would be sensitive to a mitochondrial toxin (choice B is correct).

SOLUTIONS TO MICROBIOLOGY PRACTICE PASSAGE

1. **B** Bacteria can be cultured from patient blood only when an active infection is present in the blood. This patient could have already cleared the infection and mounted an immune response, resulting in a positive ELISA but negative culture result (choice B is correct). The ELISA test is very specific (choice C is wrong), and there is no reason to believe that a human would develop the same or similar antibodies against a *B. anthracis* infection and a viral infection. Even if the patient was infected with a virus that caused symptoms similar to a *B. anthracis* infection, he or she would not have a positive ELISA given the specificity of antibodies (choice A is wrong). According to the passage, *B. anthracis* can be grown in culture (choice D is wrong).

2. **D** A positive result from a sample of cerebrospinal fluid would result in a diagnosis of meningitis, not anthrax (choice D is correct). The passage states that an infection with *B. anthracis* can manifest as cutaneous, pulmonary, or gastrointestinal anthrax, which indicates that a positive result from samples of blood, sputum, or feces could lead to an anthrax diagnosis (choices A, B, and C can be eliminated).

3.   **D**   If the patient has very recently been infected with *B. anthracis* for the first time, the body may not yet have mounted a detectable immune response (choice D is correct). A significant humoral response in the form of elevated serum antibodies will be detected approximately one week after infection. However, the already-tested blood sample would not register a positive result after seven days, since outside of the body blood lacks the machinery to produce antibodies; a fresh blood sample would be required (choice C is wrong). A positive blood culture could result from contamination, but this is less likely than an active infection (choice A is possible but less likely than choice D). *B. anthracis* is not part of the body's normal flora; it is a disease-causing agent (choice B is wrong).

4.   **D**   According to the passage, the PCR assay will amplify three loci on the bacterial chromosome and one on each of the virulence plasmids (2 total from the plasmids). This means there should be five DNA fragments amplified by PCR, and the technician should have seen a total of five bands on the electrophoresis gel (choice D is correct).

5.   **A**   Round bacterial cells are known as cocci. *Streptococcus* bacteria causing streptococcal pharyngitis, commonly called strep throat, would develop into a culture of round bacterial cells (choice A is correct). *Mycobacterium tuberculosis* is rod-shaped, as indicated by the "bacillus" in tubercle bacillus (choice B is wrong). The passage explicitly states that *Bacillus anthracis* is rod-shaped, and this can also be inferred from the genus *Bacillus* (choice C is wrong). *Spirillum minus* is a spiral-shaped bacterium (choice D is wrong).

6.   **C**   Hypotension is a reduction in blood pressure. ACTH stimulates the release of cortisol and aldosterone from the adrenal cortex, and aldosterone causes an increase in the reabsorption of Na^+ from the distal tubules of the kidneys. This would lead to an increase in blood pressure, or hypertension (choice C does not cause hypotension and is the correct answer choice). SA node depression would result in a decrease in heart rate and a subsequent decrease in blood pressure (choice A is a possible cause of hypotension and can be eliminated). Destruction of the posterior pituitary would lead to a drop in ADH and a subsequent inability to reabsorb water from the collecting ducts of the kidneys. This would result in a decrease in blood volume and thus a drop in blood pressure (choice B is a possible cause of hypotension and can be eliminated). Hemorrhage would also lead to a decrease in blood volume and result in hypotension (choice D can be eliminated).

Chapter 11
Eukaryotic Cell Biology

FREESTANDING QUESTIONS: EUKARYOTIC CELL BIOLOGY

1. An evolutionary biologist proposes the hypothesis that the nucleus originated from a prokaryotic ancestor. Which of the following lends support to this hypothesis?

A) The inner membrane possesses fatty acids found predominately in bacteria.
B) The outer membrane possesses fatty acids found predominately in bacteria.
C) The nucleus possesses only a single lipid bilayer.
D) The nuclear membrane contains cholesterol.

2. A researcher attempting to express a eukaryotic protein in a cell line discovers that rather than being secreted as he had hoped, large quantities of the protein are detected in the endoplasmic reticulum. What is the most likely explanation for this observation?

A) The researcher needs to select a different strain of bacteria to express the protein.
B) The protein lacked a signal sequence.
C) The protein failed to bind to bind a cytoplasmic carrier protein responsible for transport to the cell surface.
D) The protein did not fold appropriately.

3. Four cultures of *E. coli* are suspended in media containing different concentrations of solutes. The cultures are placed in a chamber initially at 22°C, and the temperature is slowly lowered until all cultures have frozen. The culture that will freeze first is the one suspended in:

A) 0.010 *m* NaCl.
B) 0.025 *m* UDP-glucose.
C) 0.030 *m* alanine.
D) 0.125 *m* K$^+$.

4. A nephrologist discovers a point mutation which abolishes the function of aquaporin-2, a transmembrane channel for water, in a subset of patients experiencing excessive urine output. What is the cause of these patients' symptoms?

A) Increased expression of aquaporin-2 in the collecting duct
B) Decreased active transport of water out of the collecting duct
C) Decreased osmotic flow of water out of the collecting duct
D) Increased medullary osmotic pressure

5. A researcher discovered a yeast strain with a mutation in the Sal3 promoter that causes its constitutive activation, propelling the cells into the M-phase of the cell cycle earlier than would typically occur. Cells with this mutation would be:

A) larger than wild type cells and spend more time in G$_2$.
B) smaller than wild type cells and spend more time in G$_2$.
C) larger than wild type cells and spend less time in G$_2$.
D) smaller than wild type cells and spend less time in G$_2$.

6. Which of the following could account for the change in ion flux from A to B, shown in the figure below, in a cell line expressing an ion channel?

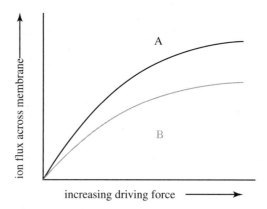

A) Simple diffusion across the membrane has decreased.
B) Protein translation has decreased.
C) The channels fail to reach saturation.
D) The channels no longer require the addition of ATP to function.

7. Which of the following would have the LEAST impact on the phagocytic ability of a neutrophil?

A) Decreased vesicular trafficking of endosomes
B) Increased lysosome pH
C) Decreased clathrin expression
D) Decreased lysosome number

8. Which of the following is not a feature of apoptosis?

A) Response to uncontrolled growth
B) Results in nuclear fragmentation
C) Mechanism of killing via caspase activation
D) Results in the uncontrolled spilling of cellular contents

9. Which of the following cells would be expected to be relatively rich in their amount of rough endoplasmic reticulum?

   I. Plasma cells (a type of B-cell)
   II. Mucus-secreting goblet cells in the small intestine
   III. Adrenal cortex cells

A) I only
B) I and II only
C) II and III only
D) I, II, and III

10. A primary spermatocyte contains 6 pg (picograms) of DNA while in the G_1 phase before undergoing meiosis. How much DNA will be present in the sperm at the completion of meiosis?

A) 3 pg
B) 6 pg
C) 12 pg
D) 24 pg

EUKARYOTIC CELL BIOLOGY PRACTICE PASSAGE

MBG-1 and MBG-2 are poorly understood human proteins, encoded on chromosomes 12*q* and 14*p,* respectively, in the human genome. Both proteins contain a mitochondrial localization domain and are known to amplify transforming growth factor beta-1 (TGF-β1) signaling. In order to determine the effects of these two proteins on mitochondria and a specific way to control MBG expression in cells, two different pools of siRNA were obtained. Each contained five different siRNA molecules. Pool 1 was designed to target MBG-1, while the second pool was for MBG-2.

Actively growing human cells were plated, and at 60–80% confluence, siRNA pools were applied separately to cells. Cells were analyzed at four different time points for protein levels (Figure 1). Additionally, mitochondrial DNA (mtDNA) and nuclear (nDNA) were separately isolated and quantified, and the ratio of mtDNA / nDNA was determined (Figure 2). Lastly, mitochondria were labeled with the fluorescent mitochondrial marker MitoTracker Red, and cells were analyzed by flow cytometric analysis (Figure 3).

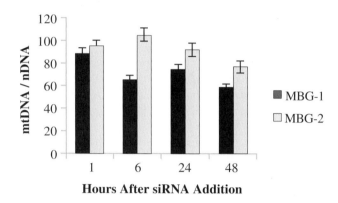

Figure 2 Amount of mtDNA in a cell population, normalized to nDNA

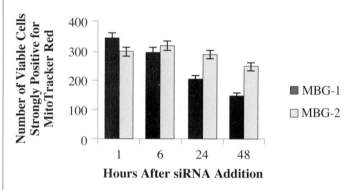

Figure 3 Number of fluorescently labeled viable cells after treatment with siRNA pool

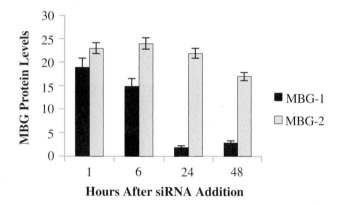

Figure 1 MBG protein levels after treatment with siRNA pools

1. Mitochondrial genes are located in:

A) only in the nuclear genome, specifically those in heterochromatin regions.

B) only in the nuclear genome, specifically those in euchromatin regions.

C) only in the mitochondrial genome, which is circular and made of double stranded DNA.

D) in both the nuclear and mitochondrial genome, both of which are made of double stranded DNA.

2. In order to better interpret the data presented in the passage, which additional experiments should have been conducted?

   I. A positive control, where scrambled siRNA was transferred into cells, to determine only the potential cell toxicity effects of the experimental outline

   II. Quantify the amount of MBG-1 and MBG-2 mRNA in the cells, via reverse transcriptase quantitative PCR

   III. Transfer siRNA molecules individually instead of in pools, to rule out synergistic effects of multiple siRNA molecules against the same target

A) II only
B) I and II only
C) I and III only
D) II and III only

3. The data presented in the passage best supports which of the following conclusions?

A) Both siRNA pools were effective at binding their target transcript and promoting its degradation.
B) siRNA pool 1 directly caused the degradation of MBG-1 protein, but siRNA pool 2 was not as effective.
C) siRNA pool 1 caused degradation of the MBG-1 transcript; siRNA pool 2 is either not effective or MBG-2 proteins have a long half-life.
D) Neither siRNA pool was effective at knocking down mRNA levels, but pool 1 was more effective at inhibiting translation.

4. The experiments in the passage would require each of the following procedures EXCEPT:

A) quantitative PCR.
B) transformation.
C) cell lysis.
D) western blot.

5. If future experiments confirm that both MBG-1 and MBG-2 promote mitochondrial biogenesis, it will be most likely true that:

A) some tissues (such as heart, muscle, pancreas and kidney) have high levels of MBG-1, MBG-2, and mitochondrial biogenesis.
B) cell stress, proliferation pathways, and pro-apoptotic pathways can promote mitochondrial biogenesis.
C) mitochondrial biogenesis occurs primarily in G_1 of the cell cycle, with negligible levels in G_2.
D) MBG-1 and MBG-2 are both synthesized by 80S ribosomes docked on the rough endoplasmic reticulum membrane.

SOLUTIONS TO FREESTANDING QUESTIONS: EUKARYOTIC CELL BIOLOGY

1. **A** The endosymbiotic theory describes a potential unicellular origin for both mitochondria and nuclei. If a researcher found that the inner lipid bilayer present in the nucleus possessed a fatty acid profile more similar to bacteria, it would lend support to the theory as the unicellular organism (which likely possesses similarities to modern prokaryotes) might have been phagocytosed and incorporated into the cell in an earlier organism (choice B is wrong, and choice A is correct). The nuclear envelope contains two lipid bilayers, and given cholesterol is found in nearly all eukaryotic membranes, it would not support the theory proposed here (choices C and D are wrong).

2. **D** When expressing a protein, problems can arise at many steps during transcription, translation, and protein trafficking. Here a protein is destined for secretion, meaning that it must first be co-translationally translocated into the endoplasmic reticulum before being transported ultimately to the cell membrane via vesicular transport (not via a cytoplasmic carrier; choice C is wrong). Accumulation of the protein in the endoplasmic reticulum indicates that it had a signal sequence (choice B is wrong), however, if the protein failed to fold appropriately, it could be prevented from further transport (choice D is correct). Since the researcher wishes to express a eukaryotic protein, it is unlikely that a bacterium would be capable of producing a functional copy of the protein, and given that the current cell line being used possesses an endoplasmic reticulum, it is not a prokaryote (choice A is wrong).

3. **A** Freezing point depression, $\Delta T_f = -k_f im$, depends upon both the van't Hoff factor and the molality of the solute in question. Note that the freezing point constant of water ($k_f = 1.9°C/m$) is the same in each instance, so it can be disregarded, and only the molality (adjusted by the van't Hoff factor) can be considered. The sodium chloride, with its van't Hoff factor of 2, is the equivalent of a 0.02 m solution. UDP-glucose and alanine do not dissociate (van't Hoff factor of 1), so they are the equivalent of 0.025 m and 0.03 m solutions, respectively. The potassium solution also has a van't Hoff factor of 1 (only one ion, K⁺ does not dissociate further!) and is the equivalent of a 0.125 m solution. The solution that will freeze first is the one with the lowest molality (and thus the least freezing point depression), 0.010 m NaCl.

4. **C** The collecting duct, which facilitates the final reabsorption of water in the kidney, expresses aquaporin-2 in response to ADH (vasopressin). This results in an increased number of aquaporin channels in the collecting duct membrane which facilitate water reabsorption into the medulla due to its high osmolality. The subset of patients described here are experiencing excessive urine output, which indicates an inability to reabsorb water. While the possible causes of such a nonspecific symptom are vast, a decrease in osmotic flow into the medulla from the collecting duct is most likely given the lack of functional aquaporin-2 in these patients (choice C is correct). Increased expression of the channel would increase water reabsorption (choice A is wrong), water is not transported actively (choice B is wrong), and increased medullary osmotic pressure would serve to increase the drive for water reabsorption, not decrease it (choice D is wrong).

5. **D** This is a 2 × 2 question; you need to decide if the cells will be smaller or larger, and if they spend more or less time in G_2. If the cells pushed through G_2 and into M-phase early, they will spend less time in G_2 (choices A and B can be eliminated). Less time in G_2 means the cells will be smaller (choice C can be eliminated, and choice D is correct). Note that a cell is unlikely to spend less time in a growth phase and be larger than wild type cells.

6. **B** The movement of ions through a channel across a membrane is facilitated diffusion (choice A is wrong). Depending on the number of channels expressed in a cell, if a sufficient amount of driving force is present, the channels can saturate (reach a transport maximum); however, failure to saturate would not change the curve overall. Curve B has a lower saturation point than Curve A, but both curves are capable of saturation. If the overall quantity of channel protein decreased in a cell, the maximal rate at which ions could cross the membrane (the saturation point) would decrease (choice B is correct). Facilitated diffusion relies on a concentration gradient as the driving force and does not require ATP (choice D is wrong).

7. **C** Clathrin-coated pits are involved in receptor-mediated endocytosis, which is a functionally different process than non-specific phagocytosis (choice C is the least likely to impact phagocytosis and is the correct answer). During phagocytosis, the membrane flows around the particle being phagocytized and forms a vesicle (known as an endosome), which travels to the lysosome where the contents are broken down (choices A and D would impact phagocytosis and are wrong). The lysosomal enzymes are acid hydrolases, and they require an acidic environment to function. An increase in pH would perturb their function (choice B is wrong).

8. **D** Apoptosis, or programmed cell death, results in stepwise destruction of a cell and release of organized apoptotic bodies without spilling cellular contents (choice D is not a feature of apoptosis and is the correct answer). Apoptosis is employed to kill cells growing uncontrollably and involves activation of caspase proteins (choices A and C are features of apoptosis and can be eliminated). One step of apoptosis is dismantling of the nucleus including fragmentation (choice B is a feature of apoptosis and can be eliminated).

9. **B** The rough endoplasmic reticulum (RER) is involved in the production and modification of secreted proteins; therefore, cells that are involved in the secretion of proteins would be expected to have a lot of RER. Start by analyzing Item III since it is found in exactly two of the answer choices; whether it is true or false, half the answers can be eliminated. Item III is false: the adrenal cortex produces steroid hormones (cortisol, aldosterone, and so on), which are derived from cholesterol, not protein. Steroid hormones are produced in the smooth endoplasmic reticulum (SER), so these cells would be expected to have a lot of SER, but not a lot of RER (choices C and D can be eliminated). Note that both remaining choices include Item I, so it must be true, and you can proceed by analyzing Item II. Item II is true: goblet cells in the small intestine produce a lot of mucus, which involves a lot of secreted proteins; therefore, these cells would also be rich in RER (choice A can be eliminated, and choice B is correct). Note that Item I is in fact true: plasma cells secrete antibodies, which are proteins.

10. **A** Meiosis results in the production of four haploid cells. Given the diploid progenitor contained 6 pg of DNA, each haploid cell will contain 3 pg of DNA (choice A is correct). The primary spermatocyte, following completion of the S-phase, would have 12 pg of DNA. During each of the following two cell divisions that number would be reduced by half; to 6 pg of DNA after meiosis I, and to 3 pg of DNA after meiosis II. The 12 pg of DNA would be divided among the four sperm cells.

SOLUTIONS TO EUKARYOTIC CELL BIOLOGY PRACTICE PASSAGE

1. **D** Mitochondrial proteins can be coded by either the nuclear or the mitochondrial genome (choice D is correct; choices A, B, and C are wrong). If coded for by the nuclear genome, the protein will contain a mitochondrial import signal. The human mitochondrial genome is small (you don't need to know these numbers, but to give you a sense of scale, it has 16,569 base pairs of double stranded DNA and codes for 37 genes). Many biochemical and cellular processes occur in the mitochondria, so this organelle must contain many other proteins (again, you don't need to know this number but mitochondria typically contain about 3000 different proteins!).

2. **D** Since Item III is found in two of the answer choices (and since it is shorter than Item I, which is also found in two answer choices), start by analyzing Item III to turn this into a 50:50 question. Item III is true: testing pools of siRNA can be a good first step, but it is possible that a few of the molecules in the mix are cooperating to cause the results presented. The passage says the experiment is being performed to "determine the effects of these two proteins on mitochondria, *and a specific way to target MBG expression in cells.*" Next then, the siRNA molecules should be applied individually (choices A and B can be eliminated). You can analyze either of the remaining items next to get the correct answer. Item I is false: the experiments in the passage are missing both positive and negative controls. Transfecting cells with scrambled siRNA to determine potential cell toxicity effects would be a good experiment to do, but this is a negative control (expected not to work), not a positive control (expected to work; choice C can be eliminated, and choice D is correct). Note that Item II is in fact true: Figure 1 shows how MBG-1 and MBG-2 protein levels change after application of the siRNA pools, but protein levels don't always correlate with mRNA levels. For example, if a certain protein has a very long half-life in the cell, siRNA may still effectively be targeting mRNA but this will not result in a change in protein levels. Knockdown experiments will ideally show the effects of siRNA on both RNA and protein. Reverse transcriptase quantitative PCR (RT-qPCR) is a good technique to quantify the amount of mRNA.

3. **C** Figure 1 shows that siRNA pool 1 effectively decreases the amount of MBG-1 protein in the cells, while siRNA pool 2 was not effective at decreasing the amount of MBG-2 protein. siRNAs bind complementary sequences on mRNAs, and this double stranded RNA is then degraded. The amount of transcript in the cell decreases and gene expression is thus negatively regulated. In the experiment in the passage, MBG-1 transcript was made and degraded when siRNA pool 1 was added. Protein levels are low because the mRNA is degraded, not because the protein is degraded (choice B is wrong) or because translation is inhibited (choice D is wrong). It is possible that MBG-2 proteins have a long half-life in the cell. In this case, even if MBG-2 siRNAs bind and degrade the transcript, there will be minimal effect of the siRNA pool on protein levels (choice C is the correct answer). Choice A is possible, but without quantifying the amount of mRNA in the cell, you cannot be sure this is happening (choice C is better than choice A).

4. **B** In the experiment, siRNA pools would be introduced into the growing cells by transfection (the transfer of nucleic acids into eukaryotic cells). Transformation is the transfer of nucleic acids into a bacterial cell, not a eukaryotic cell (choice B would not be required by the experiments and is the correct answer choice). The data in Figure 2 would require cell lysis (choice C is required and can be eliminated), extraction of DNA from different subcellular fractions, and quantitative PCR to quantify the genomes (choice A is required and can be eliminated). The cells would be lysed to generate protein lysates, and protein levels are determined via western blots (choice D is required and can be eliminated).

5. **A** Some animal tissues have a high number of mitochondria: heart and skeletal muscle require large amounts of energy for mechanical work, the pancreas is responsible for huge amounts of biosynthesis, and the kidney processes a huge volume of fluid every day. Since mitochondria generate energy (they are the "powerhouse" of the cell), these tissues will likely have many of these organelles. Mitochondria are made via biogenesis, so it makes sense that these tissues will have high levels of MBG-1, MBG-2, and mitochondrial biogenesis (choice A is correct). Pro-apoptotic pathways will promote cell death. If a cell is dying, it will not likely promote mitochondrial biogenesis (choice B is wrong). Organelle replication and general housekeeping activities of the cell are predominantly performed in the gap phases of the cell cycle (both G_1 and G_2, so choice C is wrong). The passage says that both MBG-1 and MBG-2 have mitochondrial localization signals. These proteins will not go through the secretory protein pathway (choice D is wrong).

Chapter 12
Genetics and Evolution

FREESTANDING QUESTIONS: GENETICS AND EVOLUTION

1. Duchenne Muscular Dystrophy (DMD) is an X-linked recessive trait. A normal woman who carries the DMD allele mates with a normal man. What is the probability they will have either a son with DMD or a daughter who carries DMD?

A) 100%
B) 50%
C) 25%
D) Cannot be determined with the information given

2. A thin, agouti mouse (*BbCc*) is crossed with a fat, albino mouse (*bbcc*) and several litters of pups are phenotyped. The results are: 19 thin, agouti pups, 32 thin, albino pups, 29 fat, agouti pups, and 20 fat, albino pups. Which of the following can be concluded?

A) The fat and agouti alleles are linked and on the same chromosome.
B) The fat and albino alleles are linked and on different chromosomes.
C) The gene for body size and the gene for coat color are unlinked.
D) The gene for body size and the gene for coat color are 20 mu apart on the same chromosome.

3. Which of the following best describes the principle that the change in allele frequency from one generation to the next occurs because alleles in offspring are a random sample of those in the parents, as well as from the role that chance plays in determining whether a given individual will survive and reproduce?

A) Founder effect
B) Genetic drift
C) Natural selection
D) Adaptation

4. A geneticist crosses two flowering plant lines. Plant Line #1 has green flowers (*G*) with long veins (*L*) and is crossed with Plant Line #2 that has yellow flowers (*g*) and short veins (*l*). Both lines are known to be genotypically homozygous. The resulting progeny are then back-crossed to Plant Line #2 and the resulting numbers of progeny are listed in the table below. What is the recombination frequency?

Phenotype	# Observed
green, long	410
green, short	45
yellow, long	45
yellow, short	400

A) 1%
B) 5%
C) 10%
D) 45%

5. The frequency of a recessive disease-causing allele in a randomly mating population is 0.2. What is the frequency of carriers for the disease in this population?

A) 0.04
B) 0.32
C) 0.64
D) 0.8

6. Which of the following is NOT a similarity between mitosis and meiosis?

A) Both are preceded by replication.
B) Both require the disassembly of the nuclear membrane.
C) Both utilize microtubules to negotiate the division of genetic material.
D) Both create diploid cells after one round of division.

7. A major cellular feature distinguishing cells in Kingdom Animalia from cells in other kingdoms is that animal cells:

A) lack a cell wall.
B) utilize oxidative phosphorylation.
C) have multiple linear chromosomes.
D) utilize microtubules as part of cellular motility.

8. Which of the following would best describe a scenario involving directional selection?

A) Turtles living on an island become physically separated into two groups when a tropical storm divides the habitat and eventually they are no longer able to mate.
B) Dogs are bred to produce little or no dander and thus are hypoallergenic for pet owners with allergies.
C) The ability to collect a wide variety of food is valued by a certain type of monkey, and females who exhibit this skill are able to attract more sexual partners.
D) Field mice that are able to escape into small spaces are less likely to be consumed by predators and thus larger mice are selected against over time.

9. Which of the following is/are examples of increased fitness?

   I. A female guinea pig that learns to protect her pups from consumption by the male
   II. A male rat that learns to run a maze in a shorter period of time in order to increase the size of the food reward
   III. A sterilized female rabbit whose lifespan is extended by access to plentiful food supplies

A) I only
B) II only
C) I and III only
D) II and III only

10. What pattern of inheritance would be seen in a family expressing a mitochondrial disorder?

A) All blood-related males would have the disorder and would pass it on only to male offspring.
B) All blood-related females would have the disorder if their father had it.
C) All blood-related offspring of an affected female would have the disorder.
D) All blood-related offspring of an affected individual would have the disorder.

GENETICS AND EVOLUTION PRACTICE PASSAGE

Whenever the expression of a gene is conditioned by its parental origin, geneticists say that the gene has been *imprinted*. Genetic imprinting is an inheritance process independent of the classical Mendelian inheritance, as only one parental allele is expressed. For example, paternal imprinting occurs when an allele inherited from the father is not expressed in offspring, while maternal imprinting occurs when an allele inherited from the mother is not expressed. As such, certain mechanisms must be in place to mark and silence imprinted genes.

Previous molecular analyses have repeatedly demonstrated that methylation of one or more CG dinucleotides in a gene's vicinity can affect the expression of the gene. More specifically, methylated DNA is associated with transcriptional repression. For example, in mice, the gene coding for insulin-like growth factor (Igf2) is methylated in the female germ line but not in the male germ line. As such, Igf2 is expressed when it is inherited from the father but not the mother.

During embryogenesis, the methylated and unmethylated states are preserved each time the genome replicates. However, a methylated gene that was inherited from one sex can be unmethylated when it passes through an offspring of the opposite sex. For example, a maternally imprinted gene is unmethylated when male offspring produce gametes, but remethylated when female offspring produce gametes. Thus, imprinting is re-set with each successive generation, and subsequent methylation depends on the sex of the animal.

Angelman syndrome is a classic example of an autosomal disease related to genetic imprinting. The gene implicated in the disease is deleted or mutated on the maternally inherited chromosome, while the paternal gene is silenced due to imprinting. The paternal gene cannot compensate for the loss of the gene on the maternal chromosome because imprinting has turned it off. In contrast, *Prader-Willi syndrome* (also autosomal) is caused by the combination of maternal imprinting and loss of paternally inherited genes in a nearby region of the same chromosome.

1. Is it possible for both men and women to develop Prader-Willi syndrome?

A) Yes, both sexes have an equal probability of disease.
B) Yes, both sexes can have the disease, but it is found predominantly in women because of maternal imprinting.
C) No, because it is only maternally imprinted.
D) No, because imprinting is reset with each successive generation.

2. Aberrant DNA methylation patterns (hypermethylation and hypomethylation) have been shown to be associated with human cancers. Hypermethylation typically occurs at CG islands in the promoter region and is associated with gene inactivation. Hypomethylation has also been implicated in cancer, but through different mechanisms, and may lead to the overexpression of genes. Which of the following is the most likely pattern of methylation that would lead to cancer?

A) Hypermethylation of tumor suppressor genes and hypomethylation of proto-oncogenes
B) Hypermethylation of proto-oncogenes and hypomethylation of tumor suppressor genes
C) Hypermethylation of both tumor suppressor genes and proto-oncogenes
D) Hypomethylation of both tumor suppressor genes and proto-oncogenes

3. Is it possible for a man with Prader-Willi syndrome who marries an unaffected woman to have children with *Prader-Willi syndrome*?

A) Yes, the children will either inherit a silenced (imprinted) chromosome or a mutated chromosome from him.

B) Yes, the children have a 50% chance of inheriting the father's mutated chromosome and will all inherit a silenced (imprinted) chromosome from their mother.

C) No, the mutated chromosome can only be inherited from the mother.

D) No, they could inherit the mutated chromosome from him, but could inherit a normal chromosome from their mother.

4. The gene responsible for Angelman syndrome is UBE3A. In a person with this syndrome, what is the difference between the maternal and paternal chromosome?

A) There is no difference; both homologous genes are methylated.

B) There is no difference; both homologous genes are unmethylated.

C) The maternal gene is methylated and the paternal one deleted or mutated.

D) The paternal gene is methylated and the maternal one deleted or mutated.

5. Mr. A has hemophilia; he and his wife (Ms. B, who is neither affected by hemophilia nor a carrier) produce one unaffected son (Mr. C) and one unaffected daughter (Ms. D). The son of Ms. D marries an unaffected, non-carrier woman. What is the probability they will produce a child who is a carrier of hemophilia?

A) 0

B) 1/8

C) 1/4

D) 1/2

SOLUTIONS TO FREESTANDING QUESTIONS: GENETICS AND EVOLUTION

1. **B** If D = normal and d = DMD, the mother's genotype is $X^D X^d$ and the father's is $X^D Y$. The probability of having a son with DMD ($X^d Y$) = probability of X^d from mom (0.5) multiplied by the probability of Y from dad (0.5) = 0.25. The probability of having a daughter who carries the DMD allele ($X^D X^d$) is the probability of X^D from dad (0.5) multiplied by the probability of X^d from mom (0.5) = 0.25. Since the question asks for the probability of either, these numbers must be added (Rule of Addition); however, since the two situations are mutually exclusive (they cannot have a child who is both a son and a daughter), it is not necessary to subtract the probability that the two events happen together as is normally required in the Rule of Addition. Thus, 0.25 + 0.25 = 0.5 or 50% (choice B is correct).

2. **A** This question describes the testcross of a dihybrid animal (*BbCc* × *bbcc*); the expected offspring ratios are 25% thin agouti pups (*BbCc*), 25% thin albino pups (*Bbcc*), 25% fat agouti pups (*bbCc*), and 25% fat albino pups (*bbcc*). The observed data does not match these numbers, so these genes are linked (choice C is wrong). Note that the definition of linked genes are genes that are found on the same chromosome (choice B is wrong). Thin albino pups (*Bbcc*) and fat agouti pups (*bbCc*) were the highest proportion of offspring, meaning the alleles for thin (*B*) and albino (*c*) are linked and the alleles for fat (*b*) and agouti (*C*) are linked. While it is true that the genes for body size and color are linked, they are $[(19 + 20)/100] \times 100\% \approx 40\% = 40$ mu apart, not 20 mu apart; the 19 and 20 are added together because they represent the recombinant phenotypes (choice A is correct, and choice D is wrong).

3. **B** Genetic drift is the idea that over time, some alleles become more frequent than others due to random events (choice B is correct). Natural selection is a similar idea, but the alleles do not randomly become more or less frequent. Their frequency is determined by the phenotypic advantage or disadvantage displayed in the individual organism (choice C is wrong). The founder effect describes the idea that if a small population of a species becomes isolated from the rest of the species, their allele frequency will predominate in future generations (choice A is wrong). Adaptations are structures or behaviors that enhance a specific function, causing organisms to become better at surviving and reproducing. They are produced by a combination of the continuous production of small, random changes in traits, followed by natural selection of the variants best suited for their environment (choice D is wrong).

4. **C** In the back-cross described, a *GgLl* plant is mated with a *ggll* plant. If the alleles all assorted independently, an equal ratio (1:1:1:1) of all possible phenotypes would be expected (*GgLl*, *ggLl*, *Ggll*, and *ggll*). Since the table shows that some phenotypes—specifically green short (*Ggll*) and yellow long (*ggLl*)—were present in fewer numbers, you can assume that the genes for flower color and vein length are linked (found on the same chromosome and not assorting independently). The recombination frequency (RF) is determined by dividing recombinant individuals (non-parental strains) by the total number of progeny. In this case, 90/900 = 0.10, or a RF of about 10%.

5. **B** You can assume that the population follows the Hardy-Weinberg model because it is described as exhibiting random mating. Since the disease is caused by a recessive allele, $q = 0.2$ and thus $1 - 0.2 = 0.8 = p$. The question is looking for carriers, which would mean heterozygous individuals. This is represented by $2pq = 2(0.8)(0.2) = 0.32$ (choice B is correct). Choice A represents the frequency of homozygous recessives ($0.2^2 = 0.04$) and not the frequency of carriers. Choice C represents the frequency of homozygous dominants ($0.8^2 = 0.64$), and choice D represents the frequency of the dominant allele.

6. **D** Mitosis has only one round of division and its purpose is to recreate diploid daughter cells that are copies of the parent cell. Meiosis has two rounds of division, but at the end of the first round, cells are haploid and contain two copies of that half of the genome ($1n$, $2x$); this is not the same as being diploid ($2n$, $1x$) (choice D is false and therefore the correct answer). Replication occurs before both mitosis and meiosis (choice A is true and can be eliminated), and the nuclear membrane is taken apart to allow for proper division of genetic material in both (choice B is true and can be eliminated). Once the nuclear membrane is gone, microtubules are instrumental in the physical movement to achieve proper genetic division for both (choice C is true and can be eliminated).

7. **A** All other kingdoms have cell walls except Animalia; the composition of those cell walls vary, but they are present (choice A is correct). All kingdoms have cell types that use oxidative phosphorylation (choice B is wrong). Kingdoms Protista, Fungi, Plantae, and Animalia all have multiple linear chromosomes (choice C is wrong), and all four utilize microtubules in motility structures (choice D is wrong).

8. **D** When natural selection removes those exhibiting the extremes of a trait, then the average of that trait will shift over time, creating directional selection. Choice D describes just such a situation and is the correct answer. Choice A describes the force of allopatric isolation as a trigger for speciation and can be eliminated. Choice B describes artificial selection, and choice C describes sexual selection; thus both can be eliminated.

9. **A** Since all items appear exactly twice in the answer choices, and all items are approximately the same length, it doesn't matter which item to start analyzing; start with Item I. Item I is true: by enabling more of her offspring to survive, the guinea pig is increasing her level of fitness (choices B and D can be eliminated). Since Item II is not in either of the remaining answer choices, it must be false and you can focus on Item III. Item III is false: a sterilized animal does not have fitness no matter how long it lives because it is not reproducing (choice C can be eliminated, and choice A is correct). Note that Item II is false: while learning in order to gain more food helps the individual rat, this does not inherently increase the animal's fitness.

10. **C** The ovum provides all the organelles when a zygote is formed so mitochondrial disorders are passed from mothers to all of their genetically related offspring (choice C is correct). Y-pattern inheritance is characterized by males passing the gene on to any and all (but only!) males (choice A is wrong). A female inheriting a disorder from her father would mean a connection to the X chromosome (choice B is wrong), and for all offspring to be affected, regardless of the gender of the parent, the disorder would have to express a classical dominance pattern (choice D is wrong).

SOLUTIONS TO GENETICS AND EVOLUTION PRACTICE PASSAGE

1. **A** As described in the passage, Prader-Willi is an autosomal syndrome resulting from the inheritance of a maternally-imprinted gene in combination with a deletion/mutation of the homologous paternal gene. Therefore, both genders can theoretically be afflicted with the disease equally (choices C and D are wrong). Maternal imprinting does not confer an increased risk of women being affected, particularly given that the disease is autosomal; all children have the same probability of inheriting an imprinted gene regardless of gender (choice B is wrong, and choice A is correct).

2. **A** Cancers are typically associated with inactivation of tumor suppressor genes, and the question stem states that hypermethylation can lead to gene inactivation; thus, tumor suppressor genes must be hypermethylated (choices B and D can be eliminated). It is suggested that hypomethylation may lead to the overexpression of genes; thus, the hypomethylation of a proto-oncogene could lead to its upregulation and conversion into an oncogene (choice C can be eliminated, and choice A is correct).

3. **B** The passage states that Prader-Willi syndrome is caused by the combination of maternal imprinting (gene silencing) and the inheritance of a mutated chromosome from one's father. The man in this question must have one mutated chromosome and one imprinted chromosome. However, since the gene must be maternally imprinted, he will not be able to pass the imprinting to his children; they will inherit either a mutated chromosome or a normal (unimprinted) chromosome from him (choice A is wrong). Since the gene is maternally imprinted, all children will inherit an imprinted chromosome from their mother; if they are unlucky enough to get the mutated chromosome from their father, they will also have Prader-Willi syndrome (choice B is correct). The mother does not have any mutated chromosomes (she is unaffected; choice C is wrong), and all chromosomes inherited from the mother will be imprinted and thus silenced (choice D is wrong).

4. **D** As stated in the passage, methylation is the mechanism underlying imprinted diseases, whereby methylated genes are repressed. As such, the paternal and maternal chromosomes will differ in terms of methylation patterns (choices A and B are wrong). The passage states that Angelman syndrome is a paternally imprinted disease; thus, a segment of the paternal chromosome is silenced (imprinted via methylation) and the maternal gene in this region is deleted or mutated (choice D is correct, and choice C is wrong).

5. **C** If Mr. A has hemophilia (X^hY), then his unaffected daughter, Ms. D, is a carrier of hemophilia (X^HX^h). Her son may or may not be affected depending on which X chromosome he inherits; he as a 1/2 probability of inheriting X^h. If he is affected and marries an unaffected, non-carrier woman, then all of his daughters will be carriers of hemophilia, and none of his sons would be affected. He has a 1/2 probability of being affected by hemophilia, and a 1/2 probability of producing a daughter, so the total probability of producing a carrier child is 1/4 ($1/2 \times 1/2 = 1/4$).

Chapter 13
The Nervous and Endocrine Systems

FREESTANDING QUESTIONS: THE NERVOUS AND ENDOCRINE SYSTEMS

1. Multiple sclerosis is an autoimmune disease that targets and destroys the cells that myelinate neurons. Which of the following best describes the function of a neuron that has had its myelin destroyed?

A) The neuron ceases to propagate an action potential down the axon.
B) The neuron propagates an action potential more slowly than it did when myelinated, but faster than a normal unmyelinated neuron.
C) The neuron propagates an action potential at a rate similar to a normal unmyelinated neuron.
D) The neuron fails to initiate an action potential at the axon hillock.

2. Which of the following is a possible sign of hypokalemia (low potassium concentration in the blood)?

A) Lengthened absolute refractory period
B) More positive threshold potential
C) Hyperreflexia (more rapid and more sensitive reflex responses)
D) Constipation

3. Any reflex involving skeletal muscle is considered polysynaptic. What is the best explanation for this?

A) The somatic nervous system utilizes two neurons between the CNS and the effector organ.
B) The autonomic nervous system utilizes two neurons between the CNS and the effector organ.
C) Inhibition of the opposing muscle requires the use of an interneuron.
D) Activation of the contracting muscle requires the use of an interneuron.

4. Which of the following areas of the brain is directly responsible for maintaining homeostatic mechanisms in the body?

A) Hypothalamus
B) Hippocampus
C) Cerebellum
D) Medulla oblongata

5. A researcher is designing an experiment to inhibit sympathetic nervous system effects. He decides to use a cholinergic antagonist for his experiment. Is this the best design for this experiment?

A) Yes, because the sympathetic nervous system utilizes acetylcholine at the ganglion.
B) Yes, because the sympathetic nervous system utilizes adrenergic receptors at the organ.
C) No, because a cholinergic antagonist would activate the sympathetic nervous system.
D) No, because a cholinergic antagonist would target all divisions of the peripheral nervous system.

6. Which of the following structures is involved in dynamic (rotational) equilibrium?

A) Vestibule
B) Cochlea
C) Semicircular canal
D) Tympanic membrane

7. In mammalian rod cells, the inner and outer segments function together to establish a circuit of ion flow known as dark current. Given that the outer segment is continuously depolarized in the dark, which of the following best characterizes the flow of ions in a rod cell in the dark?

A) Sodium and calcium enter the outer segment while potassium leaves the inner segment.
B) Sodium and calcium enter the inner segment while potassium leaves the outer segment.
C) Sodium leaves the inner and outer segments while potassium restores the resting membrane potential via active transport.
D) Sodium enters in the inner segment and is actively pumped out of the inner segment via a Na⁺/K⁺ ATPase.

8. Anabolic steroids mimic testosterone in the body, producing several side effects including shrinking of the testes in males. An oversecreting tumor in which of the following glands might produce a similar result?

A) Hypothalamus
B) Anterior pituitary
C) Posterior pituitary
D) Adrenal cortex

9. Which of the following is/are hormones that target the intestine?

    I. Secretin
    II. Enterokinase
    III. Calcitriol

A) I only
B) III only
C) II and III only
D) I, II, and III

10. Addison's disease is a rare endocrine disorder in which the adrenal cortex produces insufficient amounts of steroid hormones. Patients with Addison's disease may experience which of the following?

A) Low blood pressure and a craving for sweet foods
B) Low blood pressure and a craving for salty foods
C) High blood pressure and a craving for sweet foods
D) High blood pressure and a craving for salty foods

THE NERVOUS AND ENDOCRINE SYSTEMS PRACTICE PASSAGE

Anabolic-androgenic steroids were identified and synthesized in the early 1930s, and since that time have been used both therapeutically and as a blood doping agent for athletes. As their name suggests, this class of steroids have both anabolic and androgenic effects, and like other steroids, they are chemically derived from cholesterol.

The anabolic effects refer to those that result in increased protein synthesis, bone marrow production, and red blood cell production, as well as increased size and number of skeletal muscle cells. The androgenic effects, on the other hand, include those that are involved in the development of masculine characteristics. These include effects such as a thickening of the vocal cords and a deeper voice, increased androgen-sensitive hair growth (such as pubic and chest hair), increased libido, and progression of puberty in children who have not yet reached puberty. The androgenic-anabolic ratio is a measure of which effect is dominant for a certain steroid, and is listed for different steroids in Table 1.

Steroid	Ratio
Testosterone	1:1
Fluoxymesterone	1:2
Oxymetholone	1:3
Nandrolone decanoate	1:4
Oxyandrolone	1:13

Table 1   Androgenic-Anabolic Ratio in Humans

Although notoriously known as performance enhancing drugs, anabolic-androgenic steroids are also used for medicinal purposes. These can take advantage of the anabolic and androgenic effects of this class of steroids, and the type of hormone used for treatment is chosen depending on the androgenic-anabolic ratio and the desired outcome.

The use of anabolic-androgenic steroids as doping agents in athletes has been a controversial topic for several years. The desired effect of these steroids is due to their anabolic effect, which can give athletes a competitive edge. They are taken for different reasons depending on the sport; endurance athletes benefit from the increased red blood cell count, whereas athletes requiring a lot of strength benefit from the increased lean mass. However, the use of these steroids in athletes has been banned in part due to their adverse effects, which can arise due to the androgenic effects of the steroids. Additionally, anabolic-androgenic steroid use can suppress naturally produced testosterone in men. Non-androgenic side effects of these steroids include increased LDL, hypertension, acne, and liver failure. Although these steroids mimic the effects of naturally produced hormones, they continue to be one of the most detectable blood doping agents.

1. Which of the following is correct about anabolic-androgenic steroids?

A) They are difficult to detect because they are structurally similar to naturally produced hormones.
B) Marathon runners and anemic patients benefit from the same effect of anabolic-androgenic steroids.
C) Medicinal uses only take advantage of the anabolic effects.
D) Androgenic side effects only occur in men.

2. Many of the side effects of anabolic-androgenic steroids result from feedback on the hypothalamic-pituitary axis. Which of the following is true regarding the nature of this interaction?

A) It is a positive feedback cycle that results in an increase in hormone release from the anterior pituitary.
B) It is a negative feedback cycle that results in an increase in hormone release from the anterior pituitary.
C) It is a negative feedback cycle that results in a decrease in hormone release from the anterior pituitary.
D) It is a negative feedback cycle that results in a decrease in hormone release from the posterior pituitary.

3. The pharmacodynamics of steroid hormones and peptide hormones differ due to the different chemical properties of these two classes of hormones. Which of the following is true regarding these differences?

A) Steroid hormones need to be taken intravenously, whereas peptide hormones are readily taken orally.
B) Steroid hormones affect posttranslational changes, whereas peptide hormones only affect transcription.
C) Steroids begin their action with the production of second messengers, whereas peptide hormones begin their action when bound to their receptor.
D) Steroids activate their target intracellularly, whereas peptide hormones activate their target extracellularly.

4. Which of the following steroids would be best used for a cancer patient whose weight has significantly decreased?

A) Oxandrolone
B) Oxymetholone
C) Testosterone
D) Fluoxymesterone

5. Which of the following is/are medicinal use(s) of anabolic-androgenic steroids?

    I. Induction of puberty
    II. Preventing lean muscle mass loss
    III. Acne treatment

A) I only
B) II only
C) I and II only
D) I, II, and III

6. Anabolic steroids are used by some athletes to increase muscle mass. Which of the following is the best explanation for this effect?

A) They only act to increase the number of muscle fibrils.
B) They increase red blood cell count.
C) They increase protein metabolism in muscles and also increase the size and number of muscle cells.
D) They lead to an increase in testosterone production.

SOLUTIONS TO FREESTANDING QUESTIONS: THE NERVOUS AND ENDOCRINE SYSTEMS

1. **A** Myelin speeds up the propagation of an action potential down the axon by insulating areas of the axon from electrical conduction across the membrane. In a myelinated neuron, voltage-gated ion channels are clustered at the spaces between the myelin (the nodes of Ranvier), where electrical conduction can occur. As a result, the action potential appears to "leap" from node to node (saltatory conduction). When the myelin is removed, the newly unmyelinated parts of the axon do not contain enough voltage-gated ion channels to maintain the action potential, and the signal dissipates before reaching the end of the axon (choice A is correct). Because the signal dissipates before reaching the end of the axon, the neuron does not propagate the action potential more slowly; it does not propagate the signal at all (choices B and C are wrong). Myelin affects the propagation of the signal down the axon, but it does not affect the initiation of the signal at the hillock (choice D is wrong).

2. **D** A decrease in serum potassium concentration would increase the potassium gradient, causing more potassium to leave neurons. This would result in their hyperpolarization and inhibition, along with a general reduction of all neurally-mediated reflexes and functions in the body, including bowel activity; the decrease in bowel activity would lead to constipation (choice D is correct). However, this is not immediately obvious, and the best way to tackle this question is to use POE. The absolute refractory period is a product of the inactivation of the voltage-gated sodium channels and the repolarization of the cell; if anything, due to the increased potassium efflux, the cell would repolarize faster and the absolute refractory period would be shorter (choice A can be eliminated). The threshold potential is a function of the voltage-gated channels and does not depend on ion concentration (choice B can be eliminated). Hyperreflexia would be expected with neuron depolarization or a decrease in threshold potential (choice C can be eliminated). Patients with hypokalemia generally experience hyporeflexia.

3. **C** Skeletal muscles are paired for coordinated movement; when one muscle is stimulated to contract reflexively, the opposing muscle must be inhibited. The somatic nervous system utilizes a single neuron from the CNS to the muscle (choice A is wrong), and its effect is always excitatory at the neuromuscular junction. Thus, the sensory neuron can synapse directly with the motor neuron responsible for activating the contracting muscle (choice D is wrong), but it must use an interneuron to inhibit the motor neuron responsible for activating the opposing muscle (choice C is correct). Although it is true that the autonomic nervous system uses two neurons between the CNS and the effector organ, the autonomic nervous system is not responsible for the movement of skeletal muscles (choice B is wrong).

4. **A** The hypothalamus monitors homeostatic endpoints (heart rate, body temperature, etc.) in the body, and it helps to maintain set-points through its control of the pituitary gland (choice A is correct). The hippocampus is part of the limbic system, which helps with memory storage and retrieval (choice B is wrong). The cerebellum is primarily associated with the smoothing and coordination of movement (choice C is wrong). Although the medulla oblongata helps to set basic breathing rhythms and circulatory baselines, it is not directly involved in the feedback loops that regulate homeostasis (choice D is wrong).

5. **D** A cholinergic antagonist will inhibit acetylcholine (ACh), which is utilized at the ganglion in the sympathetic and parasympathetic systems and at the organ in the parasympathetic and somatic systems. Because ACh is utilized by all three divisions of the peripheral nervous system, the use of a cholinergic antagonist would not affect the sympathetic nervous system alone (choice D is correct). A cholinergic antagonist would inhibit rather than activate the

sympathetic nervous system (choice C is wrong), and it would not affect adrenergic receptors (choice B is wrong). Although it is true that the sympathetic nervous system utilizes ACh at the ganglion, the problem is that the antagonist will not be specific for the sympathetic system and is therefore not the best choice for the experiment (choice A is wrong).

6. **C** The semicircular canals, one in each of the 3-D planes, monitor body position and maintain equilibrium, particularly during rotation. The vestibule is involved in static equilibrium (choice A is wrong), the cochlea houses the hearing receptors (choice B is wrong), and the tympanic membrane (eardrum) vibrates in response to sound waves to help transmit the vibrations to the inner ear (choice D is wrong).

7. **A** If the outer segment is depolarized, then positive ions must be entering this segment. Dark current is the inward flow of sodium and calcium into the outer segment (depolarizing the outer segment) and the outward flow of potassium in the inner segment to balance the ion flow (choice A is correct, and choice B is wrong). Note also that choice A is the only answer choice that has positive ions entering the outer segment. Potassium flows passively out of the cell through leak channels (choice C is wrong), and both the inner and outer segment are involved in dark current (choice D is wrong).

8. **D** A tumor is the proliferation of abnormal cells, and in endocrine glands can result in overproduction (or underproduction) of the hormones produced by that gland. The question states that hormones are overproduced by this particular tumor. The adrenal gland produces small amounts of testosterone normally, but a tumor here could lead to large amounts being produced. The high levels of testosterone would cause feedback inhibition at the hypothalamus and anterior pituitary, resulting in dramatically reduced FSH and LH secretion. Without stimulation from these hormones, the testes will atrophy and reduce in size (choice D is correct). The hypothalamus produces GnRH, which acts on the anterior pituitary to stimulate the release of FSH and LH. These hormones would stimulate the testes, resulting in an increase in size, not a decrease (choice A is wrong). An anterior pituitary tumor would produce the same result, but without the involvement of the hypothalamus (choice B is wrong). The posterior pituitary does not produce hormones that would affect growth of the testes (choice C is wrong).

9. **B** Note that in this Roman numeral question, all of the items appear in exactly two answer choices, so it doesn't matter which item you start analyzing. Item I is false: secretin is a hormone that targets the pancreas to stimulate the release of bicarbonate (choices A and D can be eliminated). Both remaining answer choices include Item III; thus, Item III must be true, so focus on Item II. Item II is false: enterokinase is produced and acts within the intestine, but it is an enzyme, not a hormone (choice C can be eliminated, and choice B is correct). Note that Item III is true: calcitriol is a hormone derived from vitamin D that acts on the intestine to increase the absorption of calcium.

10. **B** This is a 2 × 2 question. Patients with Addison's disease have an insufficient production of steroid hormones from the adrenal cortex. These hormones include glucocorticoids (such as cortisol) and mineralocorticoids (such as aldosterone). Aldosterone causes the kidneys to retain sodium and water, which increases the systemic blood pressure. Therefore, patients with insufficient levels of aldosterone would have low blood pressure (choices C and D can be eliminated). Patients with insufficient levels of aldosterone do not retain as much sodium, thereby losing sodium in their urine. As a result, they may crave salty foods to replenish the body's sodium (choice B is correct). Aldosterone levels would not influence a person's craving for sweet foods (choice A is wrong).

SOLUTIONS TO THE NERVOUS AND ENDOCRINE SYSTEMS PRACTICE PASSAGE

1. **B** Marathon runners would want to use these steroids to enhance endurance via an increased red blood cell count, which is also why anemic patients would take these steroids (choice B is correct). The passage states that these steroids are easily detected (choice A is wrong), and that the type of steroid used medicinally depends on whether the anabolic or androgenic effects are required (choice C is wrong). It is not indicated that the androgenic side effects only occur in men; anabolic-androgenic steroid use can cause typically-male characteristics, such as growth of body hair, to be evident in females (choice D is wrong).

2. **C** Naturally occurring anabolic-androgenic steroids, including testosterone, are products of the hypothalamic-pituitary axis. The secretion of gonadotropin releasing hormone from the hypothalamus stimulates the release of LH and FSH from the anterior pituitary, which in turn stimulate testosterone production. A build-up of hormones with similar chemical structures to testosterone will induce negative feedback on the hypothalamic-pituitary axis (choice A is wrong). Negative feedback tends to inhibit the release of hormones at the target organs (choice B is wrong). In the case of anabolic-androgenic steroids, the target organ is the anterior pituitary gland, not the posterior pituitary (choice D is wrong, and choice C is correct).

3. **D** Because they are hydrophobic, steroid hormones can penetrate the cellular membrane to bind to intracellular receptors. In contrast, peptide hormones typically bind to receptors on the cell surface and produce second messengers (choice D is correct, and choice C is wrong). Also due to their hydrophobicity, steroids can be taken orally because they will readily cross the gastrointestinal membrane. Peptide hormones can be broken down by gastrointestinal peptidases and must be injected (choice A is wrong). Steroid hormones act as gene expression regulators (i.e., they affect transcription) when bound to their receptor, whereas peptides modify existing enzymes (choice B is wrong).

4. **A** Because the medicinal use would be to increase body weight, a higher anabolic effect versus androgenic effect would be desired. The steroid with the smallest androgenic-anabolic ratio is oxandrolone (choice A is correct). Oxymetholone and fluoxymesterone have intermediate ratios and should be eliminated (choices B and D are wrong). Testosterone has the highest androgenic-anabolic ratio, which is opposite of the desired effect in this case (choice C is wrong).

5. **C** Note that in this Roman numeral question, all of the items appear in exactly two answer choices, so it doesn't matter which item you start analyzing. Items I and II are true: both induction of puberty and increased lean muscle mass are effects of anabolic-androgenic steroid use, and can be used as medical treatment (choices A and B can be eliminated). Anabolic-androgenic steroids can cause acne, making Item III false (choice D can be eliminated; choice C is the correct answer).

6. **C** The passage states that the anabolic effects of steroids can lead to increased protein synthesis as well as an increase in the size and number of muscle cells (choice C is correct); this confirms that their effects go beyond only increasing the number of muscle fibrils (choice A is wrong). Although endurance athletes benefit from an increased red blood cell count, this does not increase muscle mass (choice B is a true statement but does not offer an explanation for increased muscle mass and can be eliminated). The passage states that steroid use decreases testosterone production (choice D is wrong).

Chapter 14
The Circulatory, Respiratory, Lymphatic, and Immune Systems

FREESTANDING QUESTIONS: THE CIRCULATORY, RESPIRATORY, LYMPHATIC, AND IMMUNE SYSTEMS

1. In well-trained athletes, the resting HR often ranges between 45–50 beats/min. However, their cardiac output at rest is no different from those of untrained individuals. Which of the following physiological mechanisms can account for this observation?

A) The enlarged heart size of trained athletes physically limits their HR.
B) The stroke volume of trained athletes at rest is decreased compared to untrained individuals.
C) Trained athletes have developed enlarged hearts that can pump more blood per stroke.
D) Since cardiac output and heart rate are inversely proportional, the reduced heart rate naturally causes an increased cardiac output.

2. A third-year medical student performs a physical exam on a patient and hears a third heart sound when the patient inhales deeply. A physician then examines the patient and explains to the student that this is a normal finding due to the increased chest capacity (and thus lower thoracic pressures) present on deep inhalation. What contributes to the presence of this additional heart sound?

A) Earlier closure of the pulmonary semilunar valve due to increased pulmonary artery pressure
B) Earlier closure of the pulmonary semilunar valve due to decreased pulmonary artery pressure
C) Later closure of the pulmonary semilunar valve due to increased pulmonary artery pressure
D) Later closure of the pulmonary semilunar valve due to decreased pulmonary artery pressure

3. Which of the following statements is true regarding the speed of depolarization in various areas of the heart?

A) Action potentials with rapid depolarization are found in the SA node and ventricular muscles.
B) Action potentials with rapid depolarization are found in the AV node, while action potentials with slower depolarization are found in the SA node.
C) Action potentials with slower depolarization are found in the SA node and the AV node.
D) Action potentials with slower depolarization are found in the AV node and ventricular muscles.

4. A 20-year-old patient presents to an emergency room with onset of acute asthma. He is wheezing, has shortness of breath, lacks the ability to speak an entire sentence, and has a respiratory rate of 40 per minute and nasal flaring. The family states he has been this way for about 15 minutes. The doctor draws an arterial blood gas (ABG) from the patient to assess his ability to oxygenate and ventilate. Which of the following ABGs would you expect to belong to the described patient? (Normal values: pH 7.4, P_{CO_2} 40 mm Hg, P_{O_2} 100 mm Hg, respiratory rate 10–12)

A) pH 7.40, P_{CO_2} 20 mm Hg, P_{O_2} 250 mm Hg
B) pH 9.40, P_{CO_2} 30 mm Hg, P_{O_2} 100 mm Hg
C) pH 7.50, P_{CO_2} 20 mm Hg, P_{O_2} 75 mm Hg
D) pH 6.90, P_{CO_2} 60 mm Hg, P_{O_2} 30 mm Hg

5. Which of the following is a true statement about the diaphragm?

A) It contains both skeletal and smooth muscle cells.
B) Its effector neurotransmitters are norepinephrine and acetylcholine.
C) It is innervated by both the phrenic nerve and the autonomic nervous system.
D) It receives neural signals from the cerebral cortex and the brain stem.

6. Which of the following would LEAST increase oxygen delivery to a patient suffering from anemia due to chronic renal disease?

A) Providing a nasal cannula with 100% oxygen
B) Intravenous injection of packed red blood cells
C) Administration of a drug stabilizing the oxygenated form of hemoglobin
D) Administration of erythropoietin

7. *Mycoplasma* are a type of bacteria lacking a cell wall which can cause numerous respiratory disorders. Treatment of an infection by one of these agents is complicated by their resistance to numerous antibiotics including penicillin. Which of the following forms of innate immune attack might *Mycoplasma* also be resistant to?

A) Lysozyme-induced cell death
B) Complement cytolysis
C) Neutrophilic endocytosis
D) B-cell triggered apoptosis

8. Multiple myeloma is a monoclonal plasma cell cancer originating in the bone marrow and is a common form of bone cancer observed in the elderly. What would be the most likely observation in a patient with multiple myeloma?

A) Decreased risk of bacterial infection
B) Elevated IgG production from a plasma cell targeting a single epitope
C) Elevated IgG production from a plasma cell targeting multiple epitopes
D) Increased production of red blood cells

9. A cell culture is developed with an abnormal major histocompatibility complex profile. What is the most likely profile of this cell line?

A) Neither MHC I nor MHC II
B) MHC I only
C) MHC II only
D) Both MHC I and MHC II

10. Which of the following are most likely to be found traveling in the lymphatic system?

I. Protein
II. Fat-soluble vitamins
III. Red blood cells

A) I only
B) I and II only
C) II and III only
D) I, II, and III

THE CIRCULATORY, RESPIRATORY, LYMPHATIC, AND IMMUNE SYSTEMS PRACTICE PASSAGE

Primary immunodeficiency disorders (PIDs) are categorized by the branch of the specific immune system impacted; thus, they can be cell-mediated, humoral, or combined. If a PID is characterized by defects in both B- and T-cells, it is considered to be a *severe combined immunodeficiency disorder* (SCID). Patients with this disorder are prone to infections which often spread to the blood with the first serious illness, typically occurring before one year of age.

In order to understand the mechanism of the disease and develop more effective means of treatment, a non-human mammalian model was generated. The SCID mouse lacks the ability to make B- or T-cells and thus effectively parallels the disorder seen in humans. Because of a recessive mutation on chromosome 16, these mice lack a DNA repair enzyme necessary for the recombination that occurs in the development of cells of the immune system. This animal model has provided a wealth of information about the function of the immune system in general, as well as serving as an important disease model.

Once a mouse model lacking an immune system was established, the possibility of engineering a mouse that contained a human immune system was considered. Such an animal would provide an *in vivo* model of a human system without utilizing human subjects. This led to the development of the hu-SCID chimera in which human fetal tissue, specifically that of the thymus, was placed in a SCID mouse and then followed by the introduction of human bone marrow stem cells. The result was a mouse lacking its inherent immune system but expressing functional human immune system cells, producing an excellent model in which to study immune system dynamics and disease responses.

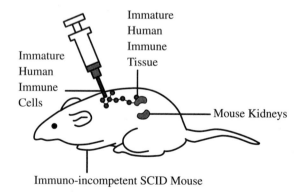

Figure 1   Representation of cellular components necessary to produce hu-SCID chimera

1. How could a cell-mediated PID contribute to impaired B-cell function?

A) B-cells would not receive stimulatory signals from helper T-cells and would not be triggered to proliferate.
B) Macrophages would be unable to present antigen to B-cells in order to induce appropriate antibody production.
C) Abnormally growing cells would fail to display intracellular peptides and would go unrecognized by B-cells.
D) The complement cascade would not be induced so B-cells would lack a necessary signal for proliferation.

2. Which of the following takes place in the lymph nodes?

A) Differentiation of B-cells
B) Release of circulating antibodies by natural killer cells
C) Nonspecific phagocytosis by macrophages
D) Removal of self-reacting B-cells

3. In the creation of the hu-SCID chimera, why is it necessary to place human thymus within the mouse?

A) The human thymus ablates any remaining immune system cells within the SCID animal.
B) The human thymus provides a source of lysozyme and thus bolsters innate immune protection.
C) The human thymus acts as the source of self-antigens, eliminating auto-reactive cells from those produced by the bone marrow progenitors.
D) The human thymus prepares the mouse's body to accept the introduction of other tissues and prevents graft rejection.

4. All of the following statements about the SCID or hu-SCID mice are true EXCEPT:

A) by utilizing human bone marrow from a wide variety of sources when creating the hu-SCID chimera, different human autoimmune diseases could be introduced into the SCID mouse.
B) helper T cells of the hu-SCID chimera are not able to be infected by HIV.
C) SCID mice have an extremely low rate of organ transplant rejection.
D) SCID mice have impaired complement immunity.

5. Which individual is most likely to present with an immune system profile like that of a person with SCID?

A) A 54-year old man who underwent a thymectomy as an infant
B) A 3-year old girl undergoing extensive radiation therapy as part of cancer treatment
C) A 27-year old woman positive for the human immunodeficiency virus (HIV)
D) A 41-year old man with Type I diabetes

6. What would be the immune system profile of the offspring of a pair of hu-SCID chimera mice?

A) Offspring would have the genetic profile for SCID and lack any human immune system cells.
B) Offspring would have the genetic profile for SCID and carry some human immune system cells.
C) Offspring might have the genetic profile for SCID and would lack any human immune system cells.
D) Offspring might have the genetic profile for SCID and would carry some human immune system cells.

SOLUTIONS TO FREESTANDING QUESTIONS: THE CIRCULATORY, RESPIRATORY, LYMPHATIC, AND IMMUNE SYSTEMS

1. **C** Cardiac output (CO, the volume of blood pumped in one minute) is the product of the stroke volume (SV, the volume of blood pumped in one beat) and the heart rate (HR, the number of beats per minute). CO = HR × SV; in other words, cardiac output is directly proportional to both heart rate and stroke volume (choice D is wrong). Thus, if heart rate decreases, the only way that CO at rest can stay constant is by a proportional increase in SV (choice C is correct, and choice B is wrong). A larger heart wouldn't necessarily limit heart rate and in any case, a limited heart rate could not account for the constant cardiac output seen in trained individuals (choice A is wrong).

2. **D** Increased pulmonary capacity upon inhalation and the resulting drop in thoracic (chest) pressure leads to decreased pressure in the pulmonary artery (choices A and C are wrong). The pulmonary semilunar valve prevents backflow of blood from the pulmonary artery to the right ventricle by closing when the pressure in the pulmonary artery exceeds the pressure of the right ventricle. With lower pulmonary artery pressure, it takes longer for the pressure in the pulmonary artery to exceed that of the right ventricle; this would delay closure of the valve (choice B is wrong, and choice D is correct). This additional heart sound, known as "normal splitting," occurs in both healthy and sick patients.

3. **C** Actions potentials with rapid depolarization are found in the atrial and ventricular myocardial cells (choices A and B are wrong). Slow action potentials (slow depolarization, slow repolarization, no plateau phase) are found in the autorhythmic cells of the SA and AV nodes only (choice D is wrong, and choice C is correct).

4. **C** During the initial phases of an asthma exacerbation, a patient breathes quickly in an effort to stay well oxygenated. In this process, he ventilates off his CO_2 to below normal levels (choice D can be eliminated). According to the Bohr effect ($H_2O + CO_2 \rightleftharpoons H_2CO_3 \rightleftharpoons H^+ + HCO_3^-$), as CO_2 falls, the pH would increase somewhat above normal (choice A can be eliminated). However, the pH would not increase to as high as 9.40; this would be toxic and lethal (choice B can be eliminated). Therefore, based on pH analysis alone, choice C is the answer. Choice C also shows that P_{CO_2} will be low, as the patient blows off carbon dioxide with a fast respiratory rate, and P_{O_2} will be lower than normal, as the patient struggles to oxygenate with constricted lungs. Of note, choice D would describe a patient that has been in respiratory distress for a longer period of time and is no longer able to compensate for the increased work of breathing (that is, he is tiring out). His CO_2 rises, and pH falls; this is a bad sign for an asthmatic.

5. **D** The diaphragm is purely skeletal muscle (choice A is false) and as such, ACh is the only neurotransmitter used (choice B is false). It's innervated only by the phrenic nerve, not autonomic nerves (choice C is false). The phrenic nerve originates both in the cerebral cortex, for voluntary breathing, and in the brain stem for involuntary control (choice D is correct).

6. **C** Erythropoietin, a hormone generated in the kidney, stimulates the production of red blood cells (RBCs). In cases of chronic renal disease, significantly lower levels of erythropoietin result in fewer RBCs being produced and decreased oxygen delivery to the tissues of the body. Administration of erythropoietin would likely increase RBC production and increase oxygen delivery (choice D would increase oxygen delivery and is the wrong answer). Injection of packed RBCs would have the same effect and increasing the concentration of inspired oxygen would slightly increase the amount of oxygen provided to the body (choices A and B increase oxygen delivery and are wrong answers). Stabilization of the oxygenated form of hemoglobin will decrease the ability for hemoglobin to unload oxygen as it travels through a capillary bed (choice C will decrease the amount of oxygen delivered and is the correct answer).

7. **A** Penicillin, and many other antibiotics, target the bacterial cell wall for destruction as a means of killing the bacterium. Lysozyme, an enzyme present in tears, saliva, and elsewhere, damages cell walls and functions similarly to penicillin; the lack of a cell wall in these bacteria would circumvent the mechanism of both penicillin and lysozyme (choice A is correct). You are provided no information to indicate that complement would be unable to target *Mycoplasma* or that neutrophils would be unable to engulf the bacteria (choices B and C are wrong). B-cells, members of the humoral immune system, are responsible for generating antibodies and are unlikely to trigger apoptosis in any cell type (choice D is wrong).

8. **B** Plasma cells are activated B-cells that secrete immunoglobulins (antibodies). Multiple myeloma involves the uncontrolled production of immunoglobulins by plasma cells. Each individual plasma cell generates antibodies which target a single epitope (choice C is wrong, and choice B is correct). While more elevated levels of antibodies may sound appealing, these patients experience an increased risk of infection (choice A is wrong), as these antibodies do not target invading microbes (they are a single clone). Expansion of this population of plasma cells in the bone marrow crowds out the healthy cells that would normally be involved in red blood cell (and other blood cell) formation (choice D is wrong).

9. **C** All nucleated cells in the body possess and express the MHC I complex on the cell surface (choice B is unlikely), and there are numerous anucleate cells that do not (choice A is unlikely). MHC II complexes are expressed on the surface of antigen presenting cells, which also possess MHC I complexes on their surface (choice D is unlikely). However, it would be incredibly unlikely for a cell to express an MHC II complex on its surface and not an MHC I complex as well (choice C is the least likely to appear in a normal cell and is the correct answer).

10. **B** Start by analyzing Item III, since it appears in exactly two of the answer choices, and whether it is true or false, you will be able to eliminate half the answers. Item III is false: under normal circumstances, red blood cells cannot exit the circulatory system and would therefore not be transported back to the blood via the lymphatic system (choices C and D can be eliminated). Note that both remaining answer choices include Item I, so it must be true, and you can continue by analyzing Item II. Item II is true: the lymphatic system also carries dietary fat, in the form of chylomicrons, including fat-soluble vitamins (choice A can be eliminated, and choice B is correct). Note that Item I is in fact true: the lymphatic system is responsible for returning water, dissolved solutes, and protein from the periphery to the blood.

SOLUTIONS TO THE CIRCULATORY, RESPIRATORY, LYMPHATIC, AND IMMUNE SYSTEMS PRACTICE PASSAGE

1. **A** The answer needs to link the function of T-cells (the cell-mediated arm of the immune system) to that of B-cells. B-cells receive co-stimulation from helper T-cells and the absence of that signal would impair B-cell proliferation and function (choice A is the best answer). While macrophages do present antigen, they present to helper T-cells, not B-cells (choice B is wrong). Abnormally growing cells are targeted by killer T-cells, but this does not involve B-cells (choice C is wrong). The complement cascade is not required for B-cell proliferation (choice D is wrong).

2. **C** The lymph nodes serve as a site for nonspecific filtration of the lymph by macrophages as well as a site for storage and activation of B- and T-cells (choice C is correct). B-cell differentiation and screening for self-reacting cells takes place in the bone marrow (choices A and D are wrong). Natural killer cells are part of the innate immune system and do not release antibodies (choice B is wrong).

3. **C** A primary role for the thymus in the immune system is to present self-antigens to developing T-cells and remove those that react to self-antigens. This helps prevent autoimmune responses (choice C is the best answer). The original SCID mouse is better able to avoid graft rejection due to its non-functional immune system (choice D can be eliminated), and there is no evidence to support the idea that the thymus will kill off native immune system cells within the mouse (choice A can be eliminated) or provide the enzyme lysozyme (choice B can be eliminated).

4. **B** Since the helper T-cells in the hu-SCID chimera come from humans in the form of a bone marrow transplant, and since human helper T-cells are capable of being infected with HIV, then the helper T-cells of the hu-SCID chimera should be able to be infected by HIV (choice B is not true and is the correct answer). One of the nice things about the hu-SCID chimera is that it can be "custom designed" by using different human bone marrow donors. If the bone marrow from a normal (non-autoimmune) individual is used, then the hu-SCID chimera would have a normal human immune system, but if the bone marrow from an individual with an autoimmune disease is used, then the hu-SCID chimera could also display that disease (choice A is true and can be eliminated). Since SCID mice lack a functional immune system, they are unable to reject transplanted organs (choice C is true and can be eliminated). Finally, the complement system can be activated by antibodies (among other ways of activation), and since the SCID mouse is unable to produce antibodies, it is likely that the SCID mouse would have some degree of compromised complement activation (choice D is true and can be eliminated).

5. **B** Since the question is looking for a condition most analogous to SCID, the correct answer needs to represent the individual with deficits in both cell-mediated and humoral immunity. Someone who had his thymus removed as a child would be expected to have deficits in cell-mediated immunity due to the lack of T-cell education and the potential for more auto-reactive T-cells, but would not have the full scale failure of SCID (choice A can be eliminated). An HIV patient will experience deficits due to infection of T helper cells. However, there is no additional information to describe the state of the patient's humoral immunity (choice C

can be eliminated). An adult with Type I diabetes has likely been living with the disorder for much of his or her life. Diabetes leads to high blood sugar (and a number of other effects such as kidney failure and poor wound healing), but this is not the same as having a non-functional immune system (choice D can be eliminated). Choice B represents the most profound lack of immune system cells in the most vulnerable patient; radiation will kill the progenitor cells that would normally be creating the immune system of a young child.

6. **A**   This is a 2 × 2 question, in which two decisions must be made to get to the correct answer. Since the mutation that leads to the SCID condition is caused by a recessive allele, SCID mice must be homozygous recessive for the mutation. Thus, if both parents have the SCID phenotype, all offspring will also be SCID (choices C and D can be eliminated). The human cells that are placed in the chimeras do not become part of the germ cell line and therefore will not be passed on (choice B can be eliminated, and choice A is the best answer).

Chapter 15
The Excretory and
Digestive Systems

FREESTANDING QUESTIONS: THE EXCRETORY AND DIGESTIVE SYSTEMS

1. *Helicobacter pylori,* a bacterium found in the stomach and duodenum, has been implicated in the formation of peptic ulcers (lesions due to inflammation and low pH). Which of the following would be the most effective initial treatment?

   A) Solid antacids to neutralize the stomach acid
   B) Parietal cell agonist to kill the *H. pylori*
   C) Oral antibiotic and solid antacids
   D) Oral antibiotic and parietal cell antagonist

2. Which of the following is NOT a way in which the absorptive capacity of the small intestine is optimized?

   A) Villi and microvilli increase the surface area of the small intestine.
   B) Smooth muscle contractions mix the chyme, allowing evenly distributed absorption.
   C) Blood flow to the small intestine is decreased during digestion.
   D) Na^+/K^+ ATPases maintain chemical and electrical gradients across cell membranes.

3. Some animals can digest cellulose, while humans cannot. What is a likely explanation for this phenomenon?

   A) Other animals have bacteria living in their digestive tracts that are capable of digesting cellulose.
   B) In humans, cellulose is physically inaccessible to the enzymes that can hydrolyze it into glucose.
   C) Humans lack a protease necessary for cellulose digestion.
   D) Cellulose blocks absorption of nutrients by microvilli.

4. Fibromuscular dysplasia is an autosomal dominant disorder that causes abnormal narrowing in the renal arteries. Which of the following explains why patients with fibromuscular dysplasia often present with systemic hypertension?

   A) The decreased diameter of the renal artery causes vessel walls to exert more pressure on the blood.
   B) The macula densa in the distal tubule responds to the increased filtrate osmolarity by stimulating renin secretion.
   C) Fibromuscular dysplasia causes systemic hypotension, so the JG cells secrete renin to compensate.
   D) The decreased glomerular filtration rate ultimately leads to the secretion of renin by the JG cells.

5. Angiotensin II receptor antagonists are a class of drugs that are commonly prescribed to treat hypertension. All of the following statements are possible explanations for why angiotensin II receptor antagonists can lower systemic blood pressure EXCEPT:

   A) they are similar in structure to angiotensin receptors, so they bind angiotensin II and prevent it from activating its endogenous receptor.
   B) they are similar in structure to angiotensin II, thereby competitively inhibiting the angiotensin II receptors.
   C) blockage of angiotensin II receptors leads to vasodilation.
   D) blockage of angiotensin II receptors reduces aldosterone and ADH secretion.

6. In Addison's disease, levels of aldosterone are much lower than normal. Which of the following symptoms would be expected in patients with this disease?

   I. Hypotension
   II. Lower urine osmolarity
   III. Decreased hematocrit

   A) I only
   B) II only
   C) I and III only
   D) II and III only

7. Many techniques have been developed in the field of bariatric surgery, but all involve minimizing the size or role of the stomach in the patient's gastrointestinal tract. Why does this accomplish the goal of weight loss while not contributing to malnutrition?

   A) Patients are counseled post-operatively to consume a high-protein diet that severely restricts the consumption of fruits or grains.
   B) The intestinal flora are still able to produce vitamin K.
   C) The techniques minimize the storage capacity of the GI tract while maintaining the brush border properties of the small intestine.
   D) Patients experience enough post-operative discomfort to discourage them from returning to their prior eating habits.

8. Which of the following are derived from cholesterol?

    I.   Vitamin D
    II.   Steroid hormones
    III. Bile

A) I only
B) I and II only
C) II and III only
D) I, II, and III

9. When blood pressure is low, which is the best description of the response in the renal arterioles?

A) Constriction of afferent arterioles, dilation of efferent arterioles
B) Constriction of both afferent and efferent arterioles
C) Dilation of afferent arterioles, constriction of efferent arterioles
D) Dilation of both afferent and efferent arterioles

10. The loop of Henle acts as a countercurrent multiplier within the kidney. What is the significance of this structural arrangement as part of the nephron?

A) Na^+ is secreted into the filtrate while K^+ is reabsorbed into the blood.
B) Urine osmolarity can exceed blood osmolarity.
C) The countercurrent multiplier triggers the release of renin from the liver.
D) Aquaporins can be inserted along the descending loop of Henle to alter its permeability to water.

THE EXCRETORY AND DIGESTIVE SYSTEMS PRACTICE PASSAGE

Following mastication, food is shifted by the tongue to the oropharynx where it is swallowed as a bolus and enters the esophagus. Here, the primary peristaltic wave begins by contracting above the bolus and relaxing beneath it in a unidirectional wave, contracting for 8–10 seconds and propelling the food toward the stomach (causing the relaxation of the upper and lower esophageal sphincters). If the entirety of the food does not reach the stomach in this primary wave, secondary peristaltic waves continue where the bolus distends the esophagus and drives the food toward the stomach.

The smooth muscle contraction seen during peristalsis in the esophagus occurs via a similar Ca^{2+}-dependent mechanism as seen in skeletal muscle, with a few notable exceptions. In place of troponin, a Ca^{2+}-dependent protein (calmodulin) activates myosin light-chain kinase. Phosphorylation leads to activation of the myosin heads, which subsequently allows for cross-bridge formation. To cease contraction, the phosphate is removed by myosin light-chain phosphatase.

Unexplained chest pain seen in patients is often attributed to esophageal spasm. While very limited information is available to characterize a diffuse esophageal spasm (DES), one study has shown that it may be linked to malfunction of endogenous nitric oxide synthesis. This was supported by the improved function of peristalsis and reduction of chest pain in patients treated with glycerin trinitrate (nitroglycerine).

1. Glycerin trinitrate likely forms which of the following in the body to treat diffuse esophageal spasm?

A) Glyceryl trinitrate
B) NO
C) NO_2
D) NO_3^-

2. A researcher creates an inducible knockout mouse designed for limiting levels of calmodulin expression in the digestive tract. Which of the following would be a likely effect in the digestive tract due to calmodulin knockout?

A) Diarrhea
B) Increased myosin light-chain phosphorylation
C) Dysphagia (painful/difficulty swallowing)
D) Increased cross-bridging

3. Researchers have characterized several compounds affecting the activity of esophageal smooth muscle activity. According to the figure, which of the following would lead to smooth muscle contraction in the esophagus?

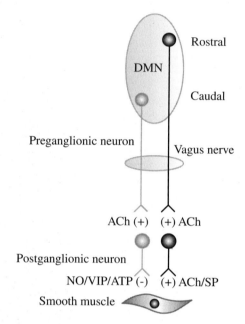

A) Increased acetylcholinesterase release
B) Destruction of the rostral potion of the dorsal motor nucleus (DMN)
C) Addition of a Substance P (SP) agonist
D) Increased vasoactive intestinal peptide (VIP)

4. Researchers have shown that peristalsis in the esophagus is preceded by a wave of smooth muscle relaxation (or inhibition of contraction) known as *deglutitive inhibition*. What is a possible reason for this wave of inhibition?

A) To eat large quantities of food in one sitting
B) To prevent potential esophageal damage associated with overuse
C) To allow for the normal drinking of water
D) To allow for increased food storage capacity in the digestive tract

5. A medical student on her internal medicine clerkship quickly eats a roll from the cafeteria but, after taking a very large final bite, feels as though she cannot move it down her entire esophagus. She is not having any difficulty breathing but is experiencing sharp pains in the center of her chest every few seconds. The pain increases for several minutes and then suddenly ends. What is the likely source of pain and why is she having difficulty swallowing the roll?

A) Primary peristaltic wave, increased pyloric sphincter tone
B) Primary peristaltic wave, increased cardiac sphincter tone
C) Secondary peristaltic wave, increased pyloric sphincter tone
D) Secondary peristaltic wave, increased cardiac sphincter tone

6. Activation of the sympathetic autonomic nervous system would have what effect on esophageal peristalsis?

A) No effect
B) Increased contractile rate
C) Decreased contractile rate
D) Decreased contractile force

SOLUTIONS TO FREESTANDING QUESTIONS: THE EXCRETORY AND DIGESTIVE SYSTEMS

1. **D** To treat peptic ulcers, you must both eliminate the infection (so that the ulcer does not recur) and neutralize the stomach acid (to reduce the inflammation and allow healing). Treatment with the appropriate antibiotic will eliminate the infection (choices A and B are wrong) and blocking release of HCl by parietal cells with an antagonist will provide a sustained higher stomach pH than will solid antacids (either alone or in combination; choice D is better than choice C). Note that choice B might be particularly harmful; an agonist would increase acid secretion, the exact opposite of what you are trying to accomplish.

2. **C** Blood flow to the intestines is increased (not decreased) during digestion, in order for the blood to pick up more nutrients from intestinal epithelium (choice C does not maximize the absorptive capacity of the small intestine and is the correct answer choice). Increasing surface area increases absorptive capacity, and villi and microvilli exist for this reason (choice A is true and can be eliminated). Mixing the chyme allows for even distribution along the intestine and more efficient absorption (choice B is true and can be eliminated). Choice D is a true statement for all cells in the body; in the intestine, the gradients allow for the secondary active transport of other nutrients, such as glucose (choice D is true and can be eliminated).

3. **A** Cellulose passes through the same digestive tract in humans as do all other nutrients, and it would be accessible to the same enzymes (choice B is wrong). Proteases cannot break down carbohydrates (choice C is wrong), and though cellulose does not interfere with the absorptive capacity of microvilli, this also does not address the question of digesting it in the first place (choice D is wrong). Choice A addresses the different digestive capability between humans and other animals, so this is the correct answer.

4. **D** The abnormal narrowing in the renal arteries results in decreased blood flow to the kidneys, thus lowering the glomerular filtration rate (GFR). When the GFR is low, the osmolarity and volume of the filtrate are decreased (choice B is wrong); the cells of the macula densa are sensitive to this decrease, and they respond by stimulating the JG cells to release renin (choice D is correct). Although systemic vasoconstriction does lead to increased blood pressure, fibromuscular dysplasia only causes local narrowing in the renal artery, which does not result in systemic hypertension (choice A is wrong). Lastly, although the JG cells normally secrete renin in response to systemic hypotension, the question text states that fibromuscular dysplasia causes systemic hypertension, not hypotension (choice C can be eliminated).

5. **A** Receptor antagonists are typically molecules that when bound to their respective receptors, elicit the opposite response as the normal ligand, or block the response of the normal ligand. Thus, angiotensin II receptor antagonists must be structurally similar to angiotensin II; they can bind to the angiotensin II receptor and block angiotensin II from binding. Since angiotensin II acts to increase blood pressure, preventing it from binding to its receptor would lower blood pressure (choice B is a possible explanation and can be eliminated). However, receptor antagonists cannot be structurally similar to the receptor itself if they are to block it (choice A cannot explain the drop in blood pressure and is the correct answer choice). Angiotensin II is a vasoconstrictor; preventing it from binding its receptor would prevent this vasoconstriction and lead to a drop in blood pressure (choice C is a possible explanation and can be eliminated). Furthermore, angiotensin II increases aldosterone and ADH release,

leading to increased sodium and water reabsorption, a higher blood volume, and a higher blood pressure. Blocking the receptor would reduce the release of these hormones and prevent their effects (choice D is a possible explanation and can be eliminated).

6.   **A**   Since all of the items appear exactly twice in the answer choices, it doesn't matter which one you start with. Item I is true: without aldosterone, much of the necessary Na$^+$ reabsorption from the distal convoluted tubule will not take place and it would be difficult to maintain a systemic rise in blood pressure; ADH will not be subsequently triggered. Thus, these patients do suffer from hypotension (choices B and D can be eliminated). Since Item II is not in either of the remaining answer choices, it must be false and you can focus on Item III. Item III is false: hematocrit is the percentage of whole blood made up of red blood cells. Aldosterone has no effect on red blood cell production (choice C can be eliminated, and choice A is correct). Note that Item II is in fact false: if Na$^+$ is not being reabsorbed, urine osmolarity would be higher, not lower.

7.   **C**   One of the primary roles of the stomach is to act as a preparatory storage tank for food that will be passed on to the small intestine. Bariatric surgery alters or bypasses the stomach, but it leaves the small intestine fully functional so that the minimal amounts of food that can be comfortably ingested will still be broken down and their nutrients absorbed (choice C is correct). Restricting major food groups would likely lead to malnutrition, not prevent it (choice A is wrong), and while the bacteria in the gut do produce vitamin K, this would also not be enough to prevent malnutrition (choice B is wrong). A patient's post-operative level of pain is never the reason to perform a procedure nor would this effect be very long-lasting, even if it was appropriate (choice D is wrong).

8.   **D**   Since Item III appears in exactly two of the answer choices, start by analyzing it. Regardless of whether it is true or false, you'll be able to eliminate half the answer choices. Item III is true: bile is derived by the liver from cholesterol (choices A and B can be eliminated). Since both remaining answer choices include Item II, it must be true and you can focus on Item I. Item I is true: vitamin D is produced in the skin photochemically from cholesterol, then activated by the liver and kidney (choice C can be eliminated, and choice D is correct). Note that Item II is in fact true: all steroid hormones are derived from cholesterol.

9.   **C**   Since blood pressure is the primary factor driving filtration, when blood pressure falls, filtration rate also falls. In order to bring the glomerular filtration rate (GFR) back up to normal, pressure must be increased in the glomerulus. One way to do that would be to increase volume in the glomerulus. Dilation of the afferent arterioles would increase influx to the glomerulus, thus increasing volume and pressure in those capillaries (choices A and B can be eliminated). Constriction of the efferent arterioles would reduce efflux from the glomerulus, effectively "trapping" blood, increasing volume and pressure, and returning GFR to normal (choice C is correct, and choice D is wrong).

10.   **B**   The switch in both directions and permeability that occurs between the descending and ascending limbs of the loop of Henle enhance the ability of the kidney to generate powerful concentration gradients within the medulla. This leads to greater fluid movement out of the collecting duct, and thus urine with an osmolarity that can exceed that of the blood (choice B is correct). The loss of Na$^+$ to the filtrate and the movement of K$^+$ into the blood is determined by aldosterone at the DCT, not the loop of Henle (choice A is wrong). Renin is not produced by the liver (choice C is wrong), and the descending limb is always permeable to water (choice D is wrong).

SOLUTIONS TO THE EXCRETORY AND DIGESTIVE SYSTEMS PRACTICE PASSAGE

1. **B** According to the passage, diffuse esophageal spasm is linked to malfunction of endogenous nitric oxide (NO) production. Since glycerin trinitrate successfully improves peristalsis and reduces chest pain, it is likely that it forms NO in the body (choice B is correct). In fact, it is a potent vasodilator and serves as a treatment for both DES and heart disease. Glyceryl trinitrate is another name for glycerin trinitrate (choice A is wrong), NO_2 is nitrous oxide ("laughing gas," choice C is wrong), and NO_3^- is nitrate (choice D is wrong).

2. **C** As described in the passage, calmodulin binds calcium and results in the activation of myosin light-chain kinase and subsequent phosphorylation of the myosin light-chain. Phosphorylation allows for cross-bridging and smooth muscle contraction. By limiting the amount of calmodulin present, smooth muscle contraction in the digestive tract cannot take place as readily, and peristalsis cannot occur regularly. This leads to discomfort when trying to swallow food (choice C is correct). Diarrhea would be expected in a situation of increased digestive tract motility (choice A is wrong). With a deficiency of calmodulin, decreased myosin light-chain phosphorylation would be expected (choice B is wrong), and thus decreased subsequent cross-bridge formation (choice D is wrong).

3. **C** An agonist produces or increases the physiological effect of interest. From the figure, SP activates smooth muscle contraction; thus, its agonist would also do so (choice C is correct). Acetylcholinesterase removes ACh from the synaptic cleft, so increasing acetylcholinesterase would decrease stimulation to the smooth muscle cell (choice A is wrong). Destruction of the rostral portion of the dorsal motor nucleus would damage the vagus nerve and would prevent smooth muscle contraction (among a list of other, far more severe problems; choice B is wrong). According to the figure, VIP inhibits smooth muscle contraction (choice D is wrong).

4. **C** From the passage, you know that esophageal peristalsis contractions last for 8–10 seconds, but drinking water occurs more rapidly than that and thus this would obstruct the next bolus of water from passing down the esophagus. By causing inhibition along the esophagus during repeated swallowing, it allows fluids to flow down the esophagus without interference from peristalsis (choice C is correct). Deglutitive inhibition will not increase the total quantity of the food that can be eaten in one sitting (although it may affect rate), nor will it increase storage capacity of the digestive tract as food is not stored in the esophagus (choices A and D are wrong). Deglutitive inhibition may prevent damage associated with food being forced down a contracted esophagus, but this would not be related to overuse (choice B is wrong).

5. **D** Given the medical student's initial inability to completely swallow the roll, primary peristaltic waves must have failed to move the roll effectively down the esophagus (choices A and B can be eliminated). Thus, secondary peristaltic waves are needed to drive the food down the esophagus and (ideally) into the stomach. Increased cardiac sphincter tone (regulating entrance of food from the esophagus into the stomach) would initially prevent food from entering the stomach and lead to discomfort with each secondary peristaltic wave (choice D is correct). The pyloric sphincter is at the end of the stomach and regulates entrance of chyme into the duodenum, thus increased tone at this sphincter is unlikely to cause the discomfort in this instance (choice C is wrong).

6. **A** While sympathetic stimulation generally results in a decrease in GI activity, esophageal peristalsis does not change with sympathetic activity; basic maintenance activities, like swallowing saliva, need to be able to continue, even if eating and drinking are not occurring as part of a fight-or-flight response (choice A is correct).

Chapter 16
The Musculoskeletal System and Skin

FREESTANDING QUESTIONS: THE MUSCULOSKELETAL SYSTEM AND SKIN

1. A researcher is measuring the movement of calcium in a cardiac muscle cell. He notes that calcium can enter the cytoplasm from either the extracellular space or the sarcoplasmic reticulum. Which of the following statements is true regarding this calcium movement?

   A) Most of the cytoplasmic calcium comes from the extracellular space.
   B) Most of the cytoplasmic calcium comes from the SR.
   C) Equal amounts of calcium enter the cytoplasm from the extracellular space and the SR.
   D) In some cardiac muscle cells, calcium comes from the extracellular space, while in others, the predominant source of the calcium is the SR.

2. When a coroner conducts a postmortem assessment, one factor he examines is the onset and progression of *rigor mortis*, which is characterized by rigidity of the skeletal muscles. What is the best explanation for this phenomenon?

   A) The body can no longer thermoregulate, and muscles become stiff due to the cold.
   B) The muscles become rigid in the early phases of decomposition.
   C) The muscles can no longer perform the power stroke, due to a lack of ATP.
   D) Myosin is unable to release actin, and the crossbridges remain intact.

3. Which of the following are characteristics of skeletal muscle fibers?

   I. Striated
   II. Uninucleate
   III. Action potential similar to a neuron

   A) I only
   B) I and III only
   C) II and III only
   D) I, II, and III

4. Immunohistochemical stains are used in order to classify cell types in biopsies of carcinomas. A stain for which of the following proteins would likely be positive in a cancer originating from cells in the epidermis (squamous epithelial cells)?

   A) Desmin
   B) Vimentin
   C) Keratin
   D) Glial fibrillary acid proteins (GFAP)

5. Acetylcholinesterase (AChE) is responsible for breaking down acetylcholine that has been released into a synapse. What would be the effect of reduced AChE at the neuromuscular junction?

   A) Acetylcholine concentrations would be lowered, and the muscle would be inhibited from contracting.
   B) Acetylcholine concentrations would be lowered, and the muscle would be stimulated to contract continuously.
   C) Acetylcholine concentrations would be increased, and the muscle would be inhibited from contracting.
   D) Acetylcholine concentrations would be increased, and the muscle would be stimulated to contract continuously.

6. Because of the distinct properties associated with different muscle fiber types, Olympic-level athletes are often interested in the fiber type composition of the muscles associated with their event. In terms of the numbers of fibers, fiber type composition of skeletal muscle remains mostly unchanged after birth; however, it is possible to increase the size of different fibers with training. Which of the following can be expected when comparing the fiber type composition in the leg muscles of Olympic runners?

   A) Sprinters should have larger Type I fibers, whereas marathon runners should have larger Type IIa fibers.
   B) Sprinters should have larger Type I fibers, whereas marathon runners should have larger Type IIb fibers.
   C) Sprinters should have larger Type IIb fibers, whereas marathon runners should have larger Type I fibers.
   D) Sprinters should have larger Type IIa fibers, whereas marathon runners should have larger Type I fibers.

7. *Bullous pemphigoid* and *pemphigus vulgaris* are both autoimmune disorders of the skin. Bullous pemphigoid is caused by IgG antibodies acting against epidermal basement membrane cellular adhesions (hemidesmosomes) and is characterized by the separation of the skin layers at that site, whereas pemphigus vulgaris is caused by IgG antibodies acting against intra-epidermal desmosomes. Which of the following is true?

A) In bullous pemphigoid the roof of the large blisters should include the dermis.
B) In pemphigus vulgaris the blisters should include disruption of blood vessels.
C) If slightly rubbed, the blisters in pemphigus vulgaris should be more flaccid and more easily ruptured than those of bullous pemphigoid.
D) Direct immunofluorescence against the IgG antibodies on a biopsy of skin showing a straight line of antibodies is more likely to be pemphigus vulgaris than bullous pemphigoid.

8. Bisphosphonates are a class of medications that function to inhibit bone resorption. They are frequently used by physicians to prevent or reduce the bone loss that occurs during osteoporosis. Which of the following is a potential mechanism of action for bisphosphonates?

A) Increase calcium absorption in the small intestine
B) Trigger apoptosis, or programmed cell death, in osteoclasts
C) Stimulate osteoblasts
D) Prevent renal losses of calcium into the urine

9. Osteopetrosis, also known as marble bone disease, is a disorder caused by a failure of normal bone resorption, which leads to thickened, dense bones. Bone cells can be found in normal numbers, and hormone levels are usually normal. Which of the following is LEAST likely to be true about osteopetrosis?

A) Decreased marrow space may lead to anemia and thrombocytopenia (deficiency of platelets).
B) Osteoclast cells are involved in the disorder.
C) The number of osteoclast cells must be decreased.
D) It may result in stunted growth.

10. In end-stage renal disease (ESRD), patients have decreased production of active vitamin D, which in turn results in decreased serum calcium levels. The low serum calcium results in hyperplasia of the parathyroid glands and leads to hyperparathyroidism. Which of the following would be expected as a result?

A) Osteitis fibrosa cystica—cystic bone lesions due to increased bone resorption
B) Osteopetrosis—thickened, dense bones due to decreased bone resorption
C) Osteitis deformans—abnormal bone architecture caused by increase in both osteoblastic and osteoclastic activity
D) Polyostotic fibrous dysplasia—bone replaced by fibroblasts, collagen, and irregular bony trabeculae

THE MUSCULOSKELETAL SYSTEM AND SKIN PRACTICE PASSAGE

In 1736, John Freke of Saint Bartholomew's Hospital described a disease in which large swellings of fused bone were felt on the back of a 14 year old patient. These swellings had been growing for three years and had formed a "fixed bony pair of bodice" on the patient's torso. Until recently, the cause of fibrodysplasia ossificans progressiva (FOP) remained a mystery, but recent research has greatly expanded the understanding of the pathophysiology behind this disease.

FOP is characterized by two clinical features: malformations of the great toes and progressive heterotropic ossification (HO). Extensive HO begins in the first decade of life and occurs with significant pain at sites of tissue damage and inflammation. Heterotropic bone replaces skeletal muscle and connective tissue, but spares the diaphragm, tongue, and extraocular muscles. Attempts to surgically remove heterotropic bone stimulate more robust bone growth. HO progresses throughout the patient's lifetime, often resulting in impaired mobility and life-threatening complications.

Recently, the gene responsible for FOP has been identified as ACVR1, which produces activin receptor protein IA; a missense mutation in the activation domain of the receptor results in the disease. ACVR1 functions as a bone morphogenetic protein (BMP) receptor and remains constitutively activated upon mutation; this results in overactive osteogenesis.

Signal transduction inhibitors (STIs) for ACVR1 are an area of significant research in the treatment of FOP. The ATP-binding site on the BMP receptor can be exploited to ensure specificity of STIs in FOP treatment and avoid cross reacting with similar BMP receptors. Because STIs are not yet available, current treatment focuses on supportive therapy and managing inflammation.

1. A pathologist examines a biopsied tissue sample under high resolution and observes numerous red, uninucleate, striated cells. Is this an appropriate tissue sample for determining whether the patient is suffering from FOP?

A) Yes, because heterotropic bone replaces skeletal muscle.
B) Yes, because heterotropic bone replaces connective tissue.
C) No, because it is not a bone sample.
D) No, because FOP does not affect cardiac muscle.

2. Which of the following is a potential molecular mechanism by which a patient could develop fibrodysplasia ossificans progressiva?

A) A mutation that generates a stop codon early in the coding region
B) A mutation in the promoter region of the gene
C) A mutation in the coding region that changes an amino acid
D) An insertion mutation in an intron

3. A patient with fibrodysplasia ossificans progressiva presents at the doctor's office. Which of the following physical exam findings would you expect to find in this patient?

A) Tongue deviates to one side when the patient is instructed to stick it out
B) Nystagmus (rapid involuntary oscillations of the eye)
C) Severe dyspnea (labored respiration)
D) Nuchal rigidity (neck stiffness)

4. According to the passage, which of the following is the most effective treatment for FOP?

A) Surgery removing the overgrown bone
B) Sonification of overgrown bone to aid in bone particle removal
C) Systemic glucocorticoids to reduce inflammation
D) Oral calcitonin

5. In the development of an STI for the treatment of FOP, a researcher discovers an increase in muscular intracellular calcium in an animal model, which results in increased muscular tone. Which of the following is the LEAST likely cause?

A) The STI acts as a receptor antagonist on the motor endplate.
B) The STI inhibits acetylcholinesterase.
C) The STI decreases the sarcoplasmic reticulum membrane integrity.
D) The STI inhibits the Ca^{2+}-ATPase of the sarcoplasmic reticulum.

SOLUTIONS TO FREESTANDING QUESTIONS: THE MUSCULOSKELETAL SYSTEM AND SKIN

1. **B** While calcium does enter the cytoplasm of cardiac muscle cells from both the extracellular space and sarcoplasmic reticulum (SR), the predominate source is the SR (choices A and C can be eliminated). Note that all cardiac muscles cells must function the same way (choice D is wrong).

2. **D** *Rigor mortis* is caused by the muscles remaining in a partially contracted state, due to the lack of ATP. During sliding filament contraction, the presence of ATP is required for the myosin head groups to release actin (choice D is correct). Although ATP is necessary for the process of muscle contraction, its presence does not directly drive the power stroke (choice C is wrong). Decomposition would result in the softening of muscle tissue as it begins to break down (choice B is wrong). Although the body does become cold in the absence of thermoregulation, temperature is not the primary factor determining mobility of the tissues (choice A is wrong), with the exception of complete freezing.

3. **B** Start by analyzing the Roman numeral item that appears in exactly two of the answer choices, since whether it is true or false, you'll be able to eliminate half the answers. Item II appears exactly twice, so start there. Item II is false: skeletal muscle cells are formed by the fusion of many smaller cells and are multinucleate syncytia (choices C and D can be eliminated). Note that both remaining answer choices include Item I, so it must be true, and you can focus on Item III. Item III is true: the skeletal muscle action potential is similar to a neural action potential (choice A can be eliminated, and choice B is correct). Note that Item I is in fact true; skeletal muscle tissue appears striated under the microscope due to the regular arrangement of actin and myosin filaments into sarcomeres.

4. **C** Keratin is a tough, hydrophobic protein that makes the skin waterproof and is found in squamous epithelial (skin) cells, thus it is likely that these cells would stain positive for keratin (choice C is correct). The other proteins are not necessary to know for the MCAT, but desmin is found in muscle (choice A is wrong), vimentin is found in connective tissue (choice B is wrong), and glial fibrillary acid proteins (GFAP) are found in neuroglia (choice D is wrong).

5. **D** This is a 2 × 2 question, which can be approached by tackling the answer choices in two parts. Because acetylcholinesterase is responsible for breaking down acetylcholine, a decrease in AChE will lead to an increase in ACh at the synapse (choices A and B are wrong). The effect of ACh at the neuromuscular junction is to depolarize the muscle cell, so an increase in ACh would stimulate muscle contraction (choice C is wrong, and choice D is correct).

6. **C** Type I fibers are slow twitch, oxidative fibers, which take longer to reach maximum tension but are very resistant to fatigue. These would increase in size with consistent endurance training, such as marathon running (choices A and B are wrong). Type IIb fibers are fast twitch, glycolytic fibers, which reach maximum tension very quickly but are fatigue sensitive. These are the most effective fibers for high intensity, short-duration exercises such as sprinting (choice C is correct). Type IIa fibers are intermediate in twitch speed and fatigue resistance; they do not provide the greatest force, which would be necessary for Olympic-level competition (choice D is wrong).

7. **C** As stated in the question stem, in bullous pemphigoid the separation occurs at the basement membrane of the epidermis and thus the roof of the blister should include all of the layers of the epidermis, but it would not include the dermis (choice A is wrong). Also, pemphigus vulgaris involves disruption of desmosomes between cells within the epidermis; since the blood vessels of the skin are contained within the dermis, it would be expected that these blisters would not disrupt the blood vessels (choice B is wrong). In fact, in pemphigus vulgaris, the blisters (or "vesicles" in this case) are fluid-filled and are very flaccid as they do not contain all of the layers of the epidermis. The "Nikolsky Sign" is when slight rubbing of the skin results in rubbing away the top layers of the skin, which occurs in pemphigus vulgaris, but classically not in bullous pemphigoid since these blisters contain all of the layers of the epidermis and thus are stronger (choice C is correct). This is one of the clinical maneuvers used in order to initially differentiate between the two disorders. Usually a skin biopsy is also obtained and often direct immunofluorescence for the IgG antibodies is utilized. Since in bullous pemphigoid the antibodies are directed against the basement membrane, the result is a relatively straight line of antibodies, whereas in pemphigus vulgaris the antibodies are more diffusely spread throughout the epidermal layer (choice D is wrong).

8. **B** The question stem states that bisphosphonates function to "inhibit bone resorption." By directly targeting the osteoclasts (the predominant cell type involved in bone resorption) for apoptosis, bone loss should be reduced (choice B is correct). Increasing calcium absorption from the intestines and preventing its loss in the urine would increase serum calcium concentrations and potentially improve bone formation. However, promoting bone formation is not equivalent to preventing bone loss, and the question text specifies that bisphosphonates act to inhibit bone resorption (choices A and D are wrong). Similarly, stimulating osteoblasts would target bone formation, not resorption (choice C is wrong).

9. **C** The question states that osteopetrosis is caused by a failure of bone resorption; thus osteoclast activity is likely decreased or impaired (choice B is true and can be eliminated). While a deficiency in the number of osteoclast cells may lead to osteopetrosis, in some cases the number of cells is normal but their function is impaired (choice C is false and the correct answer). Note also that choice C uses extreme language ("must") and contradicts the question stem. The defective bone resorption leads to thickened, dense bones, which eventually decreases the marrow space. Because the marrow space is where all blood cells and platelets are produced, this would potentially lead to anemia and thrombocytopenia (choice A is true and can be eliminated). The hardening of the bones in children with osteopetrosis can lead to stunted growth (choice D is true and can be eliminated). Note that although choice D may not be immediately obvious, choice C is clearly false.

10. **A** Parathyroid hormone causes bone resorption, thus hyperparathyroidism would lead to increased osteoclast activity and increased bone resorption (choice A is correct, and choices B and C are wrong). Polyostotic fibrous dysplasia is a form of fibrous dysplasia and does not involve osteoclasts. Based on its description in the answer choice, it might involve abnormal osteoblast activity, as bone is not being made properly (choice D is wrong).

SOLUTIONS TO THE MUSCULOSKELETAL SYSTEM AND SKIN PRACTICE PASSAGE

1. **D** This biopsy is of cardiac muscle (uninucleate, striated cells) and would not undergo heterotropic ossification (HO); therefore, you cannot conclude whether this patient is suffering from FOP (choice D is correct). Skeletal muscle is striated, but the cells are multinucleate (choice A is wrong). Connective tissue consists of cells within a matrix, and does not exhibit the striated organization of skeletal and cardiac muscle (choice B is wrong). A pathologist would be looking for ossification of tissues other than bone to diagnose FOP (choice C is wrong).

2. **C** The passage states that the gene responsible for FOP has a missense mutation in the protein's activation domain. A missense mutation is a point mutation that results in a single amino acid substitution (choice C is correct). In the case of FOP specifically, histidine is substituted for arginine at position 206 of the protein. A mutation that generates an early stop codon, which would truncate the protein, is called a nonsense mutation (choice A is wrong). A mutation in the promoter region of the gene would affect whether the gene is transcribed, but would not affect the conformation of the resulting protein (choice B is wrong). Do not be fooled by the wording in the passage, which describes a mutation in the activation domain of the protein; the promoter is a part of the DNA, not the protein. A mutation in an intron will be spliced out during RNA processing and should not affect the resulting protein; it is a silent mutation (choice D is wrong).

3. **D** According to the passage, FOP spares the diaphragm, tongue, and extraocular muscles, meaning you would expect normal physical exam findings in these areas (choices A, B, and C are not potential areas of ossification and are less likely to result in abnormal findings). Nuchal rigidity (neck stiffness) could occur due to ossification of the skeletal muscle in the neck (choice D is correct).

4. **C** According to the passage, current treatment for FOP focuses on supportive therapy and management of inflammation. Glucocorticoids reduce inflammation and could help decrease the degree of heterotropic ossification in the patient (choice C is a viable treatment). Both surgical removal of bone and sonification would likely result in trauma which may worsen the condition (choices A and B are not viable treatments). Oral calcitonin, a polypeptide, would be digested in the stomach and would not have significant therapeutic benefit; more importantly, calcitonin helps stimulate osteoblasts and bone formation which is clearly not the best option for treating FOP (choice D is wrong).

5. **A** If the STI acted as an antagonist (inhibitor) at the motor endplate, fewer ligand-gated ion channels would open and the cell may fail to depolarize enough to stimulate the opening of voltage-gated calcium channels. This would result in decreased cytosolic calcium (choice A is least likely to explain an increase in intracellular calcium and increased muscular tone and is thus the correct answer). Acetylcholinesterase (AChE) is responsible for the destruction of acetylcholine at the neuromuscular junction. Inhibiting AChE would result in increased levels of ACh, increased muscular stimulation, and increased intracellular calcium levels (choice B is a possible cause and can be eliminated). Because calcium is stored in the sarcoplasmic reticulum (SR), disruption of the SR membrane integrity could result in an increase in intracellular calcium (choice C is a possible cause and can be eliminated). The Ca^{2+}-ATPase is responsible for removing calcium from the cytosol and returning it to the sarcoplasmic reticulum. Its inhibition would result in increased intracellular calcium (choice D is a possible cause and can be eliminated).

Chapter 17
The Reproductive Systems

FREESTANDING QUESTIONS: THE REPRODUCTIVE SYSTEMS

1. A woman suffers a hemorrhage into her pituitary gland which destroys only the portion of the anterior pituitary responsible for producing luteinizing hormone. What will be the effect of this destruction on her menstrual cycle?

A) Her menstrual cycle will not be affected by the destruction.
B) She will still ovulate and release estrogen, but not progesterone.
C) She will become anovulatory.
D) She will still ovulate and release progesterone, but not estrogen.

2. Suppose that gastrulation proceeded abnormally such that the ectoderm did not develop. Which of the following organs would fail to form?

A) Heart
B) Brain
C) Liver
D) Stomach

3. When injected, an anabolic androgenic steroid (AAS) such as testosterone cypionate becomes testosterone in the blood. When this occurs, the testosterone level naturally produced by the body:

A) increases because negative feedback causes FSH to decrease.
B) increases because positive feedback causes GnRH to increase.
C) decreases because negative feedback causes FSH to decrease.
D) decreases because negative feedback causes LH to decrease.

4. If the mother of a child with an XY genotype is exposed to testosterone-blocking chemicals during the first trimester of her pregnancy, what tissues/structures will develop in the infant?

A) Ovaries, internal and external female genitalia
B) Testes, internal and external female genitalia
C) Testes and external male genitalia only
D) Testes and external female genitalia only

5. A patient attempting to get pregnant has her blood drawn and has elevated levels of progesterone. Given it has been two weeks since her last menstruation, what best describes the uterine phase she is currently in?

A) Follicular phase
B) Proliferative phase
C) Luteal phase
D) Secretory phase

6. Which of the following are appropriate analogous pairs?

    I. Labia majora, crus of the penis
    II. Labia minora, spongy urethra
    III. Ovary, testis

A) I only
B) II only
C) II and III only
D) I, II, and III

7. Which of the following correctly describes the development of the placenta?

A) zygote → morula → trophoblast → placenta
B) zygote → blastocyst → inner cell mass → placenta
C) zygote → morula → inner cell mass → placenta
D) zygote → trophoblast → morula → placenta

8. All of the following are true of the placenta EXCEPT:

A) it takes approximately three months to develop.
B) it is the site of exchange of fetal/maternal nutrients.
C) it secretes hCG to maintain the corpus luteum.
D) it contains tissue derived both from the mother and developing zygote.

9. A new fertility clinic claims to have developed a lower cost method for *in vitro* fertilization. The physician would harvest primary oocytes from immature follicles before placing them in a dish containing the donor's sperm. Any resulting ova would then be implanted into the expectant mother. Is this method viable?

A) Yes, although the risk of having fraternal twins will be significantly increased.
B) Yes, although the risk of having monozygotic twins will be significantly increased.
C) No, it is not possible to induce implantation with an *in vitro* fertilized embryo.
D) No, the oocytes would not provide viable zygotes when fertilized.

10. A researcher studying the fast block to polyspermy has narrowed down a potential mechanism to a few possibilities. Which is most likely?

A) Potassium efflux out of the ovum
B) Sodium influx into the ovum
C) Chloride influx into the ovum
D) Glucose influx into the ovum

THE REPRODUCTIVE SYSTEMS PRACTICE PASSAGE

Fetal heart rate (FHR) monitoring is a common obstetric procedure that is used in approximately 85% of live births in the United States. Typically the FHR monitor displays the fetal heart rate and the amniotic pressure as a function of time.

There are different patterns of fetal heart rate that can be important to identify and monitor. An "acceleration" is a visually apparent increase (onset to peak in less than 30 seconds) in FHR from the most recent baseline. This is typically caused by normal fetal movements. An "early deceleration" is a gradual decrease (onset to minimum in more than 30 seconds) in FHR with return to baseline that mirrors the uterine contraction. Early decelerations are usually due to head compression from the uterine contraction, which is generally normal. An abrupt (onset to minimum in less than 30 seconds) decrease in FHR below the baseline that lasts greater than 15 seconds, but less than 2 minutes, is called a "variable deceleration." Umbilical cord compression is the most common cause of variable decelerations, and is most often secondary to oligohydramnios (reduced amount of amniotic fluid). Variable decelerations are important indicators of probable fetal distress.

The baseline of the FHR tracing is also important to evaluate. A bradycardiac baseline (FHR < 110 bpm) may signify severe fetal hypoxia or congenital heart malformations. A tachycardiac baseline (FHR > 160 bpm) may also be caused by fetal hypoxia, anemia, or maternal fever.

FHR monitor outputs obtained from two different patients are provided below.

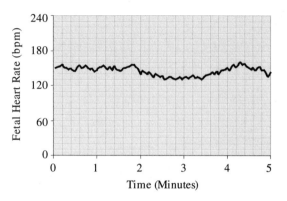

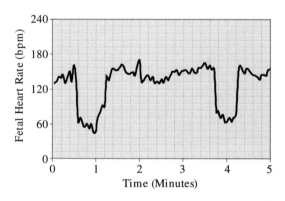

Figure 1   Normal (healthy) fetal heart trace from Patient #1

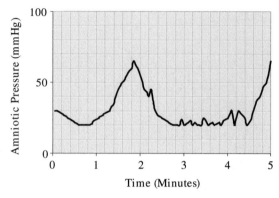

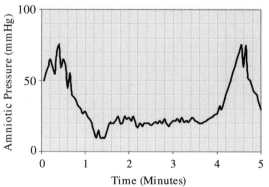

Figure 2   Fetal heart trace from Patient #2

1. Which of the following is the most probable cause of the FHR pattern seen in Figure 2?

A) Fetal movements due to increased maternal activity
B) Head compression from normal contractions
C) Maternal fever
D) Premature rupture of amniotic membranes (PROM) resulting in oligohydramnios

2. Which of the following is the most likely cause for the difference in fetal and adult heart rate?

A) Increased parasympathetic activity at the adult AV node
B) Increased norepinephrine release at the adult AV node
C) Decreased parasympathetic activity at the fetal SA node
D) Decreased norepinephrine release at the fetal SA node

3. Ventricular septal defects (VSDs) are the most common congenital heart malformations. VSD is due to a failure of the ventricular septum to fully close during development. Which of the following primary germ layers is responsible for forming the septum of the ventricles of the heart?

A) Endoderm
B) Mesoderm
C) Ectoderm
D) Cardioderma

4. Nondisjunction during anaphase of meiosis may lead to a trisomy known as Klinefelter's syndrome (XXY). The resulting individual has a male phenotype, however has testicular atrophy, a slender body shape, gynecomastia, and female hair distribution. This syndrome usually results in dysgenesis of the seminiferous tubules, as well as abnormal Leydig cell function. Which of the following hormones would be expected to be increased, compared to a normal male, in a patient with Klinefelter's syndrome?

A) Inhibin
B) Testosterone
C) FSH
D) Prolactin

5. Which of the following would most likely exacerbate early decelerations observed during FHR monitoring?

A) Administration of oxytocin to mother
B) Decreasing pressure on the cervix
C) Decreasing amniotic fluid volume
D) Injection of epinephrine (a sympathetic agonist) in the umbilical vein

6. Which of the following is NOT a trigger for labor?

A) Increased uterine stretch
B) Decreased levels of hCG
C) Increased stretch of the cervix
D) Decreased levels of estrogen

SOLUTIONS TO FREESTANDING QUESTIONS: THE REPRODUCTIVE SYSTEMS

1. **C** If the portion of the anterior pituitary that produces LH is destroyed, then LH levels will not surge during the menstrual cycle and ovulation would not occur (choice C is correct, and choices B and D are wrong). In the absence of ovulation, the corpus luteum would not develop either, although if FSH is unaffected, the follicle would most likely develop and release estrogen. Regardless, the menstrual cycle would be affected (choice A is wrong).

2. **B** The ectoderm gives rise to the nervous system and epidermis; thus, if it did not develop properly, the brain would fail to form (choice B is correct). The mesoderm gives rise to connective tissue, bone, muscles, urogenital organs, and the circulatory and lymphatic systems (choice A can be eliminated). The endoderm gives rise to the respiratory tract, gastrointestinal tract, and endocrine glands and organs (choices C and D can be eliminated).

3. **D** This is a 2 × 2 question since you first need to decide if testosterone levels will increase or decrease. When an anabolic androgenic steroid (AAS) mimics testosterone, the naturally produced testosterone level decreases (choices A and B are wrong). This is due to negative feedback; the presence of the AAS causes the hypothalamus to release less gonadotropin releasing hormone (GnRH), which in turn causes the anterior pituitary to release less luteinizing hormone (LH) and follicle stimulating hormone (FSH). Since LH typically stimulates testosterone production, the reduced levels of LH lead to a decreased production of testosterone (choice D is correct, and choice C is wrong).

4. **D** The XY genotype would produce testicles (choice A is wrong) that would subsequently release Mullerian inhibiting factor (MIF). MIF would prevent internal female genitalia from developing (choice B is wrong). Though testicles would be present and producing testosterone, the mother's chemical exposure would block the effects of testosterone during the critical developmental window. This would prevent the formation of additional male genitalia and lead to an external female phenotype (choice C is wrong, and choice D is correct).

5. **D** The menstrual cycle is a 28-day cycle that affects two organs: the ovary and the uterus. The 28 days as they apply to the ovary are referred to as the *ovarian cycle,* and include the follicular, ovulation, and luteal phases. The 28 days as they apply to the uterus are referred to as the *uterine cycle,* and include menstruation, the proliferative phase, and the secretory phase. A patient with elevated levels of progesterone two weeks after her last menstruation is in the secretory phase of her uterine cycle (choice D is correct). While she is also in the luteal phase, this term characterizes the phase of her ovarian cycle, not uterine cycle (choice C is wrong). The follicular phase is characterized by a slow increase in estrogen before ovulation; this is part of the ovarian cycle (choice A is wrong). The proliferative phase of the uterine cycle is the phase during which the endometrial lining increases its thickness (choice B is wrong).

6. **C** Start by analyzing the Roman numeral item that appears in exactly two answer choices, since whether it is true or false, you'll be able to eliminate half the answers. Both Items I and III appear exactly twice, so start with Item I. Item I is false: the labia majora are analogous to the scrotum in the male (choices A and D can be eliminated). Since both remaining

choices include Item II, it must be true, and you can focus on Item III. Item III is true: the ovary is analogous to the testis in the male (choice B can be eliminated, and choice C is correct). Note that Item II is in fact true: the labia minora are analogous to the spongy urethra in the male.

7. **A** The correct progression of development from the zygote leading to a placenta begins with cleavage to generate a ball of cells known as a morula. Blastulation then occurs, resulting in a structure called a blastocyst; this is a hollow ball of cells (the trophoblast) with a mass of cells on the inside (the inner cell mass). The inner cell mass ultimately becomes the embryo, while the trophoblast ultimately becomes the placenta (choice A is correct).

8. **C** The development of the placenta takes approximately three months and contains tissue of both fetal and maternal origin which serve as a site of exchange of nutrients between the mother and developing fetus (choices A, B, and D are true statements about the placenta and can be eliminated). The placenta begins production of progesterone to maintain the pregnancy and the corpus luteum degenerates after the first trimester of pregnancy (choice C is a false statement about the placenta and the correct answer choice).

9. **D** Primary oocytes are held in prophase I for decades until ovulation begins. Normally each month, a follicle develops and this results in the completion of meiosis I and formation of a secondary oocyte, which is then ovulated. Here the physician is harvesting oocytes from immature follicles, which have not yet completed meiosis I and would likely be incapable of generating a viable zygote (choice D is correct). Given that any fertilization is not probable, it is also unlikely that twins will be the result (choices A and B are wrong). There is no inherent reason why a fertilized embryo could not be implanted into the endometrium; in fact, in vitro fertilization is a successful industry which relies upon just that (choice C is wrong).

10. **B** The fast block to polyspermy results from the depolarization of the ovum. Of the answer choices, only the influx of sodium will result in the depolarization of a cell (choice B is correct). Efflux of potassium or influx of chloride would hyperpolarize the cell (choices A and C are wrong). Glucose, which lacks a charge, would result in no change in the membrane potential of the cell (choice D is wrong).

SOLUTIONS TO THE REPRODUCTIVE SYSTEMS PRACTICE PASSAGE

1. **D** Figure 2 shows a FHR pattern consistent with variable decelerations, since there is an erratic FHR with abrupt, deep decelerations. As the passage indicates, this is commonly caused by umbilical cord compression, which may result from oligohydramnios (decreased amniotic fluid). Thus, a premature rupture of the amniotic membranes would lead to decreased amniotic fluid and would be an explanation for the umbilical cord compression and resulting variable decelerations (choice D is correct). Fetal movements would be expected to cause normal accelerations in the pattern (choice A is wrong). Head compression from normal contractions would cause early decelerations and an expected increase in amniotic pressure, which would coincide with the contractions themselves (choice B is wrong), and maternal fever would cause a baseline tachycardia (FHR > 160 bpm, so choice C is wrong).

2. **C**   According to the passage, fetal heart rate is normally between 110–150 bpm, which is significantly elevated compared to adult heart rate. The SA node serves as the pacemaker in the healthy heart (choices A and B are wrong) and a decrease in parasympathetic activity at the fetal SA node relative to the adult SA node would result in an elevated fetal heart rate (choice C is correct). Norepinephrine serves as the most common neurotransmitter at the final synapse in the sympathetic autonomic nervous system, so a decrease in sympathetic activity would serve to slow the fetal heart rate, which does not account for the observation that it is faster than in the adult (choice D is wrong).

3. **B**   The mesoderm is responsible for all muscle, bone, connective tissue, urogenital organs, and the entire cardiovascular/lymphatic system, including blood and the heart (choice B is correct). The ectoderm is responsible for the nervous system as well as the epidermis of the skin and its derivatives (hair, nails, sweat glands, sensory receptors) and nasal, oral, and anal epithelium (choice C is incorrect). The endoderm forms the GI tract epithelium (except the mouth and anus), the GI glands (liver, pancreas, etc.), urinary bladder, and the epithelial lining of the urogenital organs and ducts (choice A is incorrect). Cardioderma is not a primary germ cell layer at all (choice D is incorrect). Cardioderma is actually the genus name of the "Heart-nosed bat" (*Cardioderma cor*).

4. **C**   A patient with Klinefelter's syndrome has testicular atrophy, thus any hormone normally produced by the testes (testosterone and inhibin) would be decreased and can be eliminated (choices A and B are wrong). The decrease in testosterone and inhibin would lead to decreased negative feedback on the anterior pituitary, causing increased levels of LH and FSH (choice C is correct). Prolactin should be unaffected in patients with Klinefelter's syndrome; the gynecomastia (excessive development of the breasts in males) in this case is due to the increased levels of estrogen (choice D can be eliminated).

5. **A**   According to the passage, early decelerations are usually due to head compression from uterine contraction. Administration of oxytocin, a hormone which increases the intensity of uterine contraction during labor, would exacerbate this effect (choice A is correct). Decreasing pressure on the cervix and decreasing amniotic fluid volume would both result in a decrease in uterine contraction and would likely decrease early decelerations (choices B and C are wrong). Epinephrine, a sympathetic agonist, would serve to increase heart rate resulting in tachycardia (choice D is wrong).

6. **B**   There are several things that can lead to an excitable uterus and possible labor. Increased stretch on the uterus can trigger its contraction (choice A could be a trigger for labor and can be eliminated). Increased stretch on the cervix, typically caused by the baby's head, can trigger the release of oxytocin, which in turn stimulates uterine contractions (choice C could be a trigger for labor and can be eliminated). Due to the deterioration of the placenta, decreased levels of estrogen can stimulate contractions (choice D could be a trigger for labor and can be eliminated). However, hCG is virtually absent from the system from about five months of gestation onward; its levels are high during early pregnancy to maintain the corpus luteum (and thus the levels of estrogen and progesterone), but hCG levels begin to fall once the placenta is formed (about 3 months gestation) and are virtually absent by full term labor (choice B is not a trigger for labor and is the correct answer choice).

Part 4

MCAT Psychology and Sociology

Chapter 18
Research Methods

FREESTANDING QUESTIONS: RESEARCH METHODS

1. A team of researchers measures a negative correlation between income and length of labor time in a group of pregnant women. It is expected that as income increases, labor time:

A) decreases.
B) increases.
C) stays the same.
D) The change in labor time cannot be determined.

2. Due to scheduling and logistical limitations, researchers could only conduct a study on Tuesdays and Thursdays between 7pm and 9pm. They were therefore limited to individuals who were available at this time. This setup would have created issues in:

A) external validity, due to the selection criteria.
B) internal validity, due to a potential Hawthorne effect.
C) external validity, due to the lack of a control group.
D) internal validity, due to impression management.

3. Researchers want to explore the experience of subjects as they engage in the Stroop task, a task in selective attention that measures the ability to distinguish between discordant stimuli. The researchers are not merely interested in response time but want to know qualitative details about the subjects' internal experiences. Which of the following methodologies should the researchers implement?

A) Correlational method
B) Observational method
C) Survey method
D) Phenomenological method

4. Which of the following is a limitation of the ethnographic method?

A) Cultural validity is low, since the observer is not a member of the society of interest.
B) External validity is low, because the experimental conditions do not match the real world.
C) External validity is low, because only one culture is sampled.
D) Construct validity is low, since the instruments have not been checked for reliability.

5. A team of researchers finds that there is a complex relationship between IQ and sociability. Measures of sociability were found to be high for individuals within one standard deviation of the mean for intelligence, and gradually decreased for individuals with both very high and very low IQ scores. Which of the following correlations would be measured in this instance?

A) Positive
B) Negative
C) No correlation
D) A correlation cannot be determined.

6. In a study of the impact of personality type on the interpretation of a social symbol, which of the following is a possible operational definition of the independent variable?

A) Personality type is the independent variable, so it can be defined as results on a questionnaire designed to measure five-factor model personality traits.
B) Personality type is the independent variable, so it can be defined as degree of sympathetic arousal and amygdala activation when seeing a symbol.
C) Symbol interpretation is the independent variable, so it can be defined as average ranking, from positive to negative, of a series of neutral symbols.
D) Symbol interpretation is the independent variable, so it can be defined as degree of sympathetic arousal and amygdala activation when seeing a symbol.

7. Attrition, or subjects dropping out of a study before its completion, is a threat to:

A) internal validity, because it introduces a potential cofounding variable.
B) internal validity, because the group may no longer be representative.
C) external validity, because it introduces a potential confounding variable.
D) external validity, because the group may no longer be representative.

8. Which of the following research methodologies would best explore the development of human memory over time?

A) Case study
B) Longitudinal study
C) Observational study
D) Archival study

RESEARCH METHODS PRACTICE PASSAGE 1

Recent adaptations in technology, such as smartphones and the Internet, have been found to have potentially negative effects on physical and psychological well-being. Sociologists refer to the time it takes to catch up to technological innovations as cultural lag. Researchers have been interested in studying the effects of cultural lag on attention, cognition, and psychopathology.

A study was conducted with 347 students from first-year introductory psychology courses at a four-year state university in the Midwest, where a large majority of students were in-state residents. They were incentivized with extra credit in their course, and of the 347 that were invited, 62 participants who chose to participate were first asked to respond on a Likert scale from 1 to 5 how often they used their cell phones, social media, and the Internet. Based on the results, participants were divided into 2 groups of 31 students each. Both groups contained more females, 21 and 23 in the low usage and high usage groups, respectively. Researchers also considered GPA, and found that the cumulative GPAs for both groups were similar, 3.16 and 3.32, respectively, a difference that was not found to be significant. It was hypothesized that the group that used various types of digital media more would manifest detrimental effects along a range of variables, measured by a battery of exams on reaction time, working memory, and ability to conduct tasks while ignoring a distractor. Participants were also given two implicit surveys to measure depression and anxiety, respectively.

Results supported the research hypotheses. Based on the results, researchers determined that the stress response may have been the link between technology use and the measurement variables, since various studies showed that stress was known to have detrimental effects on each of these areas. The group suggested to campus health experts that they should recommend students to limit their use of digital media to mitigate the effects of cultural lag.

1. Which of the following conclusions can be most reasonably drawn from the study in passage?

A) Stress plays a critical role in the relationship between technology and cognitive effects because it provides the most plausible mediating variable.

B) There was a relationship between technology use and psychopathology because the research utilized various psychometrics.

C) Cultural lag regarding digital media is an ongoing problem on college campuses because the research conducted used random assignment and random sampling to test the hypotheses.

D) Use of social media caused detrimental effects on cognition because of the strain placed on the attentional mechanism, as demonstrated by comparison with the control group.

2. If the researchers are correct in their conclusion, what is likely to happen in a second study of elderly adults who are known to be more sensitive in their response to stress?

A) They will have difficulty attending to stimuli.

B) They will score higher on depression.

C) The low digital usage group will have slower reaction times.

D) The high digital usage group will demonstrate increased anxiety.

3. A likely confounding variable created by the experimental design was:

A) school performance.

B) gender.

C) extraversion.

D) academic major.

4. The methodology described in the passage created threats to external validity due to each of the following considerations EXCEPT:

A) geographic location.

B) lack of a control group.

C) student availability.

D) age.

5. Which of the following pairs represents a qualitative and quantitative variable, respectively?

A) Reaction time and coping ability

B) Reaction time and depression score

C) Type of coping response and level of depression

D) Attending fluidity ability and reaction time

6. Each of the following could be an operational definition of the dependent variable EXCEPT:

A) depression inventory score.

B) sympathetic nervous system arousal.

C) size of social media network.

D) time attending to distracting variables.

RESEARCH METHODS PRACTICE PASSAGE 2

Video games have grown to become one of the most-used forms of entertainment media. Surveys show that the average video game player spends between 10 and 15 hours per week on video games, and educational researchers have suggested that this time would be better spent on other activities such as homework and after-school activities. Video games use classic research in behavioral psychology to provide reinforcement on schedules that activate the brain's dopamine reward circuit, the same region that is implicated in addiction and substance abuse. However, other neuroscientific research has shown that regions associated with cognitive tasks are also activated by video games. For example, improvements in visual tasks including contrast sensitivity, object tracking, and spatial attention have been measured. To test the impact of video games on cognitive visual tasks, researchers employed two types of research: correlational and experimental.

Study 1

The first study conducted correlational research and showed that individuals who spend more time playing video games are likely to also have increased spatial attention, and show greater integration between the occipital lobe and other areas of the cortex. This increased sensory integration is associated with greater response flexibility, and the ability to learn new visual cognitive tasks more quickly.

Study 2

An initial follow-up study investigated whether there is a causal relationship between video game play and object tracking. Each of 23 male participants came to a research laboratory and completed an object tracking task that was presented on a screen, and reaction time was measured according to how quickly the subjects fixed their gaze on a new object in the visual field and also how long the subjects were able to keep their gaze fixed on the target as it moved. The experimental group was then given a visual task similar to a video game that involved a first-person perspective and completing virtual tasks. Results showed that there was an increase in object tracking ability compared to the control group.

Study 3

A second follow-up study was conducted to test the impact of a set of video games on amblyopia; the researchers concluded that more research was needed to see. A phenomenological analysis was conducted on a group of four participants diagnosed with amblyopia, commonly known as lazy eye. The four subjects were observed in their homes, then given a varied regimen of video games that they played at least 2 hours a day for one month. Using measures of object tracking it was found that amblyopia improved by an average of 13% in the four subjects.

1. Compared to the first follow-up study, the second follow-up study had:

   A) high internal validity and low external validity.
   B) high internal validity and high external validity.
   C) low internal validity and low external validity.
   D) low internal validity and high external validity.

2. Which of the following pairs of correlations is consistent with the research described in the passage?

   A) +0.60 between video game play and sensory integration and –0.33 between video game play and time to learn new tasks
   B) +0.35 between video game play and sensory integration and +0.21 between video game play and time to learn new tasks
   C) +0.07 between video game play and sensory integration and –0.40 between video game play and time to learn new tasks
   D) –0.47 between sensory integration and time to learn new tasks and +0.44 between sensory integration and response flexibility

3. Which of the following describes the comparisons made in Study 2 and Study 3, respectively?

   A) Within subjects for Study 2 and within subjects for Study 3
   B) Between subjects for Study 2 and within subjects for Study 3
   C) Within subjects for Study 2 and between subjects for Study 3
   D) Between subjects for Study 2 and between subjects for Study 3

4. Which of the following is a dependent variable from the research?

   A) Amblyopia
   B) Visual cognitive tasks
   C) Object tracking
   D) Video game perspective

5. The best control condition for researchers to use in Study 2 would be a group of:

   A) 25 boys and girls assigned a movie to watch and given similar object tracking tasks.
   B) 50 boys assigned a different set of video games.
   C) 25 boys of similar age assigned a movie to watch and given the same measure of object tracking to test the effect.
   D) 50 boys and girls assigned a different set of video games.

SOLUTIONS TO FREESTANDING QUESTIONS: RESEARCH METHODS

1. **A** A negative correlation suggests that as the value measured for one variable increases, the other decreases, and vice versa. Therefore, as income increases, labor time is expected to decrease (choice A is correct). Labor time would increase if the correlation were positive (choice B is wrong). There was a result measured, so the measurement would not stay the same (choice C is wrong), and the direction of change is known because the type of correlation is given in the question stem (choice D is wrong).

2. **A** This question can be completed more quickly with the observation that the first part of the answer choices divides the set of choices in half. The first step is to determine if the situation described in the question stem is a threat to internal or external validity. The recruitment method is problematic because the experiment will not sample individuals who have different schedules and are not available at that time. A sample that is not representative of the population is a threat to external validity, not internal validity (choices B and D are wrong). Selection criteria are the processes used to select participants for an experiment. This describes the scheduling issue presented in the question stem (choice A is correct). A lack of control group is a threat to internal validity, since this attribute is related to how well-designed the study is and to what extent researchers can draw conclusions based on findings (choice C is wrong).

3. **D** The phenomenological method is a technique used to evaluate the experience of some phenomenon and often obtain more introspective details about an event than is possible with other methods. This method is also usually qualitative, or descriptive, as the question stem suggests (choice D is correct). The correlational method is a quantitative measure of the relationship between two variables (choice A is wrong). The observational method involves observation and minimal interference by the researcher. It would be very difficult to know about subjects' internal experiences by simply observing them (choice B is wrong). The survey method tends to give general characteristics of an event or experience, since it contains general questions that are tested on numerous individuals. This characteristic would make it difficult to know about subjects' unique internal experiences. The survey method is also quantitative in most cases, since subjects often provide a numerical assessment of their self-reported beliefs or feelings (choice C is wrong).

4. **C** External validity is an issue in ethnographic studies, mainly because the methodology involves deep exploration of a single culture or subculture, so it provides limited information on how the results might apply to other cultures (choice C is correct). Cultural validity is not a type of validity checked for by researchers (choice A is wrong). Experimental conditions in ethnographic research are usually very close to the real world, since the researcher makes every attempt to not disrupt the environment. The goal of ethnographic research is to observe the culture in a naturalistic setting (choice B is wrong). Ethnographic researchers do not usually use surveys, but deep analysis, in their evaluations of the cultures they study, so construct validity is very unlikely to be a consideration. Construct validity most usually applies to psychometric instruments such as surveys (choice D is wrong).

5. **C** The results described in the question are curvilinear in nature. They do not represent a linear relationship and would show up as a bell on a graph. Correlational research does not pick up nonlinear trends (choice C is correct; choices A, B, and D are wrong).

6. **A** This question can be resolved more quickly by noticing that the first part of the answer choices divides the set of choices in half. The first step is to determine whether personality type or symbolic interpretation is the independent variable. The study described is designed to measure how personality affects symbolic interpretation. Therefore, the independent variable—the variable manipulated by the researcher—is personality type (choices C and D are wrong). The five-factor model is a common measure of personality (choice A is correct). Sympathetic arousal and amygdala activation do not define personality type (choice B is wrong).

7. **A** Attrition is primarily a threat to internal validity, because there may be some non-trivial reason that subjects are dropping out. This would present a confounding variable, because if the reason for attrition were related to the hypothesis, it could provide an alternative explanation for the results (choice A is correct). Non-representative samples are a threat to external, not internal validity (choice B is wrong). Confounding variables are a threat to internal, not external validity (choice C is wrong). It is less likely that enough subjects drop out to threaten the external validity of the study. Also, if participants began to drop out, internal validity would be threatened first, such that it would be difficult to draw a conclusion that would then be applied to the external population (choice D is wrong).

8. **B** Longitudinal studies are best for exploring how variables develop over time. They involve conducting periodic measurements of the same individuals over many years to see how certain variables change. This is the ideal methodology for exploring the question presented in the stem (choice B is correct). Case studies are best for understanding individuals in a comprehensive way. This would be an ideal methodology for understanding one person's memory development, but would not allow for generalization to human memory (choice A is wrong). An observational study could meet the criteria, but observational studies do not specifically deal with the development of variables over a long period of time. This study methodology usually involves observing events in a naturalistic setting, and although this could be done over time intervals, this is not usually a feature of observational research (choice C is wrong). Archival studies would be best for exploring how a phenomenon was different many years ago, to use as a comparison with other epochs. However, archival research would not be ideal for understanding how age evolved for groups of individuals, since it is impossible to control for variables with data taken many years ago, and there are often gaps in the data available (choice D is wrong).

SOLUTIONS TO RESEARCH METHODS PRACTICE PASSAGE 1

1. **B** Psychopathology refers to mental disorders or abnormal behavior. The research described found a relationship between time spent using various forms of technology and slowed cognitive function. The psychometrics used were the battery of exams on cognitive functions (reaction time, working memory, and multitasking) as well as the Likert scale that was used to assess technology use (choice B is correct). The researchers proposed stress as a possible mediator in paragraph 3; however, the actual research to establish this relationship was not actually conducted. A mediating variable is a variable that provides a link in a causal relationship and helps to show why that relationship exists. The researchers did not conduct any tests on stress and how stress relates to technology use (choice A is wrong). The research did suggest that cultural lag was a point of concern since new technologies seemed to be related to cognitive problems. However, the study did not contain the random sampling from the population described in the answer choice, namely college campuses. The study only sampled from one university, and without follow-up research, you cannot be sure that the results apply to students on other campuses (choice C is wrong). The researchers cannot be sure that social media caused the detrimental effects because the independent variable is not manipulated directly by the researchers in this case. Instead, it is measured and the subjects are placed into groups. Also, there was no control group. There was only a high technology and low technology group (choice D is wrong).

2. **D** The researchers concluded that stress was a potential mediating result because of its known relationship with the cognitive variables. Stress and anxiety are known to be related to each other, so high digital usage would be associated with increased anxiety (choice D is correct). The research described showed a relationship between digital usage and attention, not stress response and attention. Note that stress response does not necessarily mean that the group will actually experience more stress, but that they will respond with greater sensitivity if stress occurs. Therefore, the known relationships between stress and attention and stress and depression do not necessarily apply (choices A and B are wrong). Slower reaction time was associated with the high digital use group, not the low digital use group (choice C is wrong).

3. **C** Extraversion is a characteristic related to how energizing individuals find social interactions with others. Individuals who are high in extraversion tend to be more sociable, garrulous, and spend more time interacting with others. It may therefore be more likely that they engage more with social media and technology, spending more time on their phones. This could make high extraversion individuals more susceptible to the effects of the study (choice C is correct). School performance and gender were both measured in the study, and the researchers did not find large differences between the two groups in either variable (choices A and B are wrong). Academic major is unlikely to be a confounding variable since there is not a clear link between major and digital media usage. Also, there are many academic majors, and variables with many groups are less likely to be confounded, since any effect will be distributed across a spectrum (choice D is wrong).

4. **B**   For except/not/least questions, evaluate each answer choice and eliminate ones that are true. Geographic location is a threat to external validity because the participants attend a midwestern university where most individuals are from in-state (choice A is true and can be eliminated). The study did lack a control group, but this is a threat to internal validity, because it is a flaw in the way the research is designed that affects the ability to draw conclusions from the variables (choice B is false and is therefore the correct answer choice). Student availability is a threat to external validity, because only some students participated in the study, so the research results may not apply as well to the entire student population, which includes students who may be too busy to participate in the research (choice C is true and can be eliminated). Age is a threat to external validity since most students will be in their early 20s. This means the results may not apply to older adults (choice D is true and can be eliminated).

5. **C**   The correct answer choice will pair a qualitative variable with a quantitative variable. Type of coping response suggests that coping responses will be broken into categories, a sign that it is a qualitative variable, since it would not involve a numerical continuum but rather placement into one of several different coping styles. Depression level can be measured quantitatively, since "level" suggests a score along a scale (choice C is correct). Reaction time is a quantitative variable (choices A and B are wrong). Attending fluidity ability suggests a measure along a continuum. Most variables along a continuum tend to be quantitative in nature, whereas most categorical variables tend to be qualitative. This suggests that attending fluidity is a quantitative variable (choice D is wrong).

6. **C**   For except/not/least questions, evaluate each answer choice and eliminate the answer choices that are true. A dependent variable is an outcome variable measured by the researchers to test the extent of effect of the manipulation in the study. Depression is one of the dependent, or measurement, variables (choice A is true and can be eliminated). Sympathetic nervous system arousal is related to anxiety, one of the dependent variables (choice B is true and can be eliminated). Size of social media network is related to how much time an individual spends using digital media, which is an independent, not dependent, variable in the study (choice C is false, therefore the correct answer choice). Attention and ability to tune out distracting variables is a dependent variable in the study (choice D is true and can be eliminated).

SOLUTIONS TO RESEARCH METHODS PRACTICE PASSAGE 2

1. **D**   Internal validity refers to how well a study is conducted, and it allows valid conclusions to be drawn between independent and dependent variables. Between Study 2 and Study 3, Study 2 contains a control group, and more rigorous methodology, so it has more internal validity (choices A and B are wrong). Study 3, on the other hand, has greater external validity. Researchers used a variety of video games and individuals were observed in their natural settings, compared to Study 2 participants who were observed in a laboratory setting. Study 2 also used a visual task, not actual video games (choice D is correct, and choice C is wrong).

2. **A** Study 2 states that video game play is associated with increased sensory integration, which is represented by a positive correlation. It also indicates that playing video games reduced the time to learn new tasks, which would be indicated by a negative correlation (choice A is correct, and choice B is wrong). A correlation of +0.07 is likely to be negligible since it is very close to 0, the correlational representation of no linear relationship (choice C is wrong). The connection between sensory integration and time to learn new tasks is not explicitly stated as a correlation, and it cannot be assumed that a correlation between video game play and sensory integration combined with a correlation between video game play and time to learn new tasks implies that there is also a correlation between sensory integration and time to learn new tasks (choice D is wrong).

3. **B** Study 2 compares the experimental group to a control group, which is a comparison between two different groups, that is, between subjects (choices A and C are wrong). Study 3 compares the subjects at one point to the same subjects at a point later on in time, known as within subjects because the comparison is made within the same person (choice B is correct, and choice D is wrong).

4. **C** The dependent variable is the variable that is measured. Object tracking, as described in Study 2, is one of the measured variables (choice C is correct). Amblyopia is a condition, and individuals with this condition were used in Study 3. Amblyopia itself, however, was not the variable measured; rather, improvement in the condition (choice A is wrong). Visual cognitive tasks were mentioned in Study 1, the correlational study. Correlational studies do not have independent or dependent variables because there is no causal relationship (choice B is wrong). Type of video games played is manipulated by the researchers, not measured, making it an independent variable (choice D is wrong).

5. **C** The optimal control group in an experimental study is as similar as possible to the experimental group along all potential confounding variables such that it isolates the treatment variables. In this case, the study used all boys and measured the effect of video games, so a group of boys of similar age watching a movie (a cognitively engaging task slightly different from a video game) would be best (choice C is correct). Including girls in the control group would introduce a confounding variable, gender, since this would make the control group different along a relevant variable (choices A and D are wrong). The control group should not also play video games, since that is the variable that researchers wanted to isolate and test for an effect (choice B is wrong).

Chapter 19
Social Structure, Group Identity, and Self-Identity

FREESTANDING QUESTIONS: SOCIAL STRUCTURE, GROUP IDENTITY, AND SELF-IDENTITY

1. Cooley's looking-glass self states that a person's sense of self is the result of the perception of others. The sociological theory that best captures this idea is:

   A) conflict theory.
   B) labeling theory.
   C) symbolic interaction theory.
   D) functionalist theory.

2. Each of the following is an example of groupthink, EXCEPT:

   A) members of a climate change awareness group are encouraged to independently research current debates on the issue.
   B) a family stages an intervention for an alcoholic family member.
   C) a poverty reduction group expresses confidence in their strategies and does not bother researching other strategies.
   D) a poll of private school students indicates that they believe public school students do not receive sufficient moral education.

3. Which of the following claims are most closely aligned with the principles of conflict theory?

   I. Societal structures create inequality rather than order.
   II. Analysis of social problems must focus on both personal and structural factors.
   III. Equality can be achieved through consensus.

   A) I only
   B) II only
   C) I and III only
   D) I, II, and III

4. Your classmate is about to give a speech in front of the entire class. As he walks to the podium, you notice that his hands are shaking and he's sweating. You conclude this is because your classmate must be a generally anxious individual. What term best describes why your conclusion might be incorrect?

   A) Fundamental attribution error
   B) Social facilitation
   C) Actor/observer bias
   D) Pessimism bias

5. At the beginning of the school year, a teacher is given a list describing which of his incoming students are considered to be gifted (i.e., exceptionally intelligent) and which are not. In reality, all of the students are of similar intelligence, based on standardized intelligence tests. The students are unaware of this list. Based on the self-fulfilling prophecy, what would you expect at the end of the academic year?

   A) The non-gifted students will earn higher grades.
   B) The gifted students will earn higher grades.
   C) Students will earn similar grades regardless of status.
   D) The self-fulfilling prophecy does not apply here.

6. A group has been stereotyped to do poorly on IQ tests. In order to minimize the impact of stereotype threat on the group's performance on an IQ test, telling which of the following to the group would best achieve that goal?

   A) The stereotype is untrue.
   B) The IQ test accurately measures intelligence.
   C) The IQ test is for fun and measures nothing.
   D) The IQ test is important for being accepted into college.

7. A violent mugging occurs in a residential area of a crowded city. Many people witness the act, but no one calls the police or offers assistance to the victim, even after the perpetrator leaves the scene. Which phenomenon can explain this behavior?

   A) Urbanization
   B) Social stigma
   C) The bystander effect
   D) Social loafing

8. A member of a winning basketball team has a post-victory interview in which she states, "Our team really worked hard today, and our opponents just weren't tough enough to keep up." Which attribution biases is this player exhibiting?

   I. Fundamental attribution error
   II. Self-serving bias
   III. Actor-observer bias

   A) I and II only
   B) II and III only
   C) I and III only
   D) I, II, and III

9. A sociology professor is explaining social inequality to his students. He states, "Social inequality is necessary to promote social order. It allows social mores to be instituted and normalized by way of systemic social controls, which regulate behavior throughout society." From which sociological theory are these statements derived?

A) Conflict theory
B) Symbolic interactionism
C) Functionalism
D) Social constructionism

10. In the Milgram obedience experiments, subjects given the role of "teacher" were ordered by an experimenter to administer ostensible electric shocks in increasing intensity to a supposedly restrained person given the role of "learner." Which of the following was NOT associated with a decreased level of obedience on the part of the subjects?

A) A decrease in the distance between the teacher and the learner
B) An increase in the distance between the experimenter and the teacher
C) The presence of other "teachers" who openly defied the experimenter
D) The apparently random assignment of subjects to the "teacher" and "learner" roles

11. Which hypothetical finding would pose the greatest challenge to the theory that color categories are socially constructed?

A) A study showing that native English language speakers who move to Russia, which contains two different words for blue, and learn to speak Russian quickly adopt the Russian distinction between these two colors.
B) A study showing that the racial categorization of individuals with the same skin color is often culturally dependent.
C) A study showing that all three-month-old infants, regardless of culture, have the ability to recognize red, yellow, green, blue, and purple as different and distinct color categories.
D) A study showing that color categorization of the exact same object can vary among individuals of the same culture.

12. A patient comes to therapy expressing resentment toward her older sister, having been raised in a culture in which the eldest child is traditionally favored by the parents and given preferential treatment. Since moving to the United States, however, the patient has been much nicer to her sister and now often brags about being the "baby" of her family. Based on the theory of symbolic interactionism, which of the following statements is true?

A) Her behavior in her country of origin is consistent with cultural assimilation, but her behavior in the United States is not.
B) Her behavior in her country of origin contradicts cultural assimilation, but her behavior in the United States does not.
C) Her sister was probably not part of a reference group for her until the move to the United States.
D) Her behavior with respect to her parents in her country of origin is consistent with the looking-glass self, but her behavior in the United States is not.

13. Suppose that some New Zealand migrants now living in Australia stated they had very little social contact with Australians. Which of the following concepts best describes this situation?

A) Social reproduction
B) Discrimination
C) Prejudice
D) Social isolation

14. Which sociological theory provides an appropriate framework for studying the effect that moving to a similar but different culture would have on the attitudes, behaviors, and sense of self of migrants?

A) Conflict theory
B) Functionalism
C) Social exchange theory
D) Social constructionism

15. Which of the following would best help draw a connection between genetics and the bystander effect?

A) High concordance of responsibility diffusion among identical twins with a shared environment
B) High fundamental attribution concordance among identical twins with a non-shared environment
C) High concordance of responsibility diffusion among identical twins with a non-shared environment
D) High concordance of mind guarding among identical twins with a non-shared environment

SOCIAL STRUCTURE, GROUP IDENTITY, AND SELF-IDENTITY PRACTICE PASSAGE 1

Numerous studies have demonstrated a positive correlation between violence and residential instability in lower socioeconomic status (LSES) neighborhoods. Researchers believe that, aside from demographics, social and organizational structures of LSES neighborhoods are also factors that cause crime rates to rise. The effectiveness of social controls in neighborhoods is an important component influencing the level of violence in a given area. Aside from formal social control (laws enforced by the government), informal social control should be implemented as a way for residents to work in solidarity to achieve a common goal: to live in a safe and stable neighborhood free from crime and violence.

The level of informal social control varies in each neighborhood. In addition, the well-being of the neighborhood is heavily impacted by the way neighborhoods effectively use their resources and respond to injustice in their community; if residents consistently fought to keep their public services (such as fire stations, police stations, and garbage companies), they are more likely to have less social disorder compared to neighborhoods who do not use their resources efficiently. Collective efficacy in neighborhoods is also a crucial factor in determining the level of violence and crime in a given residential area. Unlike individual efficacy, collective efficacy depends on the level of trust between neighbors. Collective efficacy is influenced by several factors, including residential mobility; a high level of residential mobility weakens collective efficacy because social ties have yet to fully develop.

In recent years, LSES neighborhoods have increased due to the deindustrialization of cities and out-migration of middle and upper class residents. As race and class segregation increase, LSES neighborhoods end up with concentrated disadvantages and greater barriers to obtaining the resources that would help achieve collective social control. Wealth is positively correlated with collective efficacy. Because there is more concentrated disadvantage and residential instability in LSES neighborhood clusters (NCs), researchers hypothesized that both concentrated disadvantage and residential instability decreases collective efficacy. To study this, researchers created 394 NCs from a collection of census tracts in Chicago and surveyed the 9409 residents in these NCs.

The survey consisted of a series of questions that assessed the level of collective efficacy in each resident's own neighborhood on a scale of 1–10 (1 being a very low level for the collective efficacy question and 10 being a very high level). Figure 1 shows the racial and ethnic composition of Chicago's NCs by SES classification from the census tracts collected. Figure 2 displays the collective responses of the surveys.

Race or ethnicity in NCs	SES		
	Low	Medium	High
Majority black	94	45	17
Majority white	0	9	78
Majority Latino	18	11	0
Latino and white	7	53	21
Latino and black	9	5	0
Black and white	2	5	7
NCs not classified above	6	3	4
Total NCs for each SES	136	131	127

Figure 1 Racial and ethnic composition by SES strata in Chicago NCs

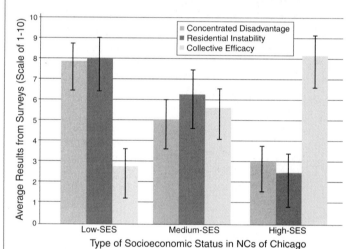

Figure 2 Average responses of residents in Chicago concerning the level of concentrated disadvantage, residential instability, and collective efficacy in their neighborhood

Adapted from R.J. Sampson, S.W. Raudenbush and F. Earls. *Neighborhoods and violent crime: a multilevel study of collective efficacy.* ©1997 by the American Association for the Advancement of Science.

1. Which of the following scenarios is NOT an example of informal social control?

   A) A bystander catches children in the act of defacing a wall and gives them a lecture on vandalism.
   B) A woman gives a disapproving look to a couple engaging in public displays of affection.
   C) A student stands up to the school bully.
   D) A police officer arrests a man for burglary.

2. In general, both formal and informal social control promote:

   A) socialization, but rejects peer pressure.
   B) socialization, but rejects the bystander effect.
   C) deviance, but rejects social loafing.
   D) deviance.

3. Based on the passage, which type of network tie would most likely build collective efficacy within neighborhoods and which type of capital does this network tie belong to?

   A) Strong ties; social capital
   B) Weak ties; social capital
   C) Strong ties; human capital
   D) Weak ties; human capital

4. When a neighborhood experiences an economic shock, such as the closure of a large nearby manufacturing company that results in the loss of hundreds of jobs, which of the following concepts most accurately defines the consequence of this type of event to the neighborhood?

   A) Social exclusion
   B) Social reproduction
   C) Social constructionism
   D) Social stratification

5. Suppose that aside from residents implementing informal social control to prevent violence and crime, residents also promote social change in neighborhoods to combat the inequality that continues to exist between social classes. Which of the following theories most accurately explains why this might occur?

   A) Functionalism
   B) Critical theory
   C) Conflict theory
   D) Traditional theory

6. Which of the following conclusions can be drawn from the data in Figure 1 and Figure 2?

   I. There are fewer heterogeneous NCs than homogeneous NCs in Chicago.
   II. NCs containing Latinos are the least likely to be high-SES, but the most likely to be medium-SES.
   III. The hypothesis is not supported by the results of the study.

   A) I and II
   B) I and III
   C) II and III
   D) I, II, and III

SOCIAL STRUCTURE, GROUP IDENTITY, AND SELF-IDENTITY PRACTICE PASSAGE 2

Immigration is a complex demographic phenomenon and has been a major source of population growth and change across the world. Recently, there has been an increasing number of New Zealanders migrating to Australia despite their high levels of satisfaction with life in New Zealand and their very positive views toward their home country. The migration of large numbers of New Zealanders to Australia has implications for the New Zealand and Australian economies, as well as their societies in general.

A recent study investigated why New Zealanders migrated to Australia, even though the migrants expressed positive views of their country. It also examined how migrants to Australia might adapt and change. To study the issue, researchers first conducted interviews with 31 New Zealand migrants to Australia. After the conclusion of the first round of interviews, a broader survey of 309 New Zealand migrants to Australia was conducted. Finally, interviews with 16 citizens of New Zealand that did not immigrate to Australia were conducted. The purpose of the study was to discover what New Zealand migrants to Australia communicate about their motivations to migrate to Australia and what effect their migration had on their national and cultural identity.

The interviews and survey led to several findings. First, migrants expressed a predominately positive, almost idealized, picture of life in New Zealand and suggested that New Zealanders were, in numerous ways, superior to Australians. Secondly, at the same time, migrants acknowledged they had changed as a result of migration and experienced a convergence with Australian identity. Even though migrants demonstrated a strong, and sometimes increased, allegiance toward New Zealand, they also came to view Australia as an accepting society that is more relaxed and affirmative than New Zealand.

Adapted from A. Greene and M. Power. *Migrating Close to Home: New Zealand Migrants' Identity in Australia.* Lambert Academic. 2010.

1. From the results described in the passage regarding New Zealand migrants to Australia one can most likely conclude that which of the following has occurred?

A) Assimilation
B) Role exit
C) Role strain
D) Ultimate attribution error

2. Which concept best explains the first result of the study?

A) Cultural relativism
B) Ethnocentrism
C) Fundamental attribution error
D) Looking-glass self

3. How might a migrant from New Zealand alter behavior and/or attitude to reduce cognitive dissonance experienced due to the findings in the study?

   I. Focus on positive aspects of Australia and that it will probably get better over time
   II. Focus on the aspects of Australian life that were dissatisfying
   III. Focus on the aspects of New Zealand life that were dissatisfying

A) III only
B) I and II only
C) I and III only
D) I, II, and III

4. The interviews conducted in the first and last part of the study may be subject to issues with:

A) attrition.
B) external validity.
C) operationalization.
D) internal validity.

SOCIAL STRUCTURE, GROUP IDENTITY, AND SELF-IDENTITY PRACTICE PASSAGE 3

Identity formation is a complex psychosocial phenomenon governed by culture, intergenerational socialization, and other factors. Developmental theories recognize that demographic variables play a critical role. The theory of symbolic interactionism asserts that the "self" is essentially a reflexive phenomenon whereby individuals see themselves as others do. One's reality is largely a product of social interaction in accordance with the meanings commonly assigned to people and things (including oneself) and is therefore subjective.

An individual's identity is therefore deeply dependent on social symbols and cultural interpretations. For example, a soldier may symbolize protection in a culture wherein the consensus views him as such, and persecution for others who imbue soldiers with a very different meaning. However, the symbolic significance of a person or thing can change; a soldier can mean "security" for a person until he is shot by one, after which soldiers symbolize pain. The perceptions of important people in one's life, who are known as "significant others," have a tremendous impact on the developing self-concept. Since one's self-image is formed and shaped primarily through this social interactive process, symbolic interactionists believe that factors such as gender, race, ethnicity, age, and cultural heritage account for profound differences in identity formation.

Researchers at a large urban university designed a study to examine the relationship between aspects of identity and demographic factors. Subjects were 387 individuals (203 females and 184 males) who were paid $10 each and were recruited through flyers posted on the university campus and at local community centers: 164 were Caucasian, 102 were African-American, 48 were Hispanic, and 73 were Asian (35 were immigrants and 38 were native-born Americans of Asian descent). These and other demographic data were collected from an application given to prospective participants.

Approximately one week after the completed application was submitted the subjects were mailed the Identity Self-Assessment Scale ("ISAS"), a questionnaire listing hundreds of words. The subject must indicate (on a 10-point Likert-type scale) the extent to which each word describes himself or herself. Some of the words (e.g., "friend") suggest a relational-oriented identity, while others (e.g., "perfectionist") suggest an achievement-oriented identity. In addition, some words (e.g., "teammate") suggest a "collective" identity, while other words (e.g., "nonconformist") suggest an "individualist" identity.

The data yielded scores on these and other subscales, which were then statistically analyzed across various demographic variables, including race, ethnicity, age, gender, and immigrant status. Native-born black, white, and Hispanic women over 50 scored significantly higher on the "relational" subscale, and significantly lower on the "achievement" subscale than did their male and younger female counterparts. No such difference between Asian women and Asian men, or among Asian women of different ages, was found along these subscales. Immigrant Asians, however, scored significantly higher on the "collective" subscale than did native-born Asian-Americans and all non-Asians.

1. Which of the following statements accurately characterizes a methodological flaw in the study?

A) The demand characteristics were prominent and likely influenced subjects' self-report responses.
B) The way in which the subjects were recruited undermines some of the reported findings that pertain to gender.
C) The ISAS had poor reliability.
D) The disproportionate number of Caucasians and African-American subjects (compared with Asians and Hispanics) undermines some of the reported findings that pertain to race and ethnicity.

2. Which of the following can be properly concluded from the results?

A) In the United States, traditional attitudes about gender cause women of some racial and ethnic groups to view themselves as less achievement-oriented than their male counterparts view themselves.
B) The study reported no significant differences between Caucasian and African-American women in the same age range with respect to achievement-orientation.
C) The Asian women who participated in the study identified as more achievement-oriented than did the Caucasian and African-American women.
D) Moving from an Eastern to a Western culture changes one's sense of collective identity.

3. Which of the following correctly describes the social roles of individuals who identifies as nonconformist, as indicated in the passage?

A) With respect to the social institution of government, promoting individuals who maintain a strong sense of individual identity is part of its manifest function.
B) Within the social institution of family, individuals who maintain a strong sense of group identity are part of its latent function.
C) Within the social institution of education, individuals who maintain a strong sense of group identity are part of its manifest function.
D) Within the social institution of the economy, promoting individuals who maintain a strong sense of individual identity is part of its latent function.

4. Suppose the researchers want to conduct a second study using ISAS scores to determine whether socioeconomic status is correlated with an achievement-oriented self-image. Which of the following changes would improve the research?

  I. Increase the amount paid to subjects for their participation.
  II. Include subjects with a more diverse set of educational backgrounds.
  III. Only recruit subjects from one Ivy League university.

A) I and II only
B) I and III only
C) II only
D) II and III only

SOLUTIONS TO FREESTANDING QUESTIONS:
SOCIAL STRUCTURE, GROUP IDENTITY, AND SELF-IDENTITY

1. **C** Symbolic interactionism argues that meaning is a social product derived from interaction. The foundation of this theory rests in the work of George Herbert Mead. Mead's belief was that people's selves are derived, in part, from social interaction. The symbolic interaction theory serves as the framework for the looking-glass self (choice C is correct). The remaining fundamental sociological theories, the conflict theory and structural functionalism, are concerned with power and social stability, respectively, which are not concepts related to Cooley's looking-glass self (choices A and D are wrong). Labeling theory is concerned with the influence of terms attributed to individuals. This theory is closely related to symbolic interactionism; however, its primary use is in relation to deviance (choice B is wrong).

2. **A** The classic characteristics of groupthink are strong group cohesiveness enforced by unquestioned belief in the morality, correctness, and invulnerability of the group. Groupthink is maintained in opposition to an identifiable out-group through stereotyping and rationalization of dissent. The correct choice (which will not be an example of groupthink) will allow for independent or critical thought within a group (choice A is correct), while the incorrect choices (which are examples of groupthink) will agree with the basic characteristics of groupthink to some degree. A poll where private school students have a unified opinion about the moral education of public school students expresses a differentiation between groups based on morality (choice D is an example of groupthink and can be eliminated). A family that stages an intervention for an alcoholic family member is an example of pressuring a group member to conform to accepted norms or face expulsion (choice B is an example of groupthink and can be eliminated). A poverty reduction group that expresses confidence in their strategies exemplifies when a group might express overconfidence and unquestioned beliefs (choice C can be eliminated).

3. **A** Start by analyzing Item III, since it appears in exactly two of the answer choices, and whether it is true or false, you can immediately eliminate half the answer (note that Item II is also found in exactly two of the answer choice, but since Item III is shorter it makes sense to start with III). Item III is false: within conflict theory, consensus is viewed as a process that operates through power and influence, and it is used to coerce agreement on social values and policies, therefore reinforcing *in*equality rather than achieving equality (choices C and D can be eliminated). Note that you only have to analyze one of the remaining items to get the correct answer. Item I is true: according to conflict theory, societal structures, rather than contributing to order, actually create and reinforce inequality (choice B can be eliminated, and choice A is correct). Note that Item II is false: conflict theory is a macro analysis of society, and it does not focus on personal factors.

4. **A** The fundamental attribution error is the error people make when they over attribute a person's behavior to internal factors (e.g., personality, etc.) while disregarding the impact of external factors, such as the impact of the stressful situation, on a person's behavior. Giving a speech is a situation that typically elicits anxiety in people regardless of their disposition. Failure to acknowledge this reality when judging someone is an example of the fundamental attribution error (choice A is correct). Social facilitation occurs when individuals perform certain behaviors better in front of an audience; this does not apply to the situation described, as the classmate appears nervous, and there is no indication that his performance is improved (choice B is wrong). The actor/observer bias occurs when we attribute our own actions to situational constraints as

opposed to dispositional ones; this does not apply to our conclusions about others (choice C is wrong). The optimism bias occurs when we believe bad things happen to others but not to us; there is no such thing as the pessimism bias (choice D is wrong).

5. **B** According to the self-fulfilling prophecy, a person's belief(s) about other people or groups will cause the person to behave in a manner that leads to an outcome consistent with his/her beliefs. Therefore, if the teacher believes that some of his students are gifted and some are normal, the self-fulfilling prophecy predicts that he will treat his students in a manner that leads to the "gifted" students performing better in the class, thereby confirming his initial belief (choice B is correct). If the non-gifted students earn higher grades, this is an outcome that serves as the polar opposite to the outcome predicted by the self-fulfilling prophecy (choice A is wrong). If students earn similar grades regardless of status, this outcome is also at odds with the self-fulfilling prophecy (choice C is wrong). Since the teacher has a pre-existing belief and an opportunity to apply it to the targets of his belief, the self-fulfilling prophecy *does* apply (choice D is wrong).

6. **C** Telling the group that the test is for fun will enable them to avoid dwelling on the negative stereotype while taking the test, and it is likely to reduce stereotype threat and improve test performance (choice C is correct). Telling the group that the stereotype is untrue wouldn't allow the group to completely avoid dwelling on the stereotype (choice A is wrong), while telling the group that the IQ test accurately measures intelligence and is important for being accepted into college would make the stereotype extremely salient, thus heightening the impact of stereotype threat on the group's performance (choices B and D are wrong).

7. **C** The bystander effect causes individuals to think that others will be likely to take action in a situation in which they might otherwise act (choice C is correct). Urbanization refers to demographic shifts and does not apply to this situation (choice A is wrong). Social stigma is a negative perception of those engaging in deviant or non-normative behavior; though not helping someone in need might be considered deviant, social stigma does not explain *why* no one helps (choice B is wrong). Social loafing occurs when individuals in groups exert less effort toward group goals. It is notably a decreased effort, not a lack of participation (choice D is wrong).

8. **A** Since none of the Items appear in exactly two answer choices, it doesn't matter which one you start analyzing. Item I is true: the fundamental attribution error causes one to attribute negative outcomes of others to internal factors, e.g., "our opponents weren't tough enough" (choice B can be eliminated). Item II is true: self-serving bias causes one to attribute their own positive outcomes to internal factors, e.g., "our team worked really hard" (choice C can be eliminated). Item III is false: actor-observer bias causes one to attribute their own negative outcome to external factors, which is not evident in the statement (choice D can be eliminated, and choice A is correct).

9. **C** Functionalism postulates that inequality is beneficial to society (choice C is correct). Conflict theory views inequality as detrimental to society (choice A is wrong). Symbolic interactionism takes a more specific approach by viewing individual social interactions as indicative of larger trends (choice B is wrong). Social constructionism examines ways in which social realities are created by groups and individuals, typically on a much smaller scale than functionalism or conflict theory (choice D is wrong).

10. **D** In the Milgram experiments, all of the subjects were asked to draw lots (along with a confederate pretending to be a naive subject) in order to determine who would be assigned to the teacher and learner roles. Accordingly, the experiment was designed so that the subjects

would believe that they could have just as easily been receiving the shocks as administering them to the "learner" (a confederate). Regardless, the majority of subjects demonstrated a high level of obedience in administering the purported shocks to the "learner" (choice D was not associated with a decrease in obedience and is the correct choice). When the "learner" was moved closer to the "teacher" in the experiment, the "teacher" was less likely to administer the shocks (choice A was associated with a decrease in obedience and can be eliminated). When the experimenter left the room and thus was no longer physically present, the "teacher" was also less likely to administer the shocks (choice B was associated with a decrease in obedience and can be eliminated). When confederates (whom the subjects believed were naive subjects like themselves also acting in the "teacher" role) refused to comply with the experimenter's instructions to shock the learner, the "teachers" were less likely to do so as well (choice C was associated with a decrease in obedience and can be eliminated).

11. **C**   Social constructionism is a theory of knowledge in sociology and communication theory that examines the development of jointly constructed understandings of the world that form the basis for shared assumptions about reality that differ across cultures and are mutable across time within each culture. This theory centers on the notion that human beings rationalize their experiences by creating models of the social world that are widely accepted as natural by individuals within a certain society. If a social constructionist were to argue that color categorization is socially constructed, this would imply a lack of any rigid universal biological basis for the way humans categorize color. Because choice C implies that all humans perceive certain basic colors in the same manner before they could reasonably be influenced by the constructs of their societies, this choice would most challenge the idea that color categorization is socially constructed (choice C is correct). In contrast, choice A suggests that the way individuals categorize certain colors is culturally dependent, so choice A would instead support the theory that color categorization is socially constructed (choice A is wrong). Choice B suggests that the way individuals categorize race is culturally dependent. Thus, choice B supports the theory that racial categories are socially constructed and is largely irrelevant to the contention that color categorization is socially constructed (choice B is wrong). Choice D suggests that the way individuals categorize the color of the same object can vary across individuals within a culture. While choice D casts doubt on the contention that color categorization is universal among all individuals within a culture, the idea that certain aspects of reality are constructs of society does not imply universal agreement on these constructs among all members of any given society. Furthermore, choice D can be easily explained by minor biological differences in individual sensory perception such as color blindness, and such differences are not disputed by social constructionist theories (choice D is wrong).

12. **D**   This question is best tackled with the Process of Elimination approach. The behavior of the patient in both countries is consistent with cultural assimilation, since the patient is acting consistently with cultural norms in both places (choices A and B are wrong). A reference group is one that individuals use for comparison and to understand oneself. Family members, especially close siblings, are likely to be part of a reference group (choice C is wrong). The looking-glass self predicts that individuals act in accordance with expectation placed on them by significant people in their lives. In this case, the parents come from a culture that favors the older sibling. The patient acts consistently with this expectation in the country of origin, but inconsistently with this expectation in the United States (choice D is correct).

13. **D** Social isolation is the complete or near-complete lack of contact with others in society. If New Zealanders had very little social contact with Australians, social isolation could be said to be occurring (choice D is correct). Discrimination is the unjust treatment of a group, based on group characteristics. In this case, it's not possible to state why the New Zealanders have little social contact with Australians, so discrimination is not supported (choice B is wrong). Similar to choice B, prejudice refers to the thoughts, attitudes, and feelings someone holds about a group that are not based on actual experience. It cannot be clearly established that prejudice is the cause of the lack of social contact (choice C is wrong). Social reproduction refers to social inequality that is transmitted from one generation to the next and would not necessarily account for a lack of social contact (choice A is wrong).

14. **D** Social constructionism is a sociological theory that argues that people actively shape their reality through social interactions. This theory looks to uncover ways in which individuals and groups participate in the construction of their perceived social reality (choice D is correct). Conflict theory views society as being in competition for limited resources. This theory would not look at the effect on attitudes, but rather would examine how different groups compete for resources (choice A is wrong). Functionalism conceptualizes society as a living organism with many different parts and organs, each of which has a distinct purpose in the establishing of social stability. As a macro level theory, this does not explain the individual change cited in the question stem (choice B is wrong). Social exchange theory suggests that individuals assign rewards and punishments to interactions and prefer those with the greatest possible benefit (choice C is wrong).

15. **C** The bystander effect is associated with diffusion of responsibility, and the best way to show a genetic connection is to study identical twins in a non-shared environment (choice C is correct). Twins in a shared environment would not allow researchers to distinguish the effects of genetics versus environment as well (choice A is wrong). The fundamental attribution error describes over attribution of behavior to personality, which is not directly related to the bystander effect (choice B is wrong). Mind guarding is associated with groupthink, not the bystander effect (choice D is wrong).

SOLUTIONS TO SOCIAL STRUCTURE, GROUP IDENTITY, AND SELF-IDENTITY PRACTICE PASSAGE 1

1. **D** According to the passage, informal social control is defined as "informal ways neighborhood residents worked together in order to proactively achieve social control." From the given scenarios, a police officer arresting a man for burglary is not an example of informal social control because it is the police officer's responsibility to maintain social order in the community. This particular scenario is considered a formal social control because the officer works in the police station, which is considered a social institution (choice D is the correct answer; choices A, B, and C can be eliminated).

2.   **B**   Socialization occurs when individuals behave in a socially acceptable manner while deviance occurs when individuals violate the social norms in society; social control promotes socialization because it encourages people to conform in ways that will maintain social stability (choices C and D can be eliminated). Peer pressure is encouraged when social control is involved because the positive peer pressure that can be exerted by an individual's peer group can allow the individual to stray away from any acts of deviance. Formal and informal social control would discourage the bystander effect because social control encourages the proactivity of residents to retain social order (choice A can be eliminated, and choice B is therefore the correct answer).

3.   **A**   Since collective efficacy "depends on the level of trust that the residents have for one another," strong ties are most likely to build collective efficacy. The stronger the tie, the more likely the residents are comfortable enough to trust one another and work in solidarity to regulate informal social controls in their neighborhood (choices B and D can be eliminated). While human capital describes the skills, knowledge, and experiences that an individual possesses and is beneficial to society, social capital is defined as benefits that individuals gain from their social network; the resources being used are ties in the residents' social network (choice C can be eliminated, and choice A is therefore the correct answer).

4.   **A**   Social exclusion is the concept of being isolated from receiving rights and opportunities that should be normally given to members in society; the passage indicates that as a result of an economic shock, residents also face an obstruction of resources in their neighborhood (choice A is correct). Social reproduction occurs when social inequality continues to be passed down to future generations; this is not related to the question stem (choice B is wrong). Social constructionism is the idea that traditional norms are created based on the consensus of the society (choice C is wrong). Social stratification is the hierarchy of status and class in a society (choice D is wrong).

5.   **C**   Conflict theory involves people who are encouraged to pursue social change due to a power struggle among the different social classes (choice C is correct). Functionalism motivates people to rely on social institutions to maintain the stability and status quo of society; social change is encouraged in the second part of the question stem (choice A is wrong). Critical theory is the concept that people consistently examine and change their society in order to achieve progress within the community; though this explains social change, it does not fully address the concept of the power struggle among social classes (choice B is wrong). Traditional theory is the idea of learning and understanding the system without proactively making improvements to society; the scenario implies that residents are trying to make changes and improvements (choice D is wrong).

6.   **A**   Since none of the Items appear in exactly two answer choices, it doesn't matter which one you start analyzing. Item I is true: based on Figure 1, there are more heterogeneous neighborhood clusters (NCs with diverse races) compared to homogeneous neighborhood clusters (NCs with similar races; choice C can be eliminated). Item II is true: Figure 1 shows that there are 21 high-SES NCs containing Latinos compared to the 24 high-SES NCs containing blacks and the 106 high-SES NCs containing whites. There are 69 medium-SES NCs containing Latinos compared to the 55 medium-SES NCs containing blacks and the 67 medium-SES NCs containing whites; therefore, NCs containing Latinos are the least likely to be high-SES, but are the most likely to be medium-SES (choice B can be eliminated).

Item III is false: the passage mentions that the level of SES is positively correlated to collective efficacy, which means that low-SES has a low level of collective efficacy. Since Figure 2 shows that concentrated disadvantage and residential instability is positively correlated to low-SES, the results of the study support the hypothesis (choice D can be eliminated, and choice A is the correct answer).

SOLUTIONS TO SOCIAL STRUCTURE, GROUP IDENTITY, AND SELF-IDENTITY PRACTICE PASSAGE 2

1. **A** The results state that New Zealanders had a predominantly positive view of life in New Zealand and believed that New Zealanders were superior to Australians. The results also state that the migrants had changed as a result of migration and experienced a convergence with Australian identity. Assimilation is the process in which an individual adopts the cultural traits of a different culture. Generally, this individual is a member of a minority group who is attempting to conform to the culture of the dominant group, as in the case of the New Zealander migrant to Australia (choice A is correct). Role exit is the process of disengaging from one role and taking on a new role, which is not clearly evident in the passage (choice B is wrong). Role strain occurs when a single status results in conflicting expectations, which is not clearly evident in the passage (choice C is wrong). The ultimate attribution error is when one judges in-group members more positively and out-group members more negatively, and it does not match the results of the study (choice D is wrong).

2. **B** Ethnocentrism is the tendency to judge people from another culture by the standards of one's own culture. Since the first reported results of the passage are that New Zealanders had a predominantly positive view of life in New Zealand and also believed that New Zealanders were superior to Australians, ethnocentrism could be said to be taking place (choice B is correct). Cultural relativism is judging another culture based on its own cultural standards and is essentially the opposite of ethnocentrism (choice A is wrong). The fundamental attribution error is when we tend to underestimate the impact of the situation and overestimate the impact of a person's character or personality on their behavior. This does not explain why there was very little social contact (choice C is wrong). The looking-glass self refers to the idea that a person's sense of self develops from interpersonal interactions with others in society and the perceptions of others. As such, people shape their self-concepts based on their understanding of how others perceive them. This does not explain why the New Zealander migrants viewed life in New Zealand positively and as superior to life in Australia (choice D is wrong).

3. **C** The first result stated in the passage is that New Zealanders had a predominantly positive view of life in New Zealand and also believed that New Zealanders were superior to Australians. The second stated result of the study is that the New Zealander migrants acknowledged they had changed as a result of migrating to Australia and experienced a convergence with Australian identity. You are asked to explain how the migrant might attempt to reduce the cognitive dissonance between these two contradictory results. Since Item II appears in exactly two of the answer choices, start by analyzing it. Item II is false. Since the migrants to Australia have had a convergence with Australian identity, it is unlikely they would focus on the aspects of Australian life that were dissatisfying. This would also have

increase cognitive dissonance by emphasizing negative beliefs about the culture where the migrants reside (choices B and D can be eliminated). Since both remaining answer choices include Item III, it must be true and you can focus on Item I. Item I is true. One way to reduce cognitive dissonance is to change attitudes or beliefs to match behavior. Focusing on the more positive aspects of Australia would align closer with the behavior of immigrating to Australia, thereby reducing dissonance (choice A can be eliminated, and choice C is correct). Item III is in fact true. Focusing on the dissatisfying aspects of New Zealand, much like focusing on the positive aspects of Australia, would justify the behavior of migrating and bring beliefs closer in line with this action.

4.   **B**   The first part of the study interviewed 31 New Zealand migrants, while the final part of the study interviewed 16 citizens of New Zealand that did not immigrate to Australia. External validity refers to the extent to which the findings of a study can be generalized to the real world. Since you are given no information regarding the make-up of the interviewees in terms of their background, demographic characteristics, etc., in addition to the small number of persons interviewed, it is highly possible that that the results of this study are not generalizable (choice B is correct). Attrition refers to the process whereby some individuals in an experiment or study are lost from the sample, potentially causing issues with representativeness. There is no evidence in the passage that any interview subjects dropped out of the interview (choice A is wrong). Operationalization refers to the process of strictly defining variables of interest in a study into measurable factors. This process takes a concept and allows it to be measured, typically either empirically and/or quantitatively. Operationalization does not describe the process of conducting interviews with small sample sizes (choice C is wrong). Internal validity refers to the extent to which we can say that the change in the dependent variable is due to the intervention or experimental manipulation. This does not match the study design described in the passage (choice D is wrong).

SOLUTIONS TO SOCIAL STRUCTURE, GROUP IDENTITY, AND SELF-IDENTITY PRACTICE PASSAGE 3

1.   **B**   The researchers reported a significant finding that older white, black, and Hispanic women were more likely than their younger counterparts to identify with "relational" words, as opposed to "achievement" words, and that the younger women were significantly more likely to do the opposite. However, subjects were recruited both from college campuses and local community centers. Since college students tend to be young, it is highly probable that most of the younger female subjects were recruited from the college campuses and most of the older female subjects were recruited from the community centers. College students are, however, a highly achievement-oriented group; the discrepancy between older and younger women can therefore be explained in terms of factors other than age (choice B is correct). Demand characteristics are subtle "cues" given to the subjects, usually inadvertently, that reveal the purpose of the study and how the subjects are expected to act or respond. While the subjects were asked questions about demographics, those questions were contained in an application that was completed separately from the ISAS a week earlier. Moreover, being asked for demographic information is typical and routine, and no further indication of the researchers' hypotheses was provided (choice A is wrong). A testing instrument is reliable

if it yields consistent scores or measurements. In this case, the subjects only took the ISAS once, so no information about the test's reliability is available (choice C is wrong). The fact that Caucasian and African-American subjects outnumbered Asians and Hispanics is not necessarily problematic, so long as there were enough subjects in each group that researchers could properly generalize from the data collected. A sample size of 387 subjects is very large; also, 73 Asians (35 immigrants and 38 native-born) and 48 Hispanics should suffice for statistical purposes, which usually require sample sizes of 30 or greater (choice D is wrong).

2. **B** The data reported in Paragraph 5 make no mention of any statistical differences between black and white women in the same age range in terms of ISAS responses pertaining to achievement (choice B is correct). While ISAS scores did show that black, white, and Hispanic women over 50 identified as less achievement-oriented than their male counterparts did, the data is correlational and one cannot properly draw any conclusions about what *causes* this discrepancy (choice A is wrong). The data show that Asian women identified as more achievement-oriented than white and black women did in relation to their male counterparts, not that Asian women identified as more achievement-oriented than the non-Asian women did in general (choice C is wrong). While Asian subjects born in the United States had a less "collective" sense of identity than their counterparts born in Asia, you do not know whether moving from one culture to another would change one's identity in this way. Moreover, once again, the study's findings are merely correlational (choice D is wrong).

3. **D** Since the question stem directs back to the passage, it is best to begin by noticing the relationship between a nonconformist mentality and identity. Paragraph 4 lists nonconformity as an example of an individualist identity. Individualist identities promote individual identity over group identity, so any answer choices that contain these identities can be eliminated (choices B and C are wrong). The economy is a type of collective activity in which individuals trade with each other and engage in group cooperation, so it is more likely that promoting individual identity is a latent, or hidden, function, than a manifest, or obvious, function (choice D is correct). Similarly, the manifest function of the government is to pass and enforce laws, which require group cooperation. Therefore, promoting an individualist identity is unlikely to be a manifest function (choice A is wrong).

4. **C** Since Item I appears in exactly two of the answer choices, start by analyzing it. Item I is false. Since the new study is measuring socioeconomic status, payment is likely to incentivize low-income individuals to participate more than high-income individuals, and is therefore likely to present a confounding variable. A greater payment increases the likelihood that the payment offered presents itself as a confounding variable (choices A and B can be eliminated). Both remaining answer choices include Item II, so it must be true, and you can focus on Item III. Item III is false. Since Ivy League schools are extremely expensive and are traditionally associated with very high SES, recruiting subjects from one such university might drastically reduce the number of participants of low or mid-range SES. In addition, individuals from disadvantaged or modest-income backgrounds who attend an Ivy League University are apt to be extremely achievement-oriented, which would confound and compromise the results of the study (choice D can be eliminated, and choice C is correct). Item II is in fact true. Since education is also an important indicator of SES, including varied educational backgrounds would allow researchers to measure how this variable relates to identity.

Chapter 20 Personality, Motivation, Attitudes, and Psychological Disorders

FREESTANDING QUESTIONS: PERSONALITY, MOTIVATION, ATTITUDES, AND PSYCHOLOGICAL DISORDERS

1. Freud's structural theory of the mind was comprised of which components?

A) Id, ego, and superego
B) Oral, anal, phallic, latency, genital
C) Libido and thanatos
D) Adaptation, assimilation, and accommodation

2. A representative for a local homeless shelter is trying to collect donations from the public for the organization. He calls local residents to ask for donations for the shelter. He begins by asking for a $200 donation. When the resident declines that amount, the representative then asks for a $20 donation, which the resident most likely will accept. What type of persuasion technique is this?

A) Foot-in-the-door technique
B) Door-in-the-face technique
C) Justification of effort
D) Role-playing

3. An environmentalist who is a passionate advocate for reducing environmental waste and greenhouse emissions is driving his hybrid car and notices a bag of empty plastic bottles on the sidewalk. He decides that something must be done with the bottles. Which of the following actions would cause the environmentalist to experience the LEAST amount of cognitive dissonance?

A) Picking the bag up and later throwing it onto the highway while driving
B) Leaving the bag on the side of the street and driving away
C) Throwing the bag into a dumpster with trash destined for the local landfill
D) Taking the bottles to a plastic recycling center

4. A patient has damage to the dopaminergic neurons of the basal ganglia, specifically a loss of dopaminergic cells in the circuit originating from the substantia nigra. The patient is most likely to be diagnosed with which one of the following diseases or disorders?

A) Schizophrenia
B) Alzheimer's disease
C) Depression
D) Parkinson's disease

5. All of the following are true for schizophrenia, EXCEPT:

A) it affects approximately 1% of the population across the globe.
B) it can manifest with positive symptoms, such as delusions or hallucinations.
C) negative symptoms, like flat affect, are also indicative of the illness.
D) it is characterized by multiple personalities.

6. Major depressive disorder and bipolar disorder differ in:

A) duration of depressive symptoms.
B) presence of manic symptoms.
C) degree of depressive symptoms.
D) presence of irritable mood.

7. According to Erik Erikson's theory of psychosocial stages, the final stage that individuals must resolve in old age is the crisis of:

A) generativity vs. stagnation.
B) integrity vs. despair.
C) intimacy vs. isolation.
D) generativity vs. integrity.

8. The psychologist most associated with the concept of the "self-actualizing tendency" is:

A) Stanley Milgram.
B) Sigmund Freud.
C) Carl Rogers.
D) Karl Marx.

9. Costa & McCrea's Big Five personality traits include all of the following EXCEPT:

A) neuroticism.
B) anxiety.
C) conscientiousness.
D) openness to experience.

10. A participant in a study on identity is found to be notably erratic. He exhibits extreme mood swings and frequent changes in personality and behavior. Friends and family often avoid him because they never know what to expect: he may be pleasant one day and then volatile and abusive the next. Which one of the following disorders is the most likely diagnosis for this individual?

A) Histrionic personality disorder
B) Antisocial personality disorder
C) Paranoid personality disorder
D) Borderline personality disorder

11. People who experience Generalized Anxiety Disorder (GAD) or Panic Disorder (PD) often try to avoid stimuli that might trigger anxiety or a panic attack. Treatment of these disorders often involves learning alternative ways to manage one's responses to such triggering stimuli. Which of the following would best characterize a stimulus that someone with GAD or PD might avoid?

A) The stimulus acts as a negative incentive.
B) The stimulus acts as an imbalance, triggering drive reduction.
C) The stimulus activates one's need for belonging.
D) The stimulus activates an optimal level of arousal.

12. A new weekly television show features households that have a family member with Alzheimer's disease. How might such a show contribute to altering attitudes toward dementia in people who themselves are caring for a family member with Alzheimer's disease?

A) The realistic role-playing of the television character could help alter viewers' attitudes, which then makes them more inclined to help their family member.
B) A public declaration made by one of the show's family members could inspire viewers to change their minds about ideas regarding stigma that might have hindered their willingness to help their family member.
C) The time viewers spend watching the show and caring for their own family member may lead viewers to feel more positively about their family member, due to a justification of effort.
D) Watching a fictional character happily care for a family member involves a small amount of effort; after watching, one might then be more willing to care for one's own family member, which involves a greater amount of effort, according to the foot-in-the-door phenomenon.

13. Researchers in a study theorized that beginning roughly in puberty, children develop the capacity to fully assess emotionally disturbing memories. Which person's work most supports their theory?

A) Sigmund Freud
B) Albert Bandura
C) Harry Harlow
D) Jean Piaget

PERSONALITY, MOTIVATION, ATTITUDES, AND PSYCHOLOGICAL DISORDERS PRACTICE PASSAGE 1

Phobias are one of the most common psychological disorders reported in the United States, afflicting approximately 10 percent of individuals at some point in their lives. The diagnostic hallmark of a phobic disorder is an intense, persistent, irrational fear of a particular object or situation that impels one to avoid it. Phobias can be debilitating if attempting to avoid the source of fear impairs occupational and social functioning or causes considerable subjective distress.

Divergent theories abound concerning the causes of phobias. The prevalence of certain phobias (e.g., the ubiquitous fear of snakes), despite the relatively minor threat that these objects typically pose in modern society, has led some to postulate evolutionary underpinnings of phobias. According to these evolutionary models, certain types of fearful behavior conferred a survival advantage upon early human beings, and these traits were genetically favored. Studies have found a strong tendency of phobias to run in families, which some researchers have interpreted as support for a genetic predisposition.

Pavlovian conditioning theories emphasize the incidental pairing of neutral and fear-producing stimuli as the primary process through which phobias develop. In sharp contrast, traditional psychoanalytic theory attributes phobic development to deep-seated unconscious mechanisms, where phobic objects serve as a symbolic "stand in" for the original source of anxiety. This idea has waned somewhat in recent years, as focus has largely shifted to biological interpretations of abnormal behavior. Considerable research has been concentrated upon phobias and their relationship to the limbic portions of the brain that control primitive fear and its processing into meaningful memories and associations.

Treatment for phobias varies, often depending upon which etiological theory the treating clinician espouses. Behavioral interventions typically involve physical exposure to the feared object in an attempt to "unlearn" the association between the neutral object and the feared one. Traditional talk therapy might entail an in-depth examination of early childhood conflicts in an attempt to grasp the intricacies of the patient's psyche and determine the latent symbolic function of the phobic object. Many clinicians now adopt a highly eclectic approach to phobia treatment that can encompass multiple theories and involve methods such as hypnosis, biofeedback, and mediation.

Pharmacological interventions have in fact become increasingly common in the treatment of phobias in recent years, reflecting a general clinical trend. Sedatives are very effective at calming a fear-stricken patient, but their tendency to be addictive requires that they be prescribed cautiously. Beta-blockers are also commonly prescribed for phobias, as they block the stimulating effects of adrenaline upon the body. The use of selective serotonin reuptake inhibitors (SSRI's), which act upon the patient's serotonin levels and can thus influence mood, has also met with some success.

1. Which one of the following disorders offers the LEAST support for the evolutionary explanation of phobias mentioned in Paragraph 2?

A) Agoraphobia (fear of open spaces and public places)
B) Arachnophobia (fear of spiders)
C) Xenophobia (fear of strangers or foreigners)
D) Aviophobia (fear of flying in an airplane or aircraft)

2. A therapist suspects that her patient's intense and debilitating fear of dogs is really a fear of his father, who is known to have been extremely abusive toward him during his early childhood. Freud would consider this an example of which ego defense mechanism?

A) Repression
B) Reaction formation
C) Displacement
D) Sublimation

3. Suppose that researchers hypothesize that the prevalence of phobic disorders among first degree relatives of those afflicted, as described in paragraph 2, is due to inherited factors (an abnormality on a particular chromosome is suspected). In order to test this hypothesis, several sets of monozygotic and dizygotic twins from a major metropolitan area are studied with respect to a variety of situational, social, and specific phobias, assessing symptomatology on a ten-point scale. The results indicate that phobic concordance between monozygotic twins was 37%, while dizygotic twin concordance was 11%. The researchers offer these findings in support of the claim that genetic factors play a substantial role in the development of phobic disorders. Which of the following is an assumption underlying the acceptance of the researchers' conclusion?

A) Assortive mating in the subject population
B) Disassortive mating in the subject population
C) Random mating in the subject population
D) Environments are more similar for dizygotic than monozygotic twins

4. Four-year-old Jane typically enjoys listening to a particular song on her parents' CD while riding in the car. One day during a car ride with her mother, they are involved in a serious accident while that particular song is playing. Subsequently, whenever Jane hears that tune she cries, trembles uncontrollably, states that she is afraid, and demands that the song be turned off. According to classical conditioning principles, the accident is the:

A) conditioned stimulus.
B) negative reinforcer.
C) unconditioned stimulus.
D) unconditioned response.

5. Suppose that computerized axial tomography scans (CT scans) of the brains of phobia subjects indicate that the subjects have lesions and/or other abnormalities in their brains at a significantly higher rate than do members of the general population. Which one of the following structures is LEAST likely to be adversely affected in the subjects' brains?

A) Amygdala
B) Wernicke's area
C) Hippocampus
D) Hypothalamus

PERSONALITY, MOTIVATION, ATTITUDES, AND PSYCHOLOGICAL DISORDERS PRACTICE PASSAGE 2

Anxiety and depression are the most prevalent psychiatric conditions affecting older adults, and both have been linked independently to risk of dementia. However, most studies have examined only anxiety-and-dementia or depression-and-dementia; few studies have looked at the co-occurrence of anxiety-and-depression as a risk factor for dementia.

A study was conducted in the Northern California medical system. Medical records of 500,000 adults with a mean age of 71 (range 60–102) were examined from a five-year period. Diagnoses of dementia, anxiety, depression, diabetes, stroke, cardiovascular disease, and traumatic brain injury were abstracted from these medical records. Associations between anxiety, depression, their co-occurrence, and risk of dementia were evaluated. Results were adjusted for age, sex, and race/ethnicity. Seven percent were diagnosed with anxiety-only, 4% with depression-only, and 5% with co-occurring anxiety-depression. Nearly 12% were diagnosed with dementia over 13 years of follow-up. Age-adjusted incidence rates of dementia were highest among those with depression-only and those with co-occurring anxiety-depression; incidence rates of dementia were lower for those with anxiety-only.

Depression-only	.80
Anxiety-only	.23
Depression-Anxiety	.85

Table 1 Correlation between the risk of dementia and depression, anxiety, and their co-occurrence

Results suggest that co-occurring anxiety-depression is associated with a higher risk of dementia in a large population-based sample of healthcare members over 13 years. Future studies aimed at understanding disparities in mental health in later life and the mechanisms linking anxiety-depression with risk of dementia are needed. Public health efforts should focus on screening and improving treatment outcomes in older populations with comorbid anxiety-depression.

A second study aimed to investigate public attitudes toward people with dementia in an urban community. Nearly 90% of the participants responded that they were able to have a good relationship with a person with dementia and help such a person if needed. However, around half of the participants would be ashamed of a family member with dementia. A multiple regression model showed that information from television and educational classes was associated with positive attitudes toward people with dementia among older adults. Increasing the availability and accessibility of information on dementia may contribute to improving public attitudes toward people with dementia.

1. Which statement is best supported by the data in Table 1?

A) Anxiety-only has a weaker correlation to dementia risk than does Depression-Anxiety.
B) Anxiety is less likely to cause dementia than depression.
C) Cognitive decline in dementia is unrelated to mood disorders.
D) Symptoms of dementia may be related to abnormal protein folding.

2. The biopsychosocial model of mental disorders considers the interaction of multiple causal factors in the expression of disorders such as depression and anxiety. Some theories of personality and therapy approach anxiety as a misplaced fear response, traceable to early life experiences but no longer remembered as such. Which of the following therapeutic approaches would most likely approach anxiety symptoms in a similar manner?

A) Cognitive-behavioral therapy (CBT)
B) Exposure therapy
C) Psychoanalytic therapy
D) Humanistic therapy

3. The second study suggests that when one has a family member with dementia, one might feel that one can have a good, helpful relationship with the family member, but that one might also feel shame. Which concept best describes the contradictory thoughts and feelings one might experience in this scenario?

A) The principle of aggregation
B) Cognitive dissonance
C) The role of self-reflection
D) Justification of effort

4. Which of the following symptoms would a person experiencing both depression and dementia most likely experience?

A) Disorganized speech
B) Flight of ideas or subjective experience that thoughts are racing
C) Insomnia or hypersomnia nearly every day
D) Diminished ability to think and concentrate

PERSONALITY, MOTIVATION, ATTITUDES, AND PSYCHOLOGICAL DISORDERS PRACTICE PASSAGE 3

In the field of early childhood development, Mary Ainsworth's seminal studies of toddlers are a cornerstone of the field now known as attachment theory. Based on observations of children's reactions to a strange situation, Ainsworth developed the classifications of secure attachment and insecure attachment, including avoidant attachment and ambivalent attachment. The U.S. foster care system was implemented to help abandoned children form healthy relationships in a way that large scale institutions could not. However, some fostered children display such poor emotional dysregulation that even when provided with a loving environment they engage in disturbing behavior such as threatening their new siblings or persistent self-urination. It has been theorized that these maladaptive emotional regulation strategies indicate insecure attachment styles—keeping the child "safe" from vulnerability to the new family through defensive rage or becoming too repulsive to approach. As a result, children in foster care can be passed from one family to another, without an improvement in their emotional regulation, until they are perceived as "unadoptable" and eventually age out of the system.

Some attempts to improve the outcomes of these children have focused on exploring their feelings of abandonment from their families of origin. Theorizing that prepubescent children may not yet have the capability to fully assess these disturbing memories, a new study focused instead on helping insecurely attached children and their foster parents learn adaptive regulation strategies, which would in turn improve their chances of forming new attachments.

These researchers surveyed families fostering children ages 6 to 10 for a yearlong study. All of the 53 children had been placed in foster care after the age of 5, due to cases of neglect, abuse, or abandonment. All had engaged in at least one of the following disruptive behaviors on a regular basis: expressing violent thoughts toward their adoptive families, stealing, hoarding food, disorders of hygiene, destroying property, or running away. At the start of the study, psychologists examined the children using the Attachment Story Completion Task (ASCT). In this task, the child is presented with stories centering on family relations in stressful situations, and is then prompted to complete the story. Based on verbal and nonverbal responses, the children were categorized as anxious-ambivalent (20) or anxious-avoidant (33).

Next, families were instructed to explore open-ended stories such as those in the ASCT twice per week, theorizing that these family group meetings would allow the foster children to practice the emotional regulation strategy of distancing, by examining stressful situations as a neutral observer, and that hopefully this practice would enable the foster children to better regulate their emotions during the course of their daily experience. Parents recorded number of disruptive behaviors

per week from the beginning of the study until its conclusion. During the course of the study, 10 families discontinued the program. The results are found in Figure 1.

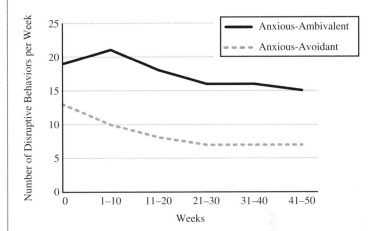

Figure 1 Average number of reported disruptive behaviors for anxious-ambivalent and anxious-avoidant attachment styles

1. Based on the results of the study, what might the researchers reasonably conclude?

A) The number of disruptive behaviors per week is negatively correlated with a difference in attachment style.
B) The type of attachment style is positively correlated with the number of disruptive behaviors per week.
C) Anxious-ambivalent children are less likely to use maladaptive emotional regulation strategies than anxious-avoidant children.
D) Anxious-avoidant children were more responsive to the ACST intervention program than the anxious-ambivalent children.

2. All of the following would improve the design of the study EXCEPT:

A) including children with secure attachment styles in the study.
B) assessing the reason that some families discontinued the study.
C) accounting for the difference in number of behaviors per week for anxious-avoidant and anxious-ambivalent children.
D) having a neutral observer record the number of disruptive behaviors per week.

3. The passage states that prior attempts to improve the outcomes of foster children focused on exploring their feelings of abandonment from of their families of origin. The shift from the focus of this prior research to the focus of the study described in the passage represents a shift between which two schools of psychology?

A) Psychoanalytic and behaviorist
B) Humanist and symbolic interaction
C) Psychoanalytic and social cognitive
D) Humanist and behaviorist

4. The ASCT as described in the study evaluates children's response to a described stressful situation, as recorded by psychologists' observations of verbal and non-verbal reactions. Which of the following would help to confirm that the children were indeed interpreting the hypothetical situation as stressful?

A) Measurements of diurnal salivary cortisol are negatively correlated with psychologists' assessments of stress response.
B) Measurements of testosterone are positively correlated with psychologists' assessments of stress response.
C) Measurements of perspiration are positively correlated with psychologists' assessments of stress response.
D) Pupil dilation is negatively correlated with psychologists' assessments of stress response.

SOLUTIONS TO FREESTANDING QUESTIONS: PERSONALITY, MOTIVATION, ATTITUDES, AND PSYCHOLOGICAL DISORDERS

1. **A** Freud's structural theory divided the mind into three structures, the id—which contains the impulses and basic drives, the superego—which he theorized was the internalized morality of the father, and the ego—which he believed developed to manage the conflicting desires and goals of the other two structures. The ego, he theorized, generally was what humans perceived as "the self" (choice A is correct). Oral, Anal, Phallic, Latency, and Genital are the stages of psychosexual development that Freud developed, not his structural theory of the mind (choice B is wrong). The concepts of Libido and Thanatos were ideas which came later to Freud, and they comprise the life and death instincts (choice C is wrong). Adaptation, assimilation, and accommodation are processes which comprise part of Piaget's developmental theory. Adaptation describes the inborn tendency to adjust to the environment, assimilation describes the process of incorporating new experiences into existing understanding, and accommodation describes modifying existing understandings to include new experiences (choice D is wrong).

2. **B** In the scenario, the representative asks for a large amount of money first (with the expectation of being turned down, or having a proverbial door slammed in his face), followed by a smaller request, that is more likely to be accepted because it seems so much less ridiculous than the large request. The door-in-the-face technique begins with a large request that is likely to be turned down, followed by a smaller request that is likely to be accepted (choice B is correct). The foot-in-the-door technique involves making a small request first, followed by a more substantial request (choice A is wrong). Justification of effort occurs when people modify their attitude to match the amount of behavior they are putting forth (choice C is wrong). Role-playing occurs when people are asked to behave in a certain way, and that role begins to influence their attitudes (choice D is wrong).

3. **D** Cognitive dissonance is the mental anguish that occurs when a person's behavior is at odds with his beliefs. An environmentalist who is passionate about reducing environmental waste and greenhouse emissions is someone who values protecting the environment. Therefore, this environmentalist will experience the least amount of cognitive dissonance if his actions (recycling the bottles) coincide with his stated beliefs (choice D is correct). On the other hand, he will experience cognitive dissonance if his actions do not align with his stated beliefs, as would be the case with: actively littering (choice A is wrong), passively littering by not doing anything (choice B is wrong), and needlessly adding the plastic to landfills (choice C is wrong).

4. **D** Parkinson's disease is associated with a loss of dopaminergic cells in the substantia nigra of the basal ganglia (choice D is correct). While schizophrenia is also associated with the dopaminergic system, the problem is an excess of dopamine production rather than a decrease (choice A is wrong). Alzheimer's disease is most strongly associated with neurofibrillary tangles and plagues in the brain, not the systematic loss of dopaminergic neurons (choice B is wrong). Depression is most associated with serotonin, not dopamine (choice C is wrong).

5. **D** Multiple personalities are characteristic of dissociative identity disorder, not schizophrenia (choice D is correct). Schizophrenia does affect approximately 1% of the population in the world (choice A is wrong), and it is characterized by both positive and negative symptoms (choices B and C are wrong).

6. **B** Major depressive disorder and bipolar disorder are both mood disorders, and while both may present similar duration and degree of depressive symptoms (choices A and C are wrong), they differ in the presence of manic symptoms; in order for a diagnosis of bipolar disorder to be made, there must be evidence of at least one manic or mixed episode (choice B is correct). Irritable mood is also potentially present in both major depressive disorder and bipolar disorder (choice D is wrong).

7. **B** During the final stage in Erik Erikson's theory, older individuals must face the crisis of integrity vs. despair (choice B is correct). The crisis of generativity vs. stagnation occurs during the prior stage, during middle age (choice A is wrong). The crisis of intimacy vs. isolation occurs during young adulthood (choice C is wrong). Generativity vs. integrity is not a crisis in Erik Erikson's theory, but rather a combination of the seventh and eighth proposed psychosocial stages (choice D is wrong).

8. **C** Carl Rogers, who is most associated with humanistic psychology, proposed that all humans possess a self-actualizing tendency that drives them to try and reach their full potential (choice C is correct). Stanley Milgram is most associated with social psychology experiments, most famously his experiments on obedience (choice A is wrong). Sigmund Freud is most associated with the psychoanalytic perspective, which does not include the self-actualizing tendency (choice B is wrong). Karl Marx is most associated with sociological theories, and he was not considered a psychologist (choice D is wrong).

9. **B** Costa & McCrea's Big Five personality traits include: extroversion, neuroticism (choice A is wrong), conscientiousness (choice C is wrong), openness to experience (choice D is wrong), and agreeableness. Anxiety is not one of the big five personality traits (choice B is correct).

10. **D** Borderline personality disorder is characterized by profound instability in identity and self-image, often resulting in labile behavior that fluctuates between extremes (choice D is correct). While histrionic personality disorder involves excessive emotionality and attention-seeking, which may resemble the individual's behavior, that pattern is typically stable and consistent, unlike that exhibited in this case (choice A is wrong). Individuals with antisocial personality disorder display a pervasive pattern of callous disregard for the rights and feelings of others and for societal rules. While such individuals are often abusive, their behavior is not characterized by instability, mood swings, or prominent changes in personality (choice B is wrong). People with paranoid personality disorder may be abusive, as they experience intense anger and unjustified feelings of persecution. However, as with the other personality disorders mentioned, their sense of identity and self-image (however inaccurate) is much more stable than would be the case with a borderline personality (choice C is wrong).

11. **A** A negative incentive is an external stimulus that helps discourage certain behaviors (choice A involves a stimulus that leads to avoidance and is therefore correct). Drive reduction theory concerns basic physiological needs, such as hunger, thirst, sex, and sleep, all of which motivate the organism to seek something, rather than avoid something, to reduce the imbalance (choice B is wrong). The need for belonging derives from Maslow's hierarchy of needs, which is irrelevant to the question scenario (choice C is wrong). The optimal level of arousal is when one's performance is at its peak, which does not seem relevant to the question scenario (choice D is wrong).

12. **C** The justification of effort involves increased valuation of an activity, person, or object due to the time and energy one has invested in it, him, or her. This is related to time invested in two activities leading to a more positive valuation (choice C is correct). In the theory of attitude and behavior, role-playing by the individual, but not another individual's role-playing, can affect changes in attitude (choice A is wrong). Public declarations by an individual, but not by another individual, involve one's attitudes following one's behavior (choice B is wrong). The foot-in-the-door phenomenon involves one being willing to comply with a larger request after having complied with a smaller request first. In order for the foot-in-the-door phenomenon to take effect, the individual must actually participate in fulfilling the smaller request (choice D).

13. **D** Jean Piaget developed a theory of cognitive development that terminated in the formal operations stage (reached during adolescence) in which children can reason abstractly and process complex emotions, and then integrate them into the self with more sophisticated schemas. This is consistent with the belief that the capacity to regulate emotionally disturbing memories would not be fully developed until puberty (choice D is correct). Sigmund Freud believed that most individuals, even fully developed adults, suppress emotionally disturbing memories and maintain them in the unconscious. It would be unlikely, according to Freud, that this capacity would exist in adolescents (choice A is wrong). Albert Bandura pioneered the Social Cognitive Perspective and Observational Learning, which did not primarily deal with emotionally disturbing memories (choice B is wrong). Harry Harlow conducted studies on social isolation in baby monkeys, which focuses on attachment and does not offer predictions about emotionally disturbing memories in humans (choice C is wrong).

SOLUTIONS TO PERSONALITY, MOTIVATION, ATTITUDES, AND PSYCHOLOGICAL DISORDERS PRACTICE PASSAGE 1

1. **D** Aviophobia is a modern phenomenon that has no survival implications for early human beings (choice D would not support an evolutionary explanation of phobias and is the correct choice). In contrast, behaviors associated with agoraphobia would indeed have conferred a survival advantage upon early human beings. The danger of falling victim to a predatory animal attack was much greater out in the open than in one's dwelling (choice A would support an evolutionary explanation of phobias and can be eliminated). Arachnophobia would confer a similar survival advantage upon those living in caves or huts who would benefit by avoiding potentially lethal venomous insects (choice B would support an evolutionary explanation of phobias and can be eliminated). Xenophobia would have also conferred a survival benefit. Encounters with those outside one's own social group were considerably more dangerous and likely to be deadly in prehistoric times (choice C would support an evolutionary explanation of phobias and can be eliminated as well).

2. **C** Displacement involves the redirection of inappropriate urges elsewhere; although the question stem involves fear instead of a sexual or aggressive urge, Freud would still likely consider the displacement of fear from father (less acceptable) to dogs (more acceptable) an application of this particular ego defense mechanism (choice C is correct). Repression

involves complete lack of recall of the painful memory, which is not indicated in the question stem (choice A is wrong). Reaction formation involves expressing the exact opposite of what one feels; since the patient is expressing fear in both instances, this ego defense mechanism doesn't seem to apply (choice B is wrong). Sublimation involves the channeling of negative emotions into something positive; there is no indication that the patient is doing this in the question stem (choice D is wrong).

3. **C**   Monozygotic twins share 100% of their genes in common, while dizygotic twins, who are no more genetically alike than ordinary siblings, share (on average) 50% of their genes in common. Therefore, if concordance for a certain trait is higher for monozygotic twins, that trait is thought to have a genetic component. However, two assumptions underlie this conclusion. The first is that mating in the subject population is random. If assortive mating occurs, wherein individuals are more likely to mate with others who have similar traits (e.g., comparable intelligence, similar body types, etc.), then dizygotic twins may actually be more genetically similar than they are typically thought to be. Accordingly, the influence of genetic factors may be overestimated (choice C is correct, and choice A can be eliminated). If a pattern of disassortive mating in the subject population occurs, wherein individuals are more likely to mate with others whose traits differ from their own, then dizygotic twins may in fact be more genetically dissimilar than typically thought. In this case, disassortive mating would actually strengthen the researchers' claim that phobias are inherited. However, disassortive mating would not necessarily have to be the case and is thus not an assumption underlying the acceptance of the researchers' claims (choice B is wrong). The second assumption underlying the belief that higher monozygotic concordance suggests an inherited trait is the presence of equally similar environments for both types of twins. If identical twins are in fact reared more similarly than their non-identical counterparts (e.g., being dressed alike, encouraged to engage in similar activities, etc.), then the influence of environmental factors may be underestimated (choice D is wrong).

4. **C**   In classical conditioning terminology, Jane's phobia developed when a neutral stimulus (the song) was paired with an unconditioned stimulus (the accident). An unconditioned stimulus is one that would ordinarily produce a particular response, in this case intense fear (which is known as the unconditioned response). The pairing of the neutral stimulus (song) and unconditioned stimulus (accident) transforms the neutral stimulus into a conditioned stimulus that can now produce fear itself (the resultant fear is now known as the conditioned response; choice C is correct, and choices A and D can be eliminated). "Negative reinforcer" is an operant conditioning term. It refers to an aversive stimulus that is removed after a certain behavior is exhibited in order to increase the occurrence of that behavior (choice B is wrong).

5. **B**   The subjects have phobias and are thus likely to have issues with limbic structures of the brain that control fear and associated memories. Wernicke's area is the portion of the brain that processes spoken language and is unlikely to be implicated in phobic disorders (choice B is least likely to be adversely affected and is the correct choice). The amygdala plays a highly important role in emotional learning and the processing of fear; it is associated with the body's "fight or flight" response to danger (choice A is likely to be adversely affected and can be eliminated). The hippocampus is greatly involved with working memory; it is thought to integrate fear signals received from the amygdala with previously existing information

in order to make them meaningful (choice C is likely to be adversely affected and can be eliminated). The hypothalamus is also largely responsible for activating the "fight or flight" response to perceived danger (choice D is likely to be adversely affected and can be eliminated).

SOLUTIONS TO PERSONALITY, MOTIVATION, ATTITUDES, AND PSYCHOLOGICAL DISORDERS PRACTICE PASSAGE 2

1. **A**   Since .23 is less than .85, Anxiety-only has a weaker correlation to dementia risk than does Depression-Anxiety (choice A is correct). Neither the table nor the passage supports claims about causality, since the study is an instance of correlational research (choice B is wrong). The table correlates dementia with anxiety and mood disorders, separately and co-morbidly (choice C is wrong). Symptoms of dementia may indeed be related to abnormal protein folding, but this statement has nothing to do with the data in the table (choice D is wrong).

2. **C**   A focus on feelings that are traceable to "early life experiences" and that are "no longer remembered as such," and are therefore unconscious, characterizes the psychodynamic or psychoanalytic approach (choice C is correct). Cognitive-behavioral therapy focuses on maladaptive thoughts in the present, rather than on buried feelings from the past (choice A is wrong). Exposure therapy derives from the behaviorist approach, which focuses on present behavior rather than past feelings (choice B is wrong). Humanistic therapy is typically more concerned with the present and especially the future than the past (choice D is wrong).

3. **B**   Cognitive dissonance describes the feeling of tension one can experience when one has two contradictory thoughts, as described in the question stem. The principle of aggregation involves predicting behavior in general on the basis of knowing one's attitudes (choice A is wrong). Self-reflection can mediate one's behavior cohering to one's attitudes, as opposed to when one acts impulsively (choice C is wrong). The justification of effort involves increased valuation of an activity or product due to the time or effort one has invested in it (choice D is wrong).

4. **D**   The DSM-5 includes diminished ability to think and concentrate as a marker of depression, and general cognitive decline as a marker of dementia (choice D is correct). The DSM-5 includes disorganized speech as a marker of dementia, but not of depression (choice A is wrong). The DSM-5 includes flight of ideas as a marker of bipolar disorder, but not of either depression or dementia (choice B is wrong). The DSM-5 includes insomnia or hypersomnia nearly every day as a marker of depression (choice C is wrong).

SOLUTIONS TO PERSONALITY, MOTIVATION, ATTITUDES, AND PSYCHOLOGICAL DISORDERS PRACTICE PASSAGE 3

1. **C** Figure 1 indicates that children in the anxious-avoidant category engaged in fewer disruptive behaviors per week than children in the anxious-ambivalent category. This is consistent with the assertion that anxious-ambivalent children are less likely to use maladaptive emotional regulation strategies. Correlation measures were not presented in the study, so it cannot be assumed that a negative slope indicates a negative correlation (choices A and B are wrong). Since there is no control group to use as comparison, it cannot be inferred whether anxious-ambivalent children were more responsive to the intervention, or whether they perhaps had better coping strategies to begin with (choice D is wrong).

2. **A** The purpose of the study, as detailed in the second paragraph, was to help insecurely attached children learn more adaptive coping mechanisms. Including securely attached children could confound the results, since they come in with a different set of attachment tendencies and emotional coping strategies, so researchers could not be confident that results would apply to the population of interest, namely children with insecure styles (choice A would NOT improve the study and is the correct answer choice). Assessing reasons that families discontinued the study could address the issue of attrition and whether participants dropping out of the study confounded the results in some way (choice B could improve the study and can be eliminated). Accounting for the difference could help to explain the reason for the observed effect (choice C could improve the study and can be eliminated). A neutral observer is optimal, since this is indicative of double-blind technique, which is universally preferred by researchers to avoid bias among the experimenters influencing the results (choice D could improve the study and can be eliminated).

3. **C** A focus on childhood and early life is indicative of the psychoanalytic method, whereas a focus on adaptive cognitive strategies of emotional regulation is indicative of the social cognitive approach (choice C is correct). The behaviorist method seeks to exclude thoughts and feelings from its model, and seeks instead to focus exclusively on observable behavior (choices A and D are wrong). The humanist method focuses on present condition and future goals, to move an individual toward more congruence between real and ideal selves. The symbolic interactionist method focuses on symbols and how their interpretation by individuals impacts interactions. Neither of these methods is consistent with the description in the question stem (choice B is wrong).

4. **C** The correct response should be consistent with the sympathetic nervous system response to stress. Increased perspiration is part of the fight-or-flight response, and sympathetic nervous system activation (choice C is correct). Diurnal salivary cortisol is also part of the sympathetic response, so this would be positively correlated with stress assessments (choice A is wrong). Testosterone increases are not associated with the stress response (choice B is wrong), and pupil dilation is positively, not negatively, correlated with stress activation (choice D is wrong).

Chapter 21
Learning, Memory, and Behavior

FREESTANDING QUESTIONS: LEARNING, MEMORY, AND BEHAVIOR

1. A psychology professor is training a puppy. She rewards the puppy with a treat each time it goes to the bathroom outside. This training approach could best be described as:

   A) classical conditioning.
   B) operant conditioning.
   C) a conditioned stimulus.
   D) spontaneous recovery.

2. People who purchase stock are most reinforced to purchase more stock when they earn money on their stock. Speculative purchasing of stock (defined as stock that may rise or fall unpredictably and does not pay out profits on a regular basis) is an example of what schedule of reinforcement for the buyer?

   A) Fixed-ratio, variable-interval
   B) Variable-ratio, variable-interval
   C) Variable-ratio, fixed-interval
   D) Fixed-ratio, fixed-interval

3. When students misbehave in class, they lose their recess privileges (meaning that they are not allowed to go outside and play with the rest of the kids). Assuming recess is desirable for students, this is an example of:

   A) positive reinforcement.
   B) negative reinforcement.
   C) positive punishment.
   D) negative punishment.

4. One controversial criticism of violent video games is that they are associated with an increase in school violence; those who oppose violent video games point out that school shootings are more common today than they were two decades ago. The idea that violent video games might cause more violent behavior in children and adolescents is supported by:

   I. Albert Bandura's observational learning principles.
   II. the principles of vicarious learning.
   III. the principles of generalization and discrimination in classical conditioning.

   A) I only
   B) II only
   C) I and II
   D) I, II, and III

5. According to the elaboration likelihood model, which of the following does NOT predict whether a message will be persuasive?

   A) The length of the message
   B) The attractiveness of the person delivering the message
   C) The truthfulness of the message
   D) The trustworthiness of the person delivering the message

6. According to reciprocal determinism, people interact with their environments in all of the following ways, EXCEPT:

   A) people choose where they want to live and work.
   B) individual personality influences how people respond to their environment.
   C) individual personality influences how people respond in a given situation.
   D) people choose to interact as social organisms.

7. According to Mary Ainsworth, an insecurely attached child is likely to:

   I. cry when his mother leaves the room but be easily consoled upon her return.
   II. cry when his mother leaves the room and continue sobbing even after her return.
   III. demonstrate no emotion when his mother leaves the room and upon her return.

   A) I only
   B) II only
   C) I and III
   D) II and III

8. The inability to encode new memories is called:

   A) anterograde amnesia.
   B) retrograde amnesia.
   C) proactive interference.
   D) retroactive interference.

9. A parrot has learned to say a greeting anytime a person rings the doorbell. The doorbell represents a:

   A) conditioned response.
   B) continuous reinforcement.
   C) conditioned stimulus.
   D) partial reinforcement.

10. Suppose that a group of parents was instructed to ignore as many of their children's disruptive behaviors as they could. If it were then discovered that, within 1–2 weeks, the average number of disruptive behaviors per week for children with anxious-ambivalent attachment style increased drastically before dropping below the baseline measurement, what concept would best explain this phenomenon?

   A) Confirmation bias
   B) Extinction burst
   C) Self-serving bias
   D) Self-fulfilling prophecy

11. Each of the following describes a token economy EXCEPT:

   A) in a psychiatric clinic, patients can earn coins that are later traded in.
   B) a teacher gives the class a pizza party when everyone in the class gets 20 homework completion stars.
   C) a tutor brings cookies when a student of foreign languages scores 90 or higher on a vocabulary test.
   D) an individual with autism can earn 5 minutes of video game time once he receives 10 stickers on a note board.

LEARNING, MEMORY, AND BEHAVIOR PRACTICE PASSAGE

Memory is the ability to store and recall information over time. Memories are encoded using visual imagery and organization. Additionally, they can be stored over time into sensory storage, short-term storage, and long-term storage. As memories are stored and retrieved, memories and recall of memories are prone to errors.

There are several errors that can occur during the storage and retrieval process. *Memory blocking* is a failure to retrieve information that has been stored despite active recall attempts. *Suggestibility* is the tendency to incorporate misleading information from external sources into personal recollections. Present information can bias the recall of previous information, which inhibits accurate retrieval from memory. *Memory misattribution* (also known as a source monitoring error) involves assignment of memories to the wrong source. This false attribution can lead to eyewitness misidentifications and serious consequences for innocent people.

In a recent study, 20 participants completed a memory task using abstract shapes. During the study phase, participants were given a study list of 100 known object shapes (such as a black shape of a phone, chair, and lamp). Each shape was presented for 3 seconds and participants were told to remember the shapes. During the test phase, there were 90 shapes randomly presented: 30 items from the original list, 30 items that were related (but not identical to) the original list, and 30 new, unrelated items. Participants were instructed to push a button every time they saw a shape from the original list.

Researchers were interested in analyzing the following potential outcomes: "correct recall" meant that the participant correctly pushed the button in response to a shape from the original list; "related, incorrect recall" meant that the participant incorrectly pushed the button for a shape that was related (but not identical) to a shape on the original list; "correct rejection" meant that the participant correctly did not push the button for a new, unrelated shape that was not on the original list.

Participants were asked to respond within a five second time limit. Using a functional Magnetic Resonance Imaging (fMRI) scan, researchers measured the brain activity of the participants during recall. Specifically, the prefrontal, parietal, motor processing, and hippocampal locations were measured for activity. Early and late visual cortical activity were also measured. Results supported that early visual processing regions exhibited greater activity during correct recognition, suggesting that implicit memory is used in correct recognition. Late visual processing regions exhibited activity during both true and false recognition, indicating that these processes contribute to the conscious experience of remembering. Figure 1 depicts the hippocampal activity associated with true and false recognition.

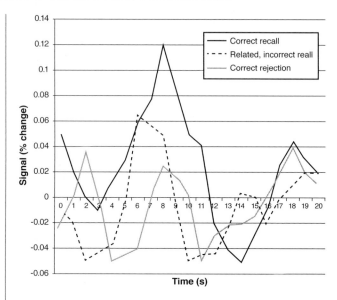

Figure 1 Brain activity in the hippocampus during true and false recognition

Adapted from S. D. Slotnick & D. L. Schacter. *A sensory signature that distinguishes true from false memories.* © 2004 by Nature Neuroscience.

1. Which of the following is an example of explicit memory?

A) Semantic memory
B) Unconscious recall
C) Procedural memory
D) Priming

2. The area of the brain responsible for visual processing is the:

A) prefrontal cortex.
B) temporal lobe.
C) parietal lobe.
D) occipital lobe.

3. According to signal detection theory, when a participant fails to push the button despite the presentation of a shape from the original list this is a:

A) hit.
B) false alarm.
C) correct rejection.
D) miss.

4. What conclusion(s) can be most reasonably drawn from the fMRI activity shown in Figure 1?

    I.   The overall change in signal activity was greatest for correct rejections because participants were recalling the shapes from their memory.
    II. The overall change in signal activity for related but incorrect recalls was less than correct recalls.
    III. The overall change in signal activity was greatest for correct recalls because participants were recalling the shapes from their memory.

A) I only
B) I and II only
C) II and III only
D) III only

5. In a follow-up experiment, scientists measured brain activity along with heart activity while participants recalled the shapes. Participants who experienced false recognition exhibited a higher heart rate than those who exhibited true recognition. How does this change the design of the study?

A) A dependent variable is added.
B) It introduces a new independent variable.
C) A control condition is added.
D) It increases the validity of the study.

6. If an individual correctly remembers a specific piece of information, but thinks she read the information in a textbook when in actuality she saw it on television, this is an example of:

A) an error in source monitoring.
B) the misinformation effect.
C) a false memory.
D) positive transfer.

SOLUTIONS TO FREESTANDING QUESTIONS: LEARNING, MEMORY, AND BEHAVIOR

1. **B** Operant conditioning uses a reward or punishment to reinforce a desired behavior; in this case, the professor provides a reward (treat) after each time her puppy demonstrates the desired behavior (going to the bathroom outside), a classic example of the application of operant conditioning principles (choice B is correct). Classical conditioning involves the pairing of a neutral stimulus (which automatically elicits the behavior) with another stimulus until the behavior occurs in response to the other stimulus (now called the conditioned stimulus); since the behavior in this example occurs first and the reward is meant to reinforce the behavior, this is not an example of classical conditioning (choice A is wrong), nor is it an example of a conditioned stimulus (choice C is wrong). Spontaneous recovery is also a principle of classical conditioning whereby a conditioned response that has become extinct over time is spontaneously recovered in response to the conditioned stimulus (choice D is wrong).

2. **B** The stock is speculative and can rise or fall at any time. Consequently, the buyer is not able to determine when his purchasing actions will be reinforced; therefore, the interval of reinforcement is variable (choices C and D can be eliminated). The buyer also cannot predict how much the stock will rise (or fall). This makes the ratio of reinforcement also variable (choice A can be eliminated). Thus, the correct answer is a variable-interval, variable-ratio schedule of reinforcement (choice B is correct).

3. **D** Negative punishment occurs when something desirable (recess) is "removed" (in this case, these children lose the desirable privilege for the day) in order to reduce a behavior (choice D is correct). Positive reinforcement is the addition or application of something desirable in order to increase a behavior; for example, if students who behaved well in class all received 20 extra minutes of recess time, this would be an example of positive reinforcement (choice A is wrong). Negative reinforcement is the removal of something undesirable to increase behavior; for example, if students who behaved well in class did not have to take the test at the end of the day, this might be an example of negative reinforcement (assuming that the test was undesirable; choice B is wrong). Positive punishment occurs when something undesirable is applied to decrease behavior; for example, if the students who behaved poorly were spanked, this would be an example of positive punishment (choice C is wrong).

4. **C** Since none of the Items appear in exactly two answer choices, it doesn't matter which Item you start analyzing. Item I is true: Albert Bandura conducted famous experiments on observational learning using a Bobo doll which suggested that when young children observe the behavior of adults, they are likely to imitate that behavior; these studies do support the idea that observed violent behavior in video games might increase the likelihood of actual violent behavior (choice B can be eliminated). Item II is true: vicarious learning, also called observational learning or social learning, suggests that humans, as social creatures, can learn from observing the behavior of others; this also supports the idea that exposure to violence in video games might increase the likelihood of violent behaviors (choice A can be eliminated). Item III is false: generalization refers to the ability of an organism that has been trained using classical conditioning principles to react to a stimulus that is similar but not identical to the conditioned stimulus, and discrimination refers to the ability of a classically trained organism to differentiate between the conditioned stimulus and other, similar stimuli; this does not support the idea that violent video games might cause more violent behavior in children (choice D can be eliminated; choice C is correct).

5. **C** According to the elaboration likelihood model, the truthfulness of the message itself is not actually a characteristic used to determine whether a message with be persuasive (choice C is correct). The message characteristics (including length) do predict persuasiveness (choice A is wrong), as do the source characteristics (including the attractiveness and the trustworthiness of the person delivering the message; choices B and D are wrong).

6. **D** People are social organisms, but this is not a tenet of reciprocal determinism (choice D is false and is the correct answer choice). On the other hand, reciprocal determinism does states that people choose their environments (choice A is true and can be eliminated); individual personality influences how people respond to their environments (choice B is true and can be eliminated); and individual personality influences how people respond to various situations (choice C is true and can be eliminated).

7. **D** Since each of the Items appears in exactly two of the answer choices, it doesn't matter which Item you start analyzing. Item I is false: according to Mary Ainsworth, a *securely* attached child will cry when his mother leaves the room but be easily consoled upon her return (choices A and C can be eliminated). Since both remaining answer choices include Item II, it must be true and you can focus on Item III. Item III is true: alternately, an insecurely attached child might also display no emotion when his mother leaves and returns (choice B can be eliminated, and choice D is correct). Note that Item II is in fact true: an insecurely attached child will remain inconsolable after his mother's return.

8. **A** The inability to encode new memories is called anterograde amnesia (choice A is correct). The inability to recall memories from the past is called retrograde amnesia (choice B is wrong). Proactive interference occurs when previously learned information interferes with the ability to recall information learned later; it does not prevent the encoding of memories but rather refers to the inability to recall them (choice C is wrong). Retroactive interference occurs when newly learned information interferes with the ability to recall previously learned information; it does not prevent the encoding of memories but rather prevents the ability to recall them (choice D is wrong).

9. **C** A conditioned stimulus is a stimulus that produces a response following learning (choice C is correct). Continuous reinforcement is when a certain behavior is reinforced every time it occurs. Partial reinforcement is when a certain behavior is reinforced at certain times. For instance, there may be a reward attached to the behavior. Continuous and partial reinforcement are based on schedules in operant conditioning, not the stimulus itself (choices B and D are wrong). A conditioned response is the response that has been learned, in this case, the greeting (choice A is wrong).

10. **B** Extinction burst describes the process in which when extinction occurs (that is, reinforcement is ceased for a specific behavior), there is a brief spike in the behavior, and rates increase before they eventually drop. This is consistent with the description in the question stem (choice B is correct). Confirmation bias describes seeking sources to support beliefs that one already holds, instead of objectively seeking information (choice A is wrong). The self-serving bias describes taking credit for positive outcomes and blaming others for negative outcomes (choice C is wrong). A self-fulfilling prophecy occurs when one holds a belief, then due to the belief engages in actions that confirm the belief, or "fulfill the prophecy," due to the set of actions conducted by the individual (choice D is wrong).

11. **C** Token economies involve the use of secondary reinforcers, which are non-intrinsic motivators that can be exchanged for other pleasurable activities or rewards. A primary reinforcer (food, water, sex, etc.) is not considered part of a token economy system (choice C is correct). Each of the other choices describes a secondary reinforcer that is given in exchange for completing a task: coins, stars, and stickers (choices A, B, and D are wrong).

SOLUTIONS TO LEARNING, MEMORY, AND BEHAVIOR PRACTICE PASSAGE

1. **A** Explicit memory refers to the act of consciously retrieving stored information and experiences. Semantic memory is a type of explicit memory that describes the retrieval of facts and knowledge (choice A is correct). Implicit memory describes when past experiences influence later behavior and performance, not the retrieval of actual facts or events. Therefore, implicit memory is unconscious (choice B is wrong). Procedural memory describes a type of implicit memory where motor and cognitive skills influence current behavior (choice C is wrong). Priming is the enhanced ability to think of a stimulus based on recent exposure to that stimulus. This is also a specific type of implicit memory (choice D is wrong).

2. **D** The occipital lobe contains the primary visual cortex and is responsible for processing visual information (choice D is correct). The prefrontal cortex is involved with many complex functions including working memory, personality, emotional processing, and decision-making; however, the prefrontal cortex does not process visual information (choice A is wrong). The temporal lobe contains the primary auditory cortex, and it is also involved with the processing of smell and emotion; it does not process visual information, however (choice B is wrong). The parietal lobe contains the primary somatosensory cortex, which processes touch information; though adjacent to the occipital lobe, it does not process visual information (choice C is wrong).

3. **D** According to signal detection theory, when someone fails to detect the intended signal, or in this case, if a participant fails to push their button despite the presentation of a shape from the original list, this would be considered a "miss" (choice D is correct). The appropriate identification of the signal (called "correct recall" in the study) would be considered a "hit" (choice A is wrong). If the signal was not present but the participant thought it was (called "related, incorrect recall" in the study), this would be considered a "false alarm" (choice B is wrong). If the signal is not present and not detected, this is a "correct rejection" (also called this is the study; choice C is wrong).

4. **C** Since each of the Items appears in exactly two of the answer choices, it doesn't matter which Item you start analyzing. Item I is false: the overall change in signal activity for correct rejections is the least (the percent change indicated by the grey line in Figure 1 demonstrates the least change; choices A and B can be eliminated). Since both remaining answer choices include Item III, it must be true, and you can focus on Item II. Item II is true: the overall change in signal activity for related but incorrect recalls was less than correct recalls, indicated by the dotted line in Figure 1 varying less than the solid black line, suggesting that

participants were not utilizing their hippocampal region as much for the incorrect recalls (choice D can be eliminated, and choice C is correct). Note that Item III is, in fact, true: the overall change in signal activity was greatest for correct recalls because participants were experiencing true recognition so they were actively retrieving memories and utilizing their hippocampi.

5.   **A**   Since scientists are measuring heart activity along with brain activity in the follow-up experiment, another dependent variable is being added because dependent variables are those being measured in the study (choice A is correct). Independent variables are those that are controlled and manipulated by the experimenters in order to determine their impact on the dependent variable (choice B is wrong). A control group is one that does not receive the experimental treatment; the addition of a new dependent variable has nothing to do with adding an experimental control (choice C is wrong). The addition of another dependent variable could, but does not necessarily, increase the validity of the study; further information would be required to make this determination (choice D is wrong).

6.   **A**   If an individual correctly remembers a specific piece of information, but thinks she read the information in a textbook when in actuality she saw it on television, she is attributing the accurate memory to an inaccurate source, which is an example of a source monitoring error (choice A is correct). The misinformation effect occurs when the information itself is incorrectly remembered, oftentimes due to exposure to other information that prevents the memory from being encoded completely accurately (choice B is wrong). A false memory is a completely inaccurate recollection of something, sometimes as a result of repeated exposure to inaccurate information, which disrupts the actual memory (choice C is wrong). Positive transfer occurs when old information or memories facilitate the learning of new information (choice D is wrong).

Chapter 22
Interacting with the Environment

FREESTANDING QUESTIONS: INTERACTING WITH THE ENVIRONMENT

1. The cocktail party effect describes our ability to detect a specific stimulus amongst competing stimuli. By definition, what type of stimulus is the cocktail party effect specifically referring to?

    A) A visual stimulus presented in the attended channel
    B) An auditory stimulus presented in the attended channel
    C) A visual stimulus presented in the unattended channel
    D) An auditory stimulus presented in the unattended channel

2. According to the resource model of attention, which of the following should prove to be the most challenging?

    A) Attempting to simultaneously study for the MCAT and pay attention to the news on television
    B) Driving a familiar route in icy conditions
    C) Trying to listen to the radio while a storm is raging outside
    D) Walking down the street while talking on the phone

3. When you go to pick up your dry cleaning you realize you've left your claim ticket, which contains the five-digit number you need to provide in order to locate your dry cleaning, on your kitchen counter. You just looked at that claim ticket ten minutes ago. Therefore, you close your eyes and try to remember the five digits on the ticket. According to Baddeley's model of working memory, to remember the digits on the claim ticket you are accessing the:

    A) central executive.
    B) visuospatial sketchpad.
    C) phonological loop.
    D) episodic buffer.

4. What EEG pattern is characteristic of the first stage of sleep (stage 1)?

    A) Theta waves
    B) K-complexes
    C) Sleep spindles
    D) Delta waves

5. After seeing several news reports of tragic auto accidents on nearby highways and thinking about it for a long time, a man decides to cancel his scheduled appointments out of town to avoid driving on those highways, because he feels certain he'll get into an accident, too. His decision can be most attributed to which of the following?

    A) Avoidance learning
    B) Intuition
    C) Functional fixedness
    D) Availability heuristic

6. The attainment of what developmental milestone separates the first and second stages in Piaget's theory of cognitive development?

    A) Sensation
    B) Object permanence
    C) Concrete operations
    D) Formal operations

7. Which scenario is most consistent with the James-Lange theory of emotion?

    A) Dan encounters a growling bear, his heart starts racing, and then he feels fearful.
    B) Dan encounters a growling bear, he appraises the situation as dangerous, and then feels fearful.
    C) Dan encounters a growling bear, his heart starts racing and he feels fearful simultaneously.
    D) Dan encounters a growling bear, he feels fearful, and then his heart starts racing.

8. Which of the following brain structures/areas is NOT involved with the experience of emotion?

    A) Medulla oblongata
    B) Amygdala
    C) Hypothalamus
    D) Frontal lobe

9. Which of the following drugs acts by depressing the central nervous system?

    I. Alcohol
    II. Marijuana
    III. Heroin

    A) I only
    B) I and III
    C) II and III
    D) I, II, and III

10. An eighteen-year-old college student switches major several times before ultimately failing out of school, then works odd jobs until at twenty-one she has no long-term plans. The individual has not successfully negotiated which developmental stage?

A) Formal operations stage
B) Genital stage
C) Identity vs. role confusion stage
D) Conventional stage

11. Which structure of the eye is most important in making the perceptual discriminations involving color spectra?

A) Choroid
B) Cornea
C) Fovea
D) Optic disc

12. If researchers were to monitor changing cortical activity to precisely localize the areas of the brain most involved with color perception, which brain imaging technology would they most likely use?

A) PET
B) fMRI
C) CT scan
D) EEG

13. Research in behavioral neuroscience shows that information from the retina travels directly to the amygdala before the same information is transmitted to the primary visual cortex. The amygdala processes a low resolution representation of the visual field, and can initiate the fight-or-flight response before full awareness of the stimulus is processed in the primary visual cortex. This finding most supports which theory?

A) Cannon-Bard
B) James-Lange
C) Schachter-Singer
D) Depth of processing

INTERACTING WITH THE ENVIRONMENT PRACTICE PASSAGE 1

Confirmation bias is the tendency to seek information that conforms to one's existing beliefs, while filtering out that which would contradict them. Ambiguous information may also be interpreted in a way that supports those beliefs. Such biases enable individuals to process information quickly but superficially. For example, subjects viewing a video of children labeled as either high or low socioeconomic status used that information to judge future academic ability, ignoring other relevant information.

Research has also shown that when new information is presented in a "disfluent" (challenging) manner, this may foster deeper and more critical thinking. For instance, high school students given study materials printed in a hard-to-read font scored higher on an exam than did their counterparts in a control group, who received the same materials in a clear font.

A pair of studies sought to determine whether disfluent information would reduce confirmation bias, with regard to both preexisting and newly formed attitudes, by making subjects work harder to read new information. The second study also hoped to determine whether deeper thinking was involved in acting without bias.

In the first study, 142 volunteer undergraduate students completed a questionnaire that included items about ethnicity, gender, age, religion, and political affiliation. Next, they read an article supporting capital punishment. Subjects were randomly given either a fluent version of the article, printed in 12-point Times New Roman font, or a disfluent version, printed in light-gray, bold and italicized 12-point Haettenschweiler font. They then answered questions about the quality, maturity, and intelligence of the writing, as well as whether they agreed with it. In the fluent condition, 90% of those who had identified themselves as strongly conservative agreed with the article, while 86% of those who had self-identified as liberal disagreed with it. However, in the disfluent condition, both conservative and liberal subjects answered significantly less in line with their stated beliefs.

In a second study, participants acted as jurors in a mock trial. Each was randomly handed a positive or negative assessment of the defendant, an assessment intended to foster bias at the experimental outset. Differences between the verdicts after reading the positive or negative assessment of the defendant were considered to be a reflection of confirmation bias. For subjects given assessments in a fluent font, there was a significant difference between the verdicts for those given a positive vs. negative assessment of the defendant, but when subjects were handed assessments printed in a disfluent font, there was no discernible confirmation bias. Some of the "disfluent" subjects, however, were also given an additional cognitive load, in the form of either having to memorize a

neutral word list (none of the words had anything to do with the mock trial or the defendant) or adhere to a time limit. Significantly more cognitive bias was measured in the memory-load / disfluent condition than in the time-limit / disfluent condition. These results are displayed in Figure 1.

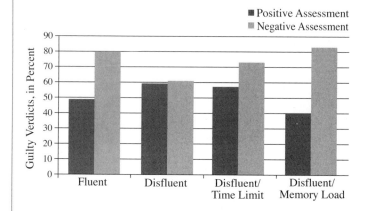

Figure 1 Percentage of guilty verdicts given in Study 2, as a function of both fluent and disfluent text, as well as disfluent text with either time limit or memory load

Adapted from I. Hernandez & J. L. Preston. *Disfluency disrupts confirmation bias.* © 2012 by Journal of Experimental Social Psychology.

1. Which of the following is NOT a reasonable conclusion, given the experiments described above?

A) Reasoning without bias requires more mental resources than reasoning based on one's expectations.
B) Memorizing lists of words constitutes the same cognitive load as does having a time limit in which to make a decision.
C) Information that is harder to process may result in its being processed more thoroughly.
D) A bias may be formed as new information is processed.

2. Which of the following is LEAST likely to involve confirmation bias?

A) Stereotyping
B) Prejudice
C) Social loafing
D) Attribution theory

3. Which of the following is the most likely explanation for why the cognitive load was included in the second experiment?

A) To make the assessments given to those in the cognitive load conditions seem more interesting
B) To determine whether effort was a factor when thinking in a less-biased manner
C) To encourage participants in the cognitive load condition to pay stricter attention
D) To conceal the true nature of the experiment

4. An apparent aim of the second experiment was to:

A) test for cognitive bias regarding longstanding prejudices.
B) expose problems in the U.S. legal system.
C) test for cognitive bias regarding newly-formed attitudes.
D) measure decision-making in the context of the stress-diathesis model.

5. Which of the following best explains the differing results between the disfluent / memory-load condition and the disfluent / time-limit condition?

A) A memory load may tie up more mental resources than does a time limit.
B) Memorizing new information may interfere with preconceived attitudes.
C) Deadlines may force some individuals to reason in a more biased manner.
D) Items in the word list may have evoked personal prejudices.

6. If the disfluency hypothesis is true, which of the following situations is likely to produce the least amount of confirmation bias?

A) Handwriting an essay with a defective pen
B) Reading a newspaper editorial in a newly-acquired language
C) Listening to a podcast while eating a meal
D) Hearing a speech given by a person with a slight foreign accent

INTERACTING WITH THE ENVIRONMENT PRACTICE PASSAGE 2

Categorical Perception (CP) is the phenomenon through which the categories understood by an observer influence that observer's perception. Many psychologists believe that CP has been demonstrated in numerous experiments in which subjects' ability to make perceptual discriminations between objects has improved when those objects belong to different categories rather than the same category, even when these experiments control for the physical difference between the objects. Experimental differences in color discrimination tasks between native speakers of languages that categorize colors differently have led many scientists to hypothesize that language plays an important role in the ability of humans to discriminate between different object categories.

A new experiment comparing Russian and English color matching has shown that [native] Russian language speakers have an advantage over [native] English language speakers in categorical perception at a boundary between two different linguistic categories of the color blue that is unique to the Russian language. As opposed to the English language, which categorizes both light and dark shades of blue as blue, the Russian language does not have any single word that encompasses all shades of blue as recognized by English speakers. Instead, the Russian words *siniy* (dark blue) and *goluboy* (light blue) divide what English speakers perceive as blue into two distinct "basic" color terms for speakers of Russian.

In the new study, when native Russian language speakers were asked to select which of two colors matched a *siniy* target, the reaction time of these participants was significantly faster if the distractor was *goluboy* than if it was a different shade of *siniy*. These results were observed even when the physical difference in hue between targets and distractors was equated. In contrast, English speakers did not show this cross-category advantage. In addition, the cross-category advantage of Russian speakers was shown to be disrupted by a competing verbal interference task, but not by a competing spatial interference task, while English speakers did not show any cross-category advantage in any condition.

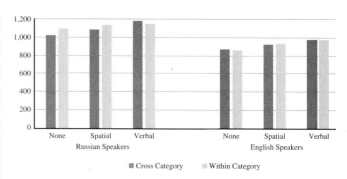

Figure 1 Russian speakers' and English speakers' mean reaction times (msec) shown for the no-interference, spatial-interference, and verbal-interference conditions

1. Which of the following concepts best explains why a competing spatial task resulted in a lower mean reaction time than did a competing verbal task for native Russian language speakers who were discriminating color shades across *siniy* and *goluboy* categories?

A) Feature detection
B) Interposition
C) Procedural memory
D) Parallel processing

2. Many scientists hypothesize that distinct linguistic categorization of continuous stimuli can help humans discriminate minor differences between such stimuli if these differences reflect different linguistic categories. All of the following results would provide evidence supporting this hypothesis EXCEPT:

A) a study that shows right-handed native Russian language speakers with severed corpora callosa discriminate more quickly across than within *siniy* and *goluboy* categories when the stimuli is presented directly in front of their right eyes rather than directly in front of their left eyes.

B) a study that shows that native Russian language speakers lose their advantage in discriminating more quickly across than within *siniy* and *goluboy* categories after they suffer significant damage to their Wernicke's areas.

C) a study that shows native English language speakers can discriminate more quickly between blue and green stimuli than can native speakers of a language that uses the same word for blue as for green.

D) a study that shows that right-handed native English language speakers can discriminate more quickly between blue and green if the stimuli is presented in their right visual field rather than their left visual field.

3. Which statement can be concluded from Figure 1?

A) Native Russian language speakers were quicker at discriminating within *siniy* and *goluboy* categories than were native English language speakers.

B) Native Russian language speakers were quicker at discriminating across *siniy* and *goluboy* categories than were native English language speakers.

C) Native Russian language speakers were quicker at discriminating across *siniy* and *goluboy* categories when they were distracted by a competing spatial task than when they were distracted by a competing verbal task.

D) Native English language speakers were quicker at discriminating within *siniy* and *goluboy* categories than they were at discriminating across *siniy* and *goluboy* categories.

4. An individual in which of the following stages of Piaget's theory of cognitive development would be LEAST likely to display the categorization advantages of native Russian language speakers demonstrated in the experiment described?

A) Pre-operational
B) Formal operations
C) Pre-conventional
D) Sensorimotor

5. Which of the following concepts best accounts for the results of the described experiment?

A) Nativist theory
B) Signal detection theory
C) Linguistic relativity
D) Interactionist theory

6. The findings described in the passage suggest that Categorical Perception:

A) depends wholly on cultural differences.
B) is innate in all humans from birth.
C) can be influenced by differences in native linguistic categories.
D) is comparable with or without interference from competing tasks.

SOLUTIONS TO FREESTANDING QUESTIONS: INTERACTING WITH THE ENVIRONMENT

1. **D** The cocktail party effect specifically describes when an auditory stimulus (choices A and C are wrong) present in the unattended channel suddenly catches our attention (choice D is correct; choice B is wrong), and our attention shifts to the unattended channel. The best example of this occurs when we are at a party engaged in conversation with one person in a loud room (we are specifically attending to one person while tuning out the rest of the noise), then suddenly we hear our name being spoken by someone a few feet away. We were not consciously attending to that other conversation, but when we hear our name, our attention shifts to the unattended conversation.

2. **A** According to the resource model of attention, we have a limited pool of resources on which to draw when performing tasks; in general, if the resources required to perform multiple tasks simultaneously exceed the available resources to do so, then the tasks will prove much more challenging to accomplish simultaneously. Three factors are associated with performance on multi-tasking: task similarity, task difficulty, and task practice. Therefore, attempting to simultaneously study for the MCAT and pay attention to the news on television would prove the most challenging because the two tasks require similar modalities of language processing, studying for the MCAT is a more difficult task, and it also requires more practice (choice A is correct). Driving a car in icy conditions would likely prove challenging, but because the route is familiar, only one task is being attended to (driving); therefore, the resource model of attention would suggest that this task would not be the most challenging (choice B is wrong). Attempting to listen to the radio during a storm would likely be annoying, but because the noise of the storm is not something that is being actively attended to, this would not prove overly challenging, according to the resource model of attention (choice C is wrong). Walking is an easy task and talking on the phone is also an easy task; furthermore, both tasks require different modalities, and both are tasks with which people tend to have a ton of practice (choice D is wrong).

3. **B** The visuospatial sketchpad, according to Baddeley's model of working memory, is relied upon to recall visual and spatial information; attempting to recall five digits that you have *seen* would then rely on your ability to access your visuospatial sketchpad (choice B is correct). In Baddeley's model, the central executive oversees the entire process of working memory, and it orchestrates the process by shifting and dividing attention (choice A is wrong). The phonological loop, according to Baddeley's model, allows you to repeat verbal or auditory information in order to remember it in the short term (choice C is wrong). The episodic buffer is where information in the working memory can interact with information in long-term memory; because there is no information in the question stem that indicates that long-term memory is being accessed, this is not an example of accessing the episodic buffer (choice D is wrong).

4. **A** The first stage of sleep is marked by low to moderate frequency theta waves (choice A is correct). K-complexes are large, slow waves and sleep spindles are high-frequency bursts of wave activity; both are characteristic of stage 2 sleep (choices B and C are wrong). Delta waves are high amplitude, low frequency waves characteristic of stage 3 sleep (choice D is wrong).

5. **D**   The availability heuristic is a tendency to make judgments based on how readily available information is in our memories. If information is readily available in our memory (like repeated reports of accidents on a specific highway), we may think something (like getting into an accident) is more common than it actually is. The man in question misinterprets the likelihood of being involved in an accident due to the availability of recent information (choice D is correct). Avoidance learning requires someone to first experience a negative outcome of a behavior in order to modify that behavior; since the question stem does not indicate that the man has had an accident on that highway in the past, avoidance learning does not explain his decision (choice A is wrong). Intuition involves understanding without conscious reasoning; since the question stem indicates that conscious thought was put into his decision, intuition is not a logical explanation (choice B is wrong). Functional fixedness is the tendency to perceive the functions of an object as fixed and unchanging, which makes it more difficult to think of different ways to use an object in solving a problem; functional fixedness does not explain the man's decision (choice C is wrong).

6. **B**   According to Piaget's theory of cognitive development, the acquisition of object permanence separates the first stage (the sensorimotor stage, which occurs from birth to roughly 1–2 years of age) and the second stage (the preoperational thought stage, which occurs from roughly 2–7 years of age); technically, object permanence marks the end of the sensorimotor stage (choice B is correct). Sensation (and motor movement) marks the sensorimotor stage (the first stage), but sensation is not the developmental milestone before the second stage (choice A is wrong). Concrete operations are a hallmark of the third stage, the concrete operational stage (choice C is wrong). Formal operations are a hallmark of the fourth and final stage, the formal operations stage (choice D is wrong).

7. **A**   According to the James-Lange theory of emotion, our physiological reactions to stimuli precede and give rise to the emotional experience; in other words, first we have a physiological reaction, then we label the situation with an emotion; therefore, the James-Lange theory would suggest that first Dan experiences physiological arousal (heart races), and then he experiences the emotion (fear; choice A is correct). The Schachter-Singer theory of emotion suggests that cognitive assessment of the situation precedes the experience of emotion (choice B is wrong). The Cannon-Bard theory of emotion suggests that the physiological response and the emotion occur simultaneously (choice C is wrong). No theories of emotion suggest that the emotion is experienced before the physiological arousal (choice D is wrong).

8. **A**   The medulla oblongata is the area of the brain that connects the spinal cord to the rest of the brain; it contains simple control centers for some of the most rudimentary functions necessary for life, including blood pressure, the vomit reflex, and the respiratory centers. The medulla is not involved with the experience of emotion, which is processed in higher brain centers (choice A is correct). In the brain, the limbic system is a collection of structures/areas that work together in processing emotional experiences. The main structure involved in emotion in the limbic system is the amygdala, which serves as the conductor of our emotional experiences (choice B is wrong). The amygdala communicates with the hypothalamus, which controls the physiological aspects of emotion, such as sweating and a racing heart (choice C is wrong), and it also communicates with the prefrontal cortex, located in the frontal lobe, which controls the conscious and behavioral aspects of emotion (choice D is wrong).

9. **B** Item II appears in exactly two of the answer choices; start by analyzing it, since whether it is true or false you can immediately eliminate half the answers. Item II is false: marijuana is in the class of drugs known as "hallucinogenics," which act by distorting sensory input into the central nervous system (choices C and D can be eliminated). Note that both remaining answer choices include Item I, so it must be true, and you can focus on Item III. Item III is true: heroin is a barbiturate, a class of drugs that also acts by slowing down the activity of the central nervous system (choice A can be eliminated, and choice B is correct). Note that Item I is in fact true: alcohol is in the class of drugs considered "depressants," which act by depressing or slowing down the activity of the central nervous system.

10. **C** Erikson's fifth stage (identity vs. role confusion) occurs during adolescence and requires the individual to establish a strong sense of self, confidence in his or her personal beliefs and desires, and a degree of comfort with various societal roles. The twenty-one year-old described appears to lack direction, has no plans or goals for her life, and has achieved little success in her academic and vocational roles (choice C is correct). Piaget's final stage (formal operations) involves the capacity to reason and think abstractly; there is no evidence that the individual failed to develop these abilities or that her lack of direction in life is due to cognitive deficiencies (choice A is wrong). Freud's genital stage of psychosexual development, which properly occurs during adolescence and adulthood, involves achieving intimacy with another person. While the individual appears confused about her societal roles and her future, there is no information provided about her interpersonal relationships (choice B is wrong). Kohlberg's fifth stage of development involves attaining a relatively high level of moral understanding in which society's laws and rules are viewed as a "social contract"; the fact that the individual appears to be a confused underachiever does not necessarily mean that she has not attained a sophisticated level of moral development (choice D is wrong).

11. **C** The 6 to 7 million cones in the human eye are concentrated mostly in and near the fovea, a small dimple in the middle of the retina. Cones provide the eye's ability to discriminate color (rods are more sensitive to low levels of visible light, but they cannot discriminate color, and are not found in the fovea; choice C is correct). The choroid is the vascular (contains blood vessels) layer of the eye found between the retina and sclera. The choroid's function is to provide nourishment to the outer layers of the retina through blood vessels, and it is not the part of the eye that discriminates color (choice A is wrong). The cornea is the transparent front part of the eye that covers the iris, pupil, and anterior chamber. While the cornea, with the anterior chamber and lens, refracts light, and accounts for approximately two-thirds of the eye's total optical power, it cannot discriminate between different shades of color (choice B is wrong). The optic disc is the point of exit for ganglion cell axons leaving the eye. Because there are no rods or cones overlying the optic disc, it creates a small blind spot in each eye (choice D is wrong).

12. **B** Functional magnetic resonance imaging (fMRI) uses a computer to combine a series of MR images taken less than one second apart to provide a functional picture of how brain activity changes over time. fMRI can display changes in oxygen levels (which indicate blood flow) in various regions of the brain in real time and can be used to produce activation maps that indicate the precise areas of the brain involved in particular mental processes (choice B is correct). Although PET (positron emission tomography) can be used to measure increased brain activity, fMRI is considered safer than PET because PET requires subjects to be injected with radioactive substances. In addition, the locational precision of fMRI data is

more precise than that of PET (choice A is wrong). CT (computed tomography) scans use a computer to combine many cross-sectional (tomographic) images generated from the differential absorption of X-rays into a three dimensional structural "snapshot" of an anatomical part, such as a human brain. CT scans do not provide functional data and thus cannot be used to examine changes in brain activity across time (choice C is wrong). Although EEG (electroencephalography) can be used to measure changes in brain activity over time with excellent temporal precision, the locational precision of fMRI data is far, far more precise than that of EEG (choice D is wrong).

13. **B** The research describes a situation in which the physiological response (a fight-or-flight reflex) occurs before the individual is aware of what is going on. This is consistent with the James-Lange theory of emotion, which states that physiological responses cause emotions (choice B is correct). Cannon-Bard theory suggests that the physiological response and awareness of the emotion occur simultaneously (choice A is wrong). Schachter-Singer theory includes a cognitive evaluation of the situation, which is not described in the question stem (choice C is wrong). Depth of processing theory is related to memory, not emotions, and suggests that the more cognitive processing memories receive and the more connections that are formed the better the individual will recall the memory (choice D is wrong).

SOLUTIONS TO INTERACTING WITH THE ENVIRONMENT PRACTICE PASSAGE 1

1. **B** Based on the results in Figure 1 and information provided in the final paragraph ("significantly more cognitive bias was measured in the memory-load/disfluent condition than in the time-limit/disfluent condition"), it is not reasonable to conclude that memorizing lists of words constitutes the same cognitive load as having a time limit in which to make a decision (choice B is correct). The idea that reasoning without bias requires more mental resources than reasoning based on one's expectations is the foundation for the design of the second experiment, which studied the effect of cognitive load (used to divert participants' mental resources) on decision-making (therefore, choice A *is* a reasonable conclusion and can be eliminated). The idea that information that is harder to process may result in its being processed more thoroughly is the hypothesis for both experiments (therefore, choice C *is* a reasonable conclusion and can be eliminated). The second experiment also tests whether a bias may be formed as new information is processed (therefore, choice D *is* a reasonable conclusion and can be eliminated).

2. **C** Social loafing occurs when an individual exerts less effort in a group than when working alone; social loafing is the least likely to involve confirmation bias (choice C is correct). Stereotyping and prejudice, on the other hand, are both forms of bias, so both are likely involved in confirmation bias (choices A and B can be eliminated). Attribution theory is a broad umbrella term, but generally describes the tendency to explain the causes of behavior or events involving others or ourselves; since attribution theory involves blaming others, it is more likely to involve confirmation bias than social loafing (choice D can be eliminated).

3. **B**   In the first paragraph, the passage states that "New information presented in a 'disfluent' (challenging) manner…may foster deeper and more critical thinking." A cognitive load may force subjects' selective attention away from the main experimental task and thus help determine whether deep thinking is a factor in reducing cognitive bias. Therefore, the cognitive load was most likely included in the second experiment in order to determine whether effort was a factor when thinking in a less-biased manner, which addresses the role of shallow thinking (possibly induced by the cognitive load; choice B is correct). Subjects' interest in the experiment is not a viable experimental reason to implement a cognitive load, since subjects' interest was not being tested (choice A is wrong). On the other hand, selective attention theory suggests that when participants are given an additional cognitive load, it will be *harder* for them to pay attention, so the cognitive load will not encourage stricter attention (choice C is wrong). Whether cognitive load was meant to conceal the nature of the experiment cannot be inferred from the paragraphs or the table (choice D is wrong).

4. **C**   The third paragraph states that "A pair of studies sought to determine whether disfluent information would reduce confirmation bias, both with regard to preexisting and *newly-formed attitudes*"; therefore, the aim of the second experiment was to test for cognitive bias regarding newly-formed attitudes (choice C is correct). Testing for cognitive bias regarding longstanding prejudices is the apparent aim of the *first* study (preexisting attitudes) not the second study (choice A is wrong). There is not enough information in the passage to suggest that the second study is aiming to expose problems in the legal system (choice B is wrong). Similarly, there is not enough information in the passage to support that the second study is aiming to test the stress-diathesis model (choice D is wrong).

5. **A**   The second paragraph states that the "second study also hoped to determine whether deeper thinking was involved in acting without bias"; therefore, the explanation that a memory load ties up more mental resources than a time limit best explains the differing results between the disfluent / memory-load condition and the disfluent / time-limit condition (the memory-load condition may have interfered more with thinking and caused subjects to base their guilt decisions on preconceptions; choice A is correct). Since memorizing new information appears to *increase* bias, the suggestion that it may interfere with preconceived attitudes does not explain why there is significantly more cognitive bias in the memory-load / disfluent condition than in the time-limit / disfluent condition (choice B is wrong). Similarly, the explanation that deadlines may force some individuals to reason in a more biased manner does not explain why there is significantly more cognitive bias in the memory-load / disfluent condition than in the time-limit / disfluent condition (choice C is wrong). The explanation that items in the word list may have evoked personal prejudices would not explain the general trend of greater cognitive bias, since each subject would have had unique personal prejudices unrelated to the experimental task (choice D is wrong).

6. **B**   The disfluency hypothesis suggests that when people work harder to absorb information, they tend to consider it more thoroughly and with less bias; therefore, reading a newspaper editorial in a newly-acquired language fits in with the hypothesis and experiments described in the passage, since reading in a newly-acquired language requires a person to process information more carefully and thoroughly (choice B is correct). In contrast, writing an essay, not taking in new information, cannot be explained by the disfluency hypothesis (choice A is wrong). While listening to a podcast involves taking in information, there is no evidence that the podcast is somehow difficult to absorb, nor that eating a meal would constitute

a difficult cognitive load (choice C is wrong). Hearing a speech given by someone with a slight accent might cause some difficulty of information absorption, but less so than reading a newspaper in a newly-acquired language (choice D is wrong).

SOLUTIONS TO INTERACTING WITH THE ENVIRONMENT PRACTICE PASSAGE 2

1. **D** Parallel processing refers to the ability of the brain to simultaneously process incoming stimuli of differing quality. For example, when combining two highly dissimilar and well-practiced tasks (e.g., repeating the same sentence while sight-reading difficult piano music), piano players are able to demonstrate parallel processing of both tasks with nearly the same speed and quality as they demonstrate when processing each task separately. When a task using auditory stimuli and manual responses is paired with a task using visual stimuli and vocal responses, dual-task costs are typically high. In contrast, very little cost is incurred when a task using auditory stimuli and vocal responses is instead paired with a task using visual stimuli and manual responses. In the experiment described, Russian language subjects incurred a much more significant reaction time penalty when discriminating colors across *siniy* and *goluboy* categories while simultaneously performing a distracting verbal task than they incurred while simultaneously performing a distracting spatial task. The advantage shown by Russian speakers and not English speakers in discriminating *siniy* and *goluboy* categories is described in the passage as resulting from the differing linguistic color categorizations of the two languages. This implies that at least some activation of linguistic processing in the brain among Russian speakers is making their reaction times quicker. Thus, the most reasonable explanation for why native Russian speakers took much longer to discriminate between *siniy* and *goluboy* categories while performing a competing verbal task than while performing a competing spatial task is the human brain's superior ability to parallel process dissimilar tasks more efficiently than it can process similar tasks (choice D is correct). Feature detection in visual perception refers to the process by which the nervous system sorts or filters complex natural stimuli to extract behaviorally relevant cues, as opposed to irrelevant background or noise (choice A is wrong). Interposition is an important monocular depth perception cue that occurs when nearer surfaces overlap more distant surfaces. This is not relevant to any of the described experimental results (choice B is wrong). Procedural memory is the part of our implicit long-term memory that is responsible for our knowing how to do things related to motor skills. While procedural memory would almost certainly be activated during any reaction time response experiment (for example, when pressing a button), it does not explain why native Russian speakers had slower reaction times while performing a competing verbal task than while performing a competing spatial task (choice C is wrong).

2. **A** At the optic chiasm, the visual pathway directs information from the right field of vision of both eyes to the left side of the human brain and from the left field of vision of both eyes to the right side of the human brain. The hemispheres of the brain of an individual with a severed corpus callosum cannot communicate with each other. Since the linguistic processing centers of all human brains are located in the dominant hemisphere (which for over 99% of right-handed individuals is the left hemisphere), right-handed split brain individuals lack the ability to name objects present only in their left field of vision because this information travels exclusively to the right hemisphere of their brains. However, visual information

presented directly in front of either eye travels to both sides of any individual's brain. Thus, the reaction time difference reported in choice A cannot be attributed to the brain's linguistic hemispheric asymmetry, and therefore this reaction time difference cannot be used to support the hypothesis that linguistic categorization helps humans to discriminate between stimuli of differing linguistic categories (choice A is correct). The study results suggested in choice B would provide further evidence that the advantage enjoyed by Russian speakers in discriminating across versus within *siniy* and *goluboy* categories is a result of linguistic categorization because Wernicke's area is the region of the brain that is most important for language comprehension. If Russian speakers were to lose their advantage in distinguishing across linguistic categories when they lose their ability to comprehend language because of damage to Wernicke's area, this would indicate that their previous advantage was due to the linguistic categories of the Russian language (choice B supports the hypothesis and can be eliminated). The study results suggested in choice C would provide further evidence that linguistic categories help humans discriminate differences between stimuli because native speakers of English, a language that differentiates blue from green, discriminated stimuli across these linguistic category boundaries more quickly than did native speakers of a language that uses the same linguistic category (word) to describe both blue and green (choice C supports the hypothesis and can be eliminated). Finally, the study results suggested in choice D would also provide further evidence that linguistic categories help humans to discriminate differences between stimuli because visual stimuli presented in the right visual field is routed to the left hemisphere of the brain, where the linguistic processing centers of the brain of over 99% of right-handed individuals also reside. Thus, the reaction time advantage described in choice D could be attributed to the nearer proximity of the language processing centers of the brain to stimuli presented in the right visual field than to stimuli presented in the left visual field (choice D supports the hypothesis and can be eliminated).

3. **C** A comparison of the second darker shaded bar with the third darker shaded bar in Figure 1 shows that the mean reaction time of Russian language speakers was much lower (quicker) across *siniy* and *goluboy* categories when they were distracted by a competing spatial task than when they were distracted by a competing verbal task (choice C is correct). A comparison of the first three lighter shaded bars with the last three lighter shaded bars in Figure 1 shows that the mean reaction times of Russian language speakers were significantly higher (slower) within *siniy* and *goluboy* categories in all distracting conditions than were the comparable reaction times of native English language speakers (choice A is wrong). A comparison of the first three darker shaded bars with the last three darker shaded bars in Figure 1 shows that the mean reaction times of Russian language speakers were also significantly higher (slower) across *siniy* and *goluboy* categories in all distracting conditions than were the comparable reaction times of English language speakers (choice B is wrong). Although the passage text may have seemed to suggest that Russian speakers had an "advantage" over English speakers across *siniy* and *goluboy* categories, inspection of Figure 1 clearly shows that this so-called "advantage" did not reflect any absolute reaction time advantage of Russian speakers over English speakers in any experimental condition. Instead, this "advantage" was a reference to the lower mean reaction time of Russian speakers across *goluboy* and *siniy* categories compared to the mean reaction time of those same Russian speakers within those linguistic color categories, an advantage that was not observed in English speakers. A

comparison of last three darker shaded bars with the last three lighter shaded bars in Figure 1 shows that the mean reaction times of native English language speakers were roughly equivalent across and within *siniy* and *goluboy* categories in all three experimental conditions (choice D is wrong).

4. **D** Jean Piaget's theory of cognitive development suggests that children move through four different stages of mental development. His theory focuses not only on understanding how children acquire knowledge, but also on understanding the nature of intelligence. Piaget's four stages are the sensorimotor stage (birth to 2 years), the preoperational stage (ages 2 to 7), the concrete operational stage (ages 7 to 11), and the formal operational stage (ages 12 and up). In Piaget's theory, children do not begin to think symbolically and learn to use words and pictures to represent objects until they pass through the sensorimotor stage and into the preoperational stage (choice D is correct). In the pre-operational stage, children begin to think symbolically and learn to use words and pictures to represent objects and thus could demonstrate categorization advantages associated with linguistic categories (choice A is wrong). In the final formal operations stage of Piaget's theory, older children and adults can not only use and understand language, but they can also think abstractly and reason about hypothetical problems (choice B is wrong). Pre-conventional does not refer to one of the four stages in Piaget's cognitive development theory. This term instead refers to the first level of Kohlberg's stages of moral development (choice C is wrong).

5. **C** Linguistic relativity assumes that languages can differ significantly in the meanings of their words and syntactic constructions, the semantics of a language can affect the way in which its speakers perceive and conceptualize the world, and speakers of different languages think differently because of the differences in their languages. The advantage shown in the experiment by Russian speakers and not English speakers in discriminating colors across the *siniy* and *goluboy* categories is described in the passage as resulting from Russian and English languages' differing linguistic categorizations, and is thus both highly relevant to and highly consistent with linguistic relativity (choice C is correct). Nativist theory, championed by Noam Chomsky, suggests that humans are genetically hardcoded to learn language (choice A is wrong). Signal detection theory describes how an observer makes decisions about weak, uncertain, or ambiguous events or signals in the presence of both environmental and internal mental noise (choice B is wrong). The interactionist theory of language stresses the environment and the context in which a language is learned. This theory focuses on the pragmatics of language rather than its grammar, which according to this theory comes later (choice D is wrong).

6. **C** Categorical perception (CP) is the phenomenon by which the mental categories possessed by an observer alter an observers' perception of sensory stimuli. CP is demonstrated when an observer's ability to make perceptual discriminations between sensory stimuli is enhanced when those stimuli belong to different possessed mental categories rather than to the same possessed mental category. In the experiment described, native Russian speakers displayed a reaction time advantage when asked to discriminate between the *siniy* (dark blue) and *goluboy* (light blue) categories compared to when they were asked to discriminate within these two linguistic categories. This advantage was not displayed by native English speakers, whose native language categorizes both stimuli as blue. This provides evidence that differences in linguistic categorization between different native languages can influence CP (choice C is correct). While the *siniy/goluboy* versus blue categorization differences between

the Russian and English language could be described as cultural, the results of a single experiment cannot suggest that all differences in CP are culturally dependent (choice A is incorrect). Similarly, the results of a single experiment cannot suggest that all differences in CP are innate in all humans. In addition, nothing described in the passage implies that the CP measured was necessarily innate (choice B is incorrect). The results described in the passage text indicated that the verbal interference significantly increased the mean reaction response times across the *siniy* and *goluboy* categories for native Russian language speakers. In addition, Figure 1 indicated that both the spatial and verbal interference tasks increased the mean reactions times both within and across categories for both Russian and English speakers (choice D is incorrect).

Part 5

MCAT
General Chemistry

Chapter 23
Atomic and Molecular Structure and Properties

FREESTANDING QUESTIONS: ATOMIC AND MOLECULAR STRUCTURE AND PROPERTIES

1. A laboratory purchases a radiation meter with a detection limit of 5×10^{-8} µCi/mL. Given the typical sample collected by this researcher initially emitted 3.3×10^{-6} µCi/mL due to ^{14}C ($t_{1/2} = 5,700$ years), what is the oldest sample that can be carbon-dated with this detector?

   A) 5,700 years
   B) 23,000 years
   C) 34,000 years
   D) 57,000 years

2. A valence electron in each of the following atoms is excited to the next unoccupied energy level. Which will emit a photon with the greatest energy upon the return of the electron to the ground state?

   A) Ne
   B) Ar
   C) Kr
   D) Xe

3. Which of the following best describes the electron configuration of a cobalt(III) ion?

   A) $[Ar] 4s^2 3d^7$
   B) $[Ar] 4s^2 3d^9$
   C) $[Ar] 3d^6$
   D) $[Ar] 4s^1 3d^5$

4. The hybridization of the central carbon in $CH_3C \equiv N$ and the C—C—N bond angle are:

   A) sp^2 and 180°.
   B) sp and 180°.
   C) sp^2 and 120°.
   D) sp^3 and 109.5°.

5. ^{95}Tc undergoes electron capture, while ^{101}Tc undergoes beta emission. Which of the following statements explains why different nuclear reactions occur for these two isotopes?

   A) The nuclei of ^{95}Tc and ^{101}Tc are both too large.
   B) ^{95}Tc has too many protons and ^{101}Tc has too few neutrons.
   C) ^{95}Tc has too many neutrons and ^{101}Tc has too few neutrons.
   D) ^{95}Tc has too many protons and ^{101}Tc has too many neutrons.

6. All of the following molecules have a bent molecular shape EXCEPT:

   A) SO_2.
   B) HCN.
   C) H_2S.
   D) O_3.

7. How many resonance structures does carbonic acid (H_2CO_3) have?

   A) 0
   B) 2
   C) 3
   D) 4

8. Which of the following statements about effective nuclear charge (Z_{eff}) is correct?

   A) Z_{eff} is smaller than Z because of shielding from filled electron shells, and it causes atomic radius to increase across a row on the periodic table.
   B) A smaller Z_{eff} results in a more positive electron affinity on the right side of the periodic table.
   C) The increase in Z_{eff} going down a periodic table column is what results in increasing atomic radius.
   D) Valence electrons of Na experience a smaller Z_{eff} than those of Cl, contributing to Na having a larger atomic radius.

9. Which molecule has the largest dipole moment?

   A) HCl
   B) CCl_4
   C) BF_3
   D) CO_2

10. A researcher studying the olfactory system attempts to isolate the components forming the scent of coffee. She isolates two compounds of interest but finds one of the two generates significantly less vapor. What potential differences could account for this difference in volatility?

   I. Molecular mass
   II. Affinity to olfactory receptors
   III. Molecular polarity

   A) I only
   B) III only
   C) I and III only
   D) I, II, and III

ATOMIC AND MOLECULAR STRUCTURE AND PROPERTIES PRACTICE PASSAGE

Dioxygen (O_2) is notable in that its ground state electronic configuration, denoted as $X^3\Sigma_g^-$, is what is known as a triplet, meaning it contains a net electronic spin of ± 1. The first two excited states of O_2 both have singlet configurations (no net electronic spin), but differ in whether the spins are paired in the same π-antibonding orbital ($a^1\Delta_g$) or different π-antibonding orbitals ($X^1\Sigma_g^+$). Molecular orbital energy diagrams corresponding to these three electronic configurations are given in Figure 1.

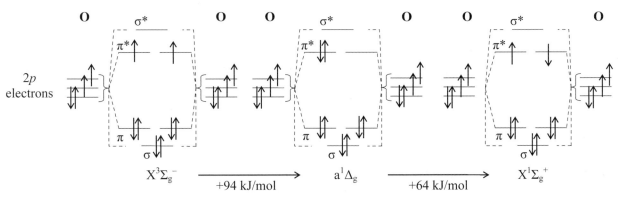

Figure 1 Electronic occupation of the molecular orbitals of O_2 in the three lowest energy states

Reactions of triplet dioxygen with organic materials, normally ground state electronic singlets, are what is known as "spin forbidden." On the other hand, the reaction of organic materials with singlet dioxygen is facile, resulting in singlet oxygen being very reactive and dangerous in the biological context. Carotenoids are a tetraterpenoid class of protective compounds known to deactivate singlet oxygen by promoting its relaxation to its triplet ground state. In particular, β-carotene has been shown in a number of studies to efficiently deactivate singlet oxygen in cultures of mammalian cells; however, more recent work using a newly developed laser technique allowing the excitation and monitoring of singlet dioxygen in the interior of individual cells failed to show any enhancement in the decay of singlet oxygen from β-carotene.

In this work, cell suspensions were treated with three different sensitizers, which absorb incident radiation and use it for the production of excited singlet oxygen. Once equilibrium was achieved, the cells were laser irradiated, and the lifetime (τ) of singlet oxygen was monitored. Three different deactivators, β-carotene, NaN_3, and BSA (bovine serum albumin), were also used in conjunction with the sensitizers. BSA is known to effectively deactivate singlet oxygen, but cannot diffuse into the interior of cells. NaN_3 is known as an effective singlet oxygen deactivator, and can easily pass into and out of living cells. The concentration of β-carotene shown previously to be necessary for the deactivation of singlet oxygen was proven to be present within cells by spectroscopic means prior to irradiation.

Sensitizer	Quenching agent	(μs) (overall cell suspension)	(μs) (individual cell interior)
Ppa	none	19	15
	BSA	20	17
	NaN_3	4	7
	β-carotene	32	16
FCh	none	20	19
	BSA	19	–
	NaN_3	–	14
	β-carotene	24	21
$AlPcS_4$	none	29	34
	BSA	13	36
	NaN_3	4	–
	β-carotene	39	31

Table 1 Measured lifetimes of singlet oxygen present in cell suspensions or interior of individual cells

1. Which of the following transitions requires the absorption of light of the shortest wavelength?

   A) $X^3\Sigma_g^- \rightarrow a^1\Delta_g$
   B) $X^1\Sigma_g^+ \rightarrow a^1\Delta_g$
   C) $a^1\Delta_g \rightarrow X^3\Sigma_g^-$
   D) $X^3\Sigma_g^- \rightarrow X^1\Sigma_g^+$

2. Which of the three sensitizers was most poorly confined within the cells?

   A) Ppa
   B) FCh
   C) $AlPcS_4$
   D) All three showed near complete confinement.

3. In which of the following electronic configurations is Hund's Rule obeyed?

   A) $a^1\Delta_g$
   B) $X^1\Sigma_g^+$
   C) $X^3\Sigma_g^-$
   D) $X^1\Sigma_g^+$ and $X^3\Sigma_g^-$

4. Despite showing no evidence for quenching singlet oxygen within mammalian cells, the presence of β-carotene was determined to extend the lifetime of irradiated cells. Which of the following is a likely explanation for this phenomenon?

   A) β-Carotene deactivates other high energy, reactive species produced in the irradiation.
   B) β-Carotene efficiently deactivates singlet oxygen in the extracellular medium, protecting the cell from attack from the outside.
   C) β-Carotene efficiently complexes singlet oxygen into other high energy singlet organic complexes, which can be eliminated from the cell by pumping or diffusion.
   D) β-Carotene concentrates in the hydrophilic domains of essential proteins, blocking the diffusion of singlet oxygen into the protein interior.

5. A hypothesis that intracellular deactivation of singlet oxygen is diffusion controlled, meaning that it is limited by the ability of singlet oxygen and deactivators to find one another in solution by random diffusion, is supported by which of the following?

   A) The relative lifetimes of singlet oxygen within the cell and in the suspension as a whole
   B) The fact that singlet oxygen diffuses much more slowly than triplet oxygen in solution
   C) The lack of intracellular deactivation of singlet oxygen by the large BSA protein
   D) The relative singlet oxygen lifetimes in the presence of β-carotene and NaN_3

SOLUTIONS TO FREESTANDING QUESTIONS: ATOMIC AND MOLECULAR STRUCTURE AND PROPERTIES

1. **C** Given each sample began with 3.3×10^{-6} μCi/mL of emitted radiation, the amount of radiation released following each half-life is as follows: 3.3×10^{-6} μCi/mL $\rightarrow$ 1.6×10^{-6} μCi/mL $\rightarrow$ 8.0×10^{-6} μCi/mL $\rightarrow$ 4.0×10^{-7} μCi/mL $\rightarrow$ 2.0×10^{-7} μCi/mL $\rightarrow$ 1.0×10^{-7} μCi/mL $\rightarrow$ 5.0×10^{-8} μCi/mL. Therefore, the oldest sample that can be dated by this detector will have decayed a total of six half-lives, or about 34,000 years (choice C is correct).

2. **A** Energy differences between electron levels become progressively smaller as the energy levels increase. For the simplified example of the Bohr atom, this relationship can be described by the equation: $E_n = -2.178 \times 10^{-18}$ J/n^2 where n represents the energy level of the electron. The atom with fewest electrons would therefore possess electrons in the lowest energy level and would undergo the largest transition (absorbing or releasing the most energy) when moving between energy levels (choice A is correct).

3   **C** Cobalt metal has an electron configuration of [Ar] $4s^2 3d^7$ (eliminate choice A). However, Co^{3+} has lost three electrons compared to the neutral atom, so it should have fewer electrons (eliminate choice B). While a few special elements in the Cr and Cu families adopt electron configurations with a half-filled s and half-filled d subshell, the cobalt ion does not follow this exception (eliminate choice D). Cobalt will lose its $4s$ valence electrons first to give a Co^{2+} ion, followed by one of its d electrons to give choice C as the correct answer.

4. **B** The central carbon has two bonding partners and no lone pairs of electrons. This indicates that the hybridization at this carbon is sp; as all sp hybridized carbons have linear (180°) bonding arrangements, choice B is the correct answer. Choice A is internally inconsistent, as sp^2 carbons have trigonal planar (120°) bonding arrangements, and therefore is incorrect. Choices C and D are not internally inconsistent, but simply give the wrong hybridizations.

5. **D** Nuclei that are unstable because they are too large typically undergo α decay (eliminate choice A). The end result of electron capture is the production of a neutron from a proton in the nucleus and a captured electron, which lowers the number of protons and increases the number of neutrons. Since ^{95}Tc undergoes electron capture, it has too many protons (eliminate choice C). Beta emission involves the conversion of a neutron into a proton and electron, which lowers the number of neutrons and increases the number of protons. ^{101}Tc undergoes β emission because it has too many neutrons (eliminate choice B).

6. **B** The shapes of all the molecules are depicted as follows. Only HCN is linear.

7. **C** Carbonic acid has the following resonance structures:

8. **D** Z_{eff} is the effective nuclear charge felt by an electron due to the repulsion of negative electrons in the filled shells between the valence electrons and the nucleus. From left to right on the periodic table, the number of protons increases but the number of filled shells remains constant, thus Z_{eff} increases and atomic radius decreases. This eliminates choice A and makes choice D the best answer. A larger Z_{eff} results in a more negative electron affinity on the right side of the periodic table, eliminating choice B. Finally, if Z_{eff} increased down a periodic table column, this would result in a smaller radius, making choice C incorrect.

9. **A** HCl (choice A) is a linear molecule with a very large dipole moment. While CCl_4 contains polar bonds, the tetrahedral shape of the molecule means all dipoles cancel one another, rendering the molecule nonpolar. The same is true for BF_3 (trigonal planar) and CO_2 (linear). As such, choice A is the only molecule with a dipole moment, so it is the correct answer.

10. **C** Since none of the Items appear in exactly two of the answer choices, it doesn't matter which Item you start analyzing. Item I is true: the difference in vapor (or vapor pressure) results from differences in the strength of the intermolecular forces of the two compounds, which is directly related to the molecular mass. Larger molecules have stronger London dispersion forces and therefore lower vapor pressures (eliminate choice B). Item II is false: while affinity for an olfactory receptor impacts our sense of smell, it will not influence the quantity of vapor present above a liquid (eliminate choice D). Item III is true: intermolecular forces are also affected by molecular polarity. More polar compounds have stronger IMFs and therefore lower vapor pressures (eliminate choice A; choice C is correct).

SOLUTIONS TO ATOMIC AND MOLECULAR STRUCTURE AND PROPERTIES PRACTICE PASSAGE

1. **D** The absorption of light indicates a transition from low energy to high energy. Choices B and C both describe the opposite kinds of transitions, going from high to low energy. Light with short wavelength is more energetic than light of long wavelengths, so the question asks for the transition of the highest energy. This corresponds to the $X^3\Sigma_g^- \rightarrow X^1\Sigma_g^+$ transition (158 kJ/mol) rather than the $X^3\Sigma_g^- \rightarrow a^1\Delta_g$ transition, which only requires 94 kJ/mol.

2. **C** The passage states that BSA effectively quenches singlet oxygen, but cannot pass into cells. Therefore, conditions where singlet oxygen is only produced within cells (meaning that the sensitizer is sequestered within the cell) should show little effect from BSA. The cell suspension lifetimes from PPa and FCh are essentially the same in the presence and absence of BSA, indicative of the singlet oxygen being produced within the cells. However, the data for $AlPcS_4$ shows a drop in lifetime in the cell suspension with the addition of BSA, meaning that singlet oxygen is being produced outside the cell, which indicates that this indicator moves freely into and out of cells.

3. **C**   Hund's Rule states that when filling degenerate energy levels (levels with exactly the same energy), the most stable configuration is one that maximizes the total amount of unpaired spin. This results in the "half-filled before whole-filled" motto associated with the law, and likewise means that that the half-filling must occur with electrons of the same spin (all arrow-up or all arrow-down). The only configuration of the three that fits this rule is $X^3\Sigma_g^-$.

4. **A**   The passage states that carotenoids are known as a protective class of compounds, the mechanism of which is certainly not limited to deactivating singlet oxygen. Irradiation with a high energy laser, causing the excitation of the sensitizer molecule, can result in energy transfer to any number of species in the vicinity of the sensitizer. While singlet oxygen is the excited state monitored here, a large number of possible harmful species may be produced in the process. Choice B may be eliminated, as the lifetime of extracellular singlet oxygen is longer in the presence of β-carotene than in its absence. Choice C may be eliminated, as such a complexation would remove singlet oxygen from the system, which would result in a decrease in its lifetime. Choice D may be eliminated because, as a terpenoid, β-carotene is a large hydrophobic molecule and as such would not segregate to hydrophilic environments.

5. **D**   There is no consistency between the relative values of singlet oxygen lifetimes inside the cell and in the suspension. This eliminates choice A. The laws of diffusion are governed by molecular motion, which in turn rely heavily on molecular speed. Molecular speed is, in turn, a function of mass, and as both kinds of oxygen (singlet and triplet) have the same mass, there will be no difference in their respective diffusion rates (eliminate choice B). The passage states that BSA cannot diffuse into the cell, a fact that eliminates choice C. Choice D is correct, as a tetraterpenoid such as β-carotene is much larger than NaN_3. This means that NaN_3 can diffuse faster than β-carotene, and since it shows better deactivation properties, this supports the hypothesis presented in the question.

Chapter 24
Thermodynamics

FREESTANDING QUESTIONS: THERMODYNAMICS

1. A mixture of ice and liquid water is placed in a thermally-conductive container and allowed to come to equilibrium with its surroundings in a room at 298 K. Which of the following is true if the system under consideration is the initial liquid water/ice mixture?

A) Heat flows from the system to the surroundings, and the entropy of the system increases.
B) Heat flows from the system to the surroundings, and the entropy of the system stays the same.
C) Heat flows from the surroundings to the system, and the entropy of the system increases.
D) Heat flows from the surroundings to the system, and the entropy of the system stays the same.

2. During the addition of 1 Joule to 1 kilogram of water, ice, or steam, which of the following statements is true given the specific heat of water (c) for each of these phases?

Phase	J/kg·°C
Liquid (water)	4186
Solid (ice)	2093
Gas (steam)	2009

A) The temperature change for steam will be the least.
B) The temperature change for ice will be the least.
C) The temperature change for steam will be the greatest.
D) The temperature change for liquid water will be the greatest.

3. The mathematical description of the Second Law of Thermodynamics allows the quantification of entropy for any transformation for which the temperature and heat input is known:

$$\Delta S = q/T$$

Which of the following statements is true regarding the entropy change associated with $H_2O(s) \rightarrow H_2O(l)$? ($\Delta H_{fus} = 334$ J/g, $\Delta H_{vap} = 2257$ J/g)

A) The entropy change associated with melting is positive and greater than that of vaporization.
B) The entropy change associated with melting is negative and smaller than that of vaporization.
C) The entropy change associated with vaporization is negative and smaller than that of melting.
D) The entropy change associated with vaporization is positive and greater than that of melting.

4. The metabolism of alcohol is aided by the enzyme alcohol dehydrogenase. If this enzyme successfully catalyzes the conversion of alcohol to acetaldehyde, which of the following statements is true?

A) ΔH of the catalyzed reaction is less than ΔH of the uncatalyzed reaction.
B) ΔH of the reaction is unaffected by the presence of a catalyst.
C) The free energy of the reactants is decreased.
D) The free energy of the products is increased.

5. In the formation of ethanol, yeast breaks a glucose molecule into two molecules of pyruvic acid via glycolysis, which are subsequently converted to alcohol via the decarboxylation reaction below:

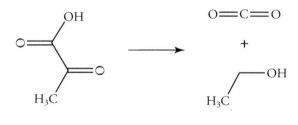

pyruvic acid　　　　　ethanol

Bond	Average Bond Dissociation Energy (kJ/mol)
C—C	335
C—H	413
C—O	327
O—H	467
C=O	799

If the conversion of one mole of glucose to two moles of pyruvic acid releases 61 kJ, which of the following is the correct ΔH_{rxn} for the overall conversion of glucose into ethanol and carbon dioxide?

A) −491 kJ
B) −1043 kJ
C) +491 kJ
D) −552 kJ

6. When ice is added to water above 0°C, it extracts energy from the water until thermal equilibrium is achieved. Considering the initial solid ice to be the thermodynamic system, which of the following best approximates the ΔH_{rxn} involved in the conversion of 100 g of ice at –5°C to liquid water at 10°C? [Note: ΔH_{fusion} = 334 kJ/kg, c_{ice} = 2.108 kJ/kg·°C, c_{liquid} = 4.184 kJ/kg·°C]

A) –38.5 kJ
B) +38.5 kJ
C) –33.4 kJ
D) +33.4 kJ

7. Which of the following reactions has the greatest increase in entropy?

A) $CH_4(g) + 2\ O_2(g) \rightarrow CO_2(g) + 2\ H_2O(g)$
B) $CH_3CH_2OH(aq) + NAD^+(aq) \rightarrow CH_3CHO(aq) + NADH(aq) + H^+(aq)$
C) $C_6H_{12}O_6(aq) + 6\ O_2(g) \rightarrow 6\ CO_2(g) + 6\ H_2O(g)$
D) $H_3CCOCOO^-(aq) + HSCoA(aq) + NAD^+(aq) \rightarrow H_3CCOSCoA(aq) + CO_2(aq) + NADH(aq)$

8. The decomposition of quartz (SiO_2) proceeds by the following reaction: $SiO_2 \rightarrow Si + O_2$. If ΔH_{rxn} = 910 kJ/mol and ΔS = 182 J/K·mol, which of the following statements must be true at 298 K?

A) ΔG is positive, and the reaction is nonspontaneous.
B) ΔG is positive, and the reaction is spontaneous.
C) ΔG is negative, and the reaction is nonspontaneous.
D) ΔG is negative, and the reaction is spontaneous.

9. Combustion reactions are typically thermodynamically favorable. For this class of reaction, which of the following must be true?

I. The reaction will take place rapidly.
II. ΔG for the reaction is negative.
III. The activation energy (E_a) for the reverse reaction is greater than the E_a for the forward reaction.

A) II only
B) I and III only
C) II and III only
D) I, II, and III

10. The combustion of glucose that occurs during cellular respiration is shown in the following series of equations:

$$C_6H_{12}O_6 \rightarrow 2\ C_2H_5OH + 2\ CO_2 \qquad \Delta H_1 = -74.4\ \text{kJ/mol}$$

$$2\ C_2H_5OH + 6\ O_2 \rightarrow 4\ CO_2 + 6\ H_2O \qquad \Delta H_2 = -2734\ \text{kJ/mol}$$

What is the heat of the reaction for the complete combustion of 90 grams of glucose to CO_2 in excess oxygen?

A) –2808.4 kJ
B) +2808.4 kJ
C) –1404.2 kJ
D) +1404.2 kJ

THERMODYNAMICS PRACTICE PASSAGE

Neonatal asphyxia, oxygen deficit during parturition, can lead to hypoxic ischemic organ damage and potentially a fatal outcome. This medical condition is caused by a combination of factors including hypotension and low blood oxygen in the mother from anesthesia. Treatment is achieved by using breathing machines to send rapid puffs of air into the newborn infant's lungs. To reduce asphyxic lesions to the brain, the infant is additionally placed under hypothermic conditions. This is achieved by cooling the infant to 33.5°C and maintaining this temperature for 72 hours.

Conventional cooling chambers utilize phase change materials (PCM), substances that possess high heats of fusion (ΔH_{fus}), and are capable of storing and releasing large amounts of heat at a constant temperature when they freeze or melt. When the surrounding temperature rises above the melting temperature of the material, heat is absorbed by the material as it undergoes the solid to liquid transition.

The primary consideration in choosing a PCM is ensuring that its melting point is close to the desired temperature of the system or process to which it is being applied, since the isothermal heat transfer during phase change will occur at this temperature. Other considerations include the magnitude of ΔH_{fus}, density, thermal conductivity, toxicity, flammability, and cost. Advances in packaging have overcome non-optimal toxicity or flammability profiles and the addition of highly conducting additives has enhanced the thermal conductivity of many PCMs.

Figure 1 below is a heating curve for a PCM, depicting how temperature (T) varies with the addition of heat (q). A related concept is how the specific heat of a substance varies with its phase. For example, the specific heat of $H_2O(s)$ is 2.108 kJ/kg·K, while that of $H_2O(l)$ is 4.184 kJ/kg·K.

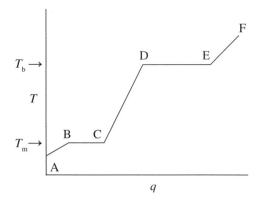

Figure 1 Heating curve

1. Most practical applications of phase change materials exploit the energy transfer during the solid-liquid transition rather than the liquid-vapor transition. Which of the following is the most reasonable explanation for this?

A) Substances exhibit a smaller change in temperature during their solid-liquid phase transition than during their liquid-vapor phase transition.
B) Substances typically absorb or release more heat during their solid-liquid phase transition than during their liquid vapor phase transition.
C) The volume change associated with the solid-liquid phase transition is much less than the volume change associated with the liquid-vapor phase transition.
D) The critical point for many materials occurs at relatively extreme temperatures and pressures.

2. Which of the following is true concerning the graph in Figure 1?

   I. The heat capacity of the solid phase can be obtained by measuring the area under the segment between points A and B.
   II. The heat capacity of the substance is smallest while it is a liquid.
   III. The average kinetic energy of the material increases while heat is transferred to it between points D and E.

A) I only
B) II only
C) II and III only
D) I, II, and III

3. A clothing designer manufactures a new line of thermoregulatory apparel using a PCM microencapsulated in flame retardant pellets woven into the fabric. Which of the following was the most critical property considered in choosing the PCM?

A) A melting point in the range of 30°C to 45°C
B) Low thermal conductivity
C) High density
D) Low solubility in aqueous solution

4. An ice cube weighing 18 grams is removed from a −10°C freezer. How much heat energy would be required to transform this ice cube into liquid water with a temperature of 10°C (ΔH_{fus} of water = 6.01 kJ/mol)?

A) 1.1 kJ
B) 5.0 kJ
C) 7.1 kJ
D) 109 kJ

5. In contrast to microencapsulation, initial attempts at macroencapsulation (containment of PCMs in large volume units) were largely unsuccessful. This led to the realization that PCMs function best in small volume cells. Which of the following is the most likely explanation?

A) The corrosive nature of many PCMs makes it difficult to identify suitable materials to contain them.
B) The increase in weight experienced when PCMs solidify makes large volume containment unfeasible.
C) The high cost of many PCMs makes high volume containment unfeasible.
D) The poor thermal conductivity of most PCMs causes them to solidify at the edges of large volume containers, preventing efficient heat transfer to the interior of larger cells.

SOLUTIONS TO FREESTANDING QUESTIONS: THERMODYNAMICS

1. **C** For this 2 × 2 type question, choices A and B may be eliminated, as heat is transferred from the ambient surroundings into the system. The final equilibrium will be 100% liquid water at room temperature. The liquid phase is higher in entropy (more random) than the solid phase, so melting the solid will increase the entropy of the system (eliminate choice D). In general, the addition of heat to a system increases molecular motion (rotational and vibrational motion, as well as translational motion), which results in an increase in randomness and higher entropy.

2. **C** The inverse relationship between c and ΔT, as expressed in the relationship $q = mc\Delta T$, indicates that the phase with the lowest c (steam; choice C) will have the highest ΔT. Even without the equation above, examining the units of specific heat can lead to the correct answer. The units of c are J/kg·°C, or the number of Joules required to raise 1 kg by 1°C. The value for ice is in the middle, so any choice including this phase is unlikely to be correct (eliminate choice B). Liquid water has the highest value, meaning it takes the most energy to raise the temperature 1°C (eliminate choice D), while steam has the lowest. If this is true, then the temperature change induced by the addition of energy will be the greatest for steam amongst the choices (eliminate choice A).

3. **D** Choices B and C can be eliminated because the entropy changes associated with both melting and vaporization are positive, not negative. Choice D is correct because vaporization involves an increase in entropy that is far greater in magnitude than the entropy change associated with melting. For 1 gram of water, $\Delta H_{fus} = 334$ J and $\Delta H_{vap} = 2257$ J. Accordingly, the $\Delta S_{fus} = (334 \text{ J})/(273 \text{ K}) = 1.22$ J/K and $\Delta S_{vap} = (2257 \text{ J})/(373 \text{ K}) = 6.05$ J/K. As shown here, the entropy change associated with vaporization is almost six times that of melting. This difference is due to the relatively more disordered state of water molecules in the gas phase than in the liquid phase.

4. **B** Choice B is correct; catalysts only affect kinetic factors of the reaction, most notably the activation energy, and thereby increase the rate at which a reaction proceeds. Free energy and enthalpy are thermodynamic quantities, and hence are unaffected by the addition of a catalyst.

5. **B** The breakdown of pyruvic acid can be considered to take place by looking at the net change of the types of bonds broken versus the types of bonds formed, namely, breaking one C—C bond and replacing it with two C—H bonds (to C-2 of pyruvic acid). The following equation may be written for a rough estimate of the enthalpy of reaction:

$$\Delta H_{rxn} = \Sigma(\text{BDE bonds broken}) - \Sigma(\text{BDE bonds formed})$$

$$\Delta H_{rxn} = (1 \text{ C—C}) - (2 \times \text{C—H})$$

$$\Delta H_{rxn} = (335) - (2 \times 413) = -491 \text{ kJ/mol}$$

This result must be multiplied by two (–982 kJ/mol glucose) because each molecule produces two pyruvic acid molecules. On top of this, the initial breakdown of glucose must be included (–61 kJ/mol), to give a final enthalpy change of –1043 kJ/mol glucose.

6. **B**   Choice B is correct because it represents the sum of the three heats that comprise the warming and melting process described. The pertinent heats are as follows:

$$q_{ice} = (0.1\ kg)(\sim2\ kJ/kg\cdot°C)(5°C) = \sim1\ kJ$$

$$q_{fus} = (0.1\ kg)(334\ kJ/kg) = 33.4\ kJ$$

$$q_{water} = (0.1\ kg)(4.184\ kJ/kg\cdot°C)(10°C) = \sim4\ kJ$$

The sum of these represents the heat of the phase change as follows:

$$q_{ice} + q_{fus} + q_{water} = \sim1\ kJ + 33.4\ kJ + \sim4\ kJ = +38.4\ kJ.$$

Choices A and C can be eliminated, as they suggest that the solid ice loses heat in an exothermic process while melting and increasing temperature. The amount of energy in choice D only accounts for the phase change portion of the process, and it neglects the two warming stages.

7. **C**   The entropy change of a reaction is dependent on the relative numbers of moles of reactants versus products, and it is also greatly affected by a change in state from a solid or liquid to the gas phase. Choice A can be eliminated since all species are in the gas phase, and there are three moles of both reactants and products. Similarly, choice D can be eliminated since all species are in the aqueous phase, and there are three moles of both reactants and products. While choice B does show an increase in entropy by going from two moles of aqueous reactants to three, choice C is a better answer because there are six moles of gaseous reactants and twelve moles of gaseous products. The change of state will result in a much larger change in entropy than the change in the numbers of aqueous moles in the reaction described in choice B.

8. **A**   For this 2 × 2 style question, first eliminate the two choices that are inconsistent with the relationship between the sign for ΔG and the spontaneity of a reaction. Since spontaneous reactions have $\Delta G < 0$, choices B and C are false. To find the Gibbs free energy for any reaction, the following equation can be used: $\Delta G = \Delta H - T\Delta S$. At 298 K, the rough calculation should look like:

$$\Delta G = \sim900\ kJ/mol - (\sim300\ K)(\sim0.2\ kJ/K\cdot mol) = 840\ kJ/mol$$

Since $\Delta G > 0$, the reaction will be nonspontaneous, and choice A is correct.

9. **C**   Start by analyzing Item I, since it appears in exactly two answer choices; whether it is true or false, you can eliminate half the answers. Item I is false: how quickly a reaction occurs is related to reaction kinetics, and it has nothing to do with thermodynamics (choices B and D can be eliminated). Since Item II appears in both of the remaining answer choices, it must be true, and you can focus on Item III. Item III is true: despite the fact that E_a is formally a kinetic quantity, the difference between the values of E_a for the forward and reverse reactions will be ΔG. If the free energy of the products is less than the free energy of the reactants, as it must be in a reaction with $\Delta G < 0$, E_a of the reverse reaction will be greater than E_a of the forward reaction (choice A can be eliminated, and choice C is correct). Note that Item II is in fact true: the question described the reaction as favorable, implying that the ΔG of the reaction is negative.

10.   **C**   The complete combustion of glucose is the combination of both equations 1 and 2. These two can be combined and written as the overall equation shown below:

$$C_6H_{12}O_6 + 6\ O_2 \rightarrow 6\ CO_2 + 6\ H_2O \quad \Delta H_{rxn} = -2808.4 \text{ kJ/mol}$$

The molecular weight of glucose is ~180 g/mol. As 90 g is 0.5 mol glucose, the total energy change will be half of the molar heat of reaction, or –1404.2 kJ. Choice A assumes the combustion of 1 mol of glucose. Both choices B and D indicate an endothermic reaction and can therefore be eliminated.

SOLUTIONS TO THERMODYNAMICS PRACTICE PASSAGE

1.   **C**   Given that the gas phase of a substance occupies a much larger volume than its liquid phase, high volume or high pressure containment would be required if the liquid-vapor phase transition were to be exploited. The volume change accompanying a liquid-solid transition is much more modest by contrast (choice C is correct). A phase change is an isothermal process (eliminate choice A). Substances have higher heats of vaporization than heats of fusion because more intermolecular interactions need to be formed or broken in the liquid-vapor transition than in the solid-liquid transition (eliminate choice B). The critical point is the temperature and pressure above which a substance takes on the characteristic of a supercritical fluid, which is neither gas nor liquid, and is not relevant to the question (eliminate choice D).

2.   **B**   Start by analyzing Item I, since it appears in exactly two of the answer choices; whether it is true or false, you can eliminate half the answers. Item I is false: the equation relating temperature to heat, $q = Cp\Delta T$, can be rearranged to give $Cp = q/\Delta T$. This does not equal the area underneath the curve on a T vs. q graph (choices A and D can be eliminated). As both remaining answer choices contain Item II, it must be correct, and you can focus on Item III. Item III is false: the segment described represents a phase change, which is isothermal. This is confirmed by the zero slope of this graph segment. Since temperature is a measure of average kinetic energy, an isothermal process implies no change in average kinetic energy. During phase changes, energy is used to overcome intermolecular forces, not contribute to increased molecular motion (choice C can be eliminated, and choice B is correct). Note that Item II is in fact true: the segment corresponding to heating of the liquid phase has the steepest slope, meaning that a small amount of heat is required to cause a large change in temperature.

3.   **A**   The passage points out that the primary consideration in choosing a PCM is ensuring that its melting point is close to the desired temperature of the system or process to which it is being applied. Since 30°C to 45°C is a range straddling normal body temperature (37°C), this was the defining criterion for choosing the material (choice A is correct). Low thermal conductivity would reduce the ability of the PCM to absorb or release energy (eliminate choice B), and high density would not be practical for a garment (eliminate choice C). No mention is made of phase change materials needing to be in aqueous solution or be water soluble (eliminate choice D).

4. **C** The solution to this question involves calculating and summing the heat transfer in 3 parts. The first (q_1) accounts for the heat needed to warm the ice from $-10°C$ to $0°C$:

$$q_1 = mc_{ice} \Delta T = (0.018\text{kg})(\sim 2 \text{ kJ/kg} \cdot \text{K})(10 \text{ K}) \approx 0.36 \text{ kJ}$$

The second (q_2) accounts for the heat absorbed during the melting transition:

$$q_2 = n(\Delta H_f) = [(18 \text{ g})/(18 \text{ g/mol})](\sim 6 \text{ kJ/mol}) \approx 6 \text{ kJ}$$

The third (q_3) accounts for the heat needed to warm the resulting water from $0°C$ to $10°C$:

$$q_3 = mc_{water} \Delta T = (0.018\text{kg})(\sim 4 \text{ kJ/kg} \cdot \text{K})(10 \text{ K}) \approx 0.72 \text{ kJ}$$

Summing the heats for each step yields $q_1 + q_2 + q_3 = 0.36 \text{ kJ} + 6 \text{ kJ} + 0.72 \text{ kJ} \approx 7 \text{ kJ}$, which is closest to choice C. Note that calculating only the energy required during melting eliminates choices A and B, and given the magnitude of choice D, it can also be eliminated.

5. **D** The correct answer to this question should explain specifically why phase change materials function more effectively in small volume cells than large volume units. If a material were corrosive, it would be equally difficult to find suitable materials to make either small or large cells (eliminate choice A). The mass of a substance does not change when undergoing a phase transition (eliminate choice B). While many phase change materials are costly, this does not explain why small cells function more effectively than large cells (eliminate choice C). Thermal conductivity must directly affect the ability of the PCM to exchange heat with the surroundings (choice D is correct by Process of Elimination).

Chapter 25
Phases and Gases

FREESTANDING QUESTIONS: PHASES AND GASES

1. According to the following phase diagram, which combination of pressure and temperature (P,T) would result in the diamond phase of tin?

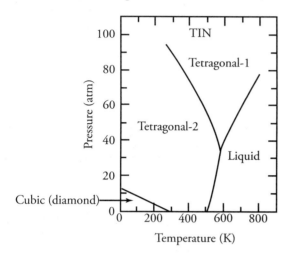

Temperature (K)

A) 10 atm, 200 K
B) 5 atm, 600 K
C) 5 atm, 100 K
D) 32 atm, 600 K

2. A balloon is filled with 2 L of He at sea level. If the temperature of the gas is increased from 23°C to 123°C, what is the resultant volume of the balloon?

A) ~1.3 L
B) ~2.7 L
C) ~6.3 L
D) ~12 L

3. Which of the following statements regarding H_2O is false?

A) A decrease in pressure can turn solid water into a liquid.
B) A decrease in temperature can cause conversion of a gas to a liquid, then solid state.
C) A decrease in temperature can cause conversion of a gas immediately to a solid state.
D) A decrease in pressure cannot induce a phase change of a gas into a solid.

4. If samples of the following gases are held at the same temperature, which of the following will be true regarding the average molecular velocity of the gas molecules?

Gas 1: B_2Cl_4

Gas 2: UF_6

Gas 3: BCl_3

Gas 4: ICl

A) All four gases will have the same molecular velocity.
B) B_2Cl_4 and BCl_3 will have the most similar molecular velocities of the four.
C) UF_6 will have the largest molecular velocity of the four.
D) B_2Cl_4 and ICl will have the most similar molecular velocities of the four.

5. Extracted natural gas is 95 mol% methane (CH_4), but it also contains ethane (2.5%), dinitrogen (1.6%), and carbon dioxide (0.7%). The pressure of natural gas in the Earth's crust can be up to 600 bar. At this pressure, what is the partial pressure of ethane?

A) 15 bar
B) 10 bar
C) 30 bar
D) 2.5 bar

6. Purification of uranium isotopes (^{234}U, ^{236}U, ^{238}U, and ^{239}U) by a sensitive separation using finely tuned diffusion across an inert membrane has been successfully carried out using $UF_6(g)$ as the mobile uranium species. A similar experiment using $UBr_4(g)$ as the mobile compound yielded very poor isotopic separation. Which is a plausible explanation for this result?

A) Bromine may only form strong bonds with the heaviest uranium isotopes.
B) Bromine is environmentally present as ^{79}Br and ^{81}Br in approximately equal amounts.
C) Residual Br^- is more basic than F^-, leading to degradation of the membrane.
D) Uranium in UF_6 is present in the +5 oxidation state, while in UBr_4 it is present in the +4 oxidation state.

7. Which of the following gases behave most ideally?

A) CO_2 at high T and low P
B) CO_2 at low T and high P
C) H_2S at high T and low P
D) H_2S at low T and high P

8. What would the expected molar volume of an ideal gas be under typical Martian winter conditions of $-100°C$ and 6×10^{-3} atm?

A) 2.3×10^2 L
B) 2.3×10^3 L
C) 7.5×10^3 L
D) 7.5×10^4 L

9. The liquid and gas phases of any substance are unique, but many substances are capable of existing in different solid phases, depending on the equilibrium stacking of molecules at a specific temperature and pressure. Which of the following is common to all solid phases of a given material?

A) All solid phases maximize dipole-dipole interactions.
B) All solid phases are arranged to alternate discrete positive and negative charges within the crystal lattice.
C) Incremental increases in temperature change every solid phase directly to the liquid phase, regardless of pressure.
D) All solid phases have a lower value of entropy ($S°$) than the liquid or gas phases.

10. Which of the following would have the greatest effect on the vapor pressure of 1 L of diethyl ether, $CH_3CH_2OCH_2CH_3$?

A) Increasing the temperature of the diethyl ether
B) Increasing the surface area of diethyl ether
C) Reducing the surface area of diethyl ether
D) Reducing the external pressure on diethyl ether

PHASES AND GASES PRACTICE PASSAGE

In the study of gases, the assumption of ideal behavior significantly simplifies calculations. This does not yield sufficiently accurate results in many cases, as gases violate the assumed aspects of ideal behavior to varying degrees. To correct for real gas behavior, scientists use several methods including evaluating the compressibility factor (Z) for a gas, and using a modified ideal gas equation. The compressibility factor, a measure of deviation from ideal gas behavior, can be calculated using Equation 1.

$$Z = \frac{PV}{nRT}$$

Equation 1

The compressibility factor for an unknown gas at varying temperatures is shown in Figure 1. At low temperatures, gas molecules move more slowly. At high pressures, gas molecules are closer together leading to more pronounced intermolecular interactions.

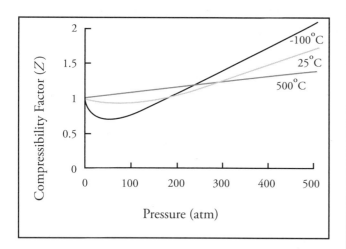

Figure 1 Compressibility factor variation with temperature and pressure

The van der Waals equation (Equation 2), a modification of the ideal gas equation adjusted to account for deviations from ideal behavior, allows for corrections to be made for real gases based on measured pressures and volumes.

$$\left(P + \frac{an^2}{V^2}\right)(V - nb) = nRT$$

Equation 2

In hopes of characterizing the deviations from ideal behavior for several gases, a researcher performs a series of experiments. She takes several measurements of each gas under varied conditions to determine the constants (a and b) found in the van der Waals equation, in which P is the measured pressure, V is the measured volume, n is the number of moles, and T is temperature. Her results are recorded in Table 1.

Gas (T = 273 K)	a (atm·L^2·mol^{-2})	b (L·mol^{-1})
He	0.03	0.03
Ar	1.3	0.04
O$_2$	1.3	0.04
CO	1.5	0.05
CH$_4$	2.4	0.05
H$_2$O	5.6	0.04

Table 1 Experimentally determined van der Waals constants for several gases

1. From the ideal gas equation, the following relationship can be established:

$$\overline{E}_{trans} = \frac{3}{2}k_B T$$

where $\overline{E}_{trans}$ is the average kinetic energy of the gas and k_B is the Boltzmann constant. All of the following are true regarding this relationship EXCEPT:

A) temperature is related to molecular momentum.
B) gases with equal temperature possess equal average molecular velocities.
C) k_B does not vary with temperature change.
D) decreased $\overline{E}_{trans}$ at high pressures results in an increased compressibility factor (Z).

2. Which of the following compressibility factor vs. pressure curves best characterizes an ideal gas?

A)

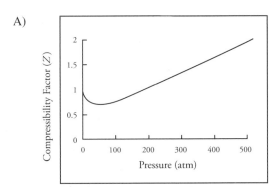

B)

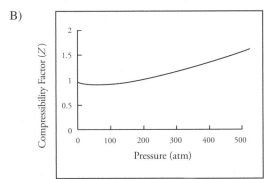

C)

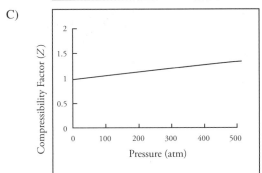

D)

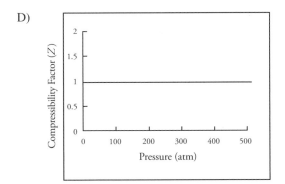

3. In the van der Waals equation, which properties are most likely accounted for by a and b, respectively?

A) Attractive forces and molecular volume
B) Attractive forces and molecular speed
C) Molecular volume and attractive forces
D) Molecular volume and boiling point

4. The researcher performs an additional set of experiments where she quantifies the compressibility factor for several known gases at room temperature and 100 atm.

Gas	Z
H_2	1.1
N_2	0.9
CO_2	0.4

A fourth gas was measured with a compressibility factor of 0.8. What is the most likely identity of this fourth gas?

A) Br_2
B) NH_3
C) CH_4
D) H_2O

5. A 50 L gas canister is filled with 0.50 mol of gaseous He and 0.50 mol of gaseous UF_6, and is heated to 500 K. Barometric measurements found the partial pressure of UF_6 to be 0.50 atm. Which of the following represents the most likely value measured for the total pressure in the canister?

A) 1.00 atm
B) 0.90 atm
C) 0.50 atm
D) 1.15 atm

6. Thermodynamic compressibility is a measure of the change in V induced by changes in P as expressed in the ratio $\Delta V / \Delta P$. Equal volumes of water equilibrated at which of the following temperatures will have the smallest thermodynamic compressibility?

A) 570 K
B) 500 K
C) 420 K
D) 370 K

SOLUTIONS TO FREESTANDING QUESTIONS: PHASES AND GASES

1. **C** Below is the placement of 5 atm and 100 K on the phase diagram, falling inside the area of the phase diagram marked for the diamond phase of tin.

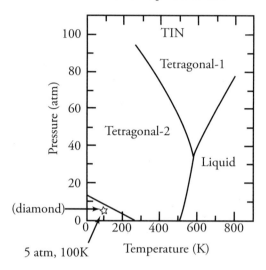

Choice A falls in the range for the tetragonal-2 phase, choice B falls in the liquid region, and choice D falls at the triple point of the phase diagram.

2. **B** So long as the balloon is held at sea level, the pressure is fixed at 1 atm. At constant pressure, Charles's Law applies to changes in T and V by the following relation (temperatures expressed in Kelvins):

$$(V_1/T_1) = (V_2/T_2)$$

$$(2/{\sim}300) = (V_2/{\sim}400)$$

$$V_2 \approx 800/300 \approx 2.66$$

3. **A** Since the phase diagram for water has a uniquely "backward-sloping" line dividing the solid and liquid states, it is impossible for a decrease in pressure (y-axis) to cause conversion of solid water into a liquid (choice A is correct). Depending on the pressure, a decrease in temperature (x-axis) can cause conversion of a gas to a liquid and ultimately to a solid, or the direct conversion of a gas to a solid (choices B and C are true and thus incorrect for this question). Depending on the temperature, an *increase* in pressure can cause conversion of gaseous water to a solid state (choice D is true and therefore incorrect).

4. **D** Kinetic molecular theory says that the molecular velocities of gas molecules can be derived from their kinetic energy, given by $(1/2)mv^2$, where m is the molecular mass and v is the molecular velocity. All four gases have the same average kinetic energy, as they all share the same temperature. Since their masses are not all the same, they will not all have the same molecular velocity (eliminate choice A). UF_6 is the heaviest of the four gases presented,

meaning it will have the lowest value of v (eliminate choice C). The molecular masses of the four gases are as follows: B_2Cl_4, ~163; UF_6, ~352; BCl_3, ~117; ICl, ~162. From comparison of B_2Cl_4, BCl_3 and ICl, it is apparent that choice D is the correct answer.

5. **A**   Dalton's Law of Partial Pressures says that $P_{total} = P_{gas1} + P_{gas2} + P_{gas3}...$, and so on. Therefore, assuming all the gases act ideally, if ethane is 2.5 mol% of the total composition of the gas, it will comprise 2.5% of the total pressure. Compute the partial pressure of ethane as follows:

$$(600 \text{ bar})(0.025) =$$

$$(600 \text{ bar})(2.5 \times 10^{-2}) =$$

$$(6)(2.5) = (6)(2 + 0.5) = 12 + 3 = 15 \text{ bar}$$

6. **B**   Choice A can be eliminated, as different isotopes do not generally present discernible differences in reaction chemistry. F^- is a more basic anion than Br^- (eliminate choice C), and the uranium in UF_6 is in the +6 oxidation state, which furthermore will not affect diffusion properties (eliminate choice D). Bromine exists as ^{79}Br (50.6%) and ^{81}Br (49.3%), while fluorine is only naturally available as ^{19}F. This complicates the weight distribution in a sample of UBr_4. For example, molecules consisting of ^{238}U, two ^{79}Br, and two ^{81}Br will have the same overall mass as a molecule made up of ^{236}U, one ^{79}Br, and three ^{81}Br. Many other combinations are available which yield equal masses for compounds with different U isotopes. Since purification by diffusion relies on differences in the molecular velocities of compounds, which in turn are functions of molecular mass, diffusion will not yield an effective separation of different U isotopes. Fluorine, with only one mass, does not present this issue, and it allows efficient separation by diffusion of UF_6.

7. **A**   Gases behave most ideally at high T and low P (eliminate choices B and D). Ideal gases do not experience forces of attraction between molecules; thus gases with weaker intermolecular forces are more ideal. CO_2 is nonpolar, while H_2S is polar and experiences dipole-dipole interactions. Thus, CO_2 behaves more ideally (eliminate choice C; choice A is correct).

8. **B**   This question calls for solving the Ideal Gas Law for volume with the value of the Ideal Gas Law constant R being approximately 0.08 L·atm·mol^{-1}·K^{-1}

$$PV = nRT$$

$$V = nRT/P$$

$$V = (1 \text{ mol})(0.08 \text{ L·atm·mol}^{-1}\text{·K}^{-1})(173 \text{ K})/(6 \times 10^{-3} \text{ atm})$$

$$V \approx (1 \text{ mol})(8 \times 10^{-2})(1.75 \times 10^2)/(6 \times 10^{-3} \text{ atm})$$

$$V \approx (14/6) \times 10^3 \text{ L}$$

$$14/6 \approx 2.3$$

Therefore, choice B is correct.

9. **D** Solid phases involve very limited mobility of molecules, and they are often very orderly arrangements of molecules into crystal lattices. When compared to the comparatively greater mobility available to molecules in the liquid and gas phases, the freezing and ordering of molecules results in low values of entropy. Choices A and B can be eliminated, as nonpolar molecules are capable of forming solid phases, as are non-ionic materials. Choice C can be eliminated with the knowledge that many solids sublimate directly to the gas phase with increasing temperatures, particularly at low pressures.

10. **A** Vapor pressure is dependent solely on the intermolecular forces a compound has and its temperature (choice A is correct). The amount of surface area has no impact (eliminate choices B and C), and while external pressure affects the boiling point, it does not affect the vapor pressure of a liquid (eliminate choice D).

SOLUTIONS TO PHASES AND GASES PRACTICE PASSAGE

1. **B** Choice B is the correct answer choice because it is a false statement: gases at equal temperatures have equal average kinetic energies ($\frac{1}{2}mv^2$), but not necessarily equal velocities (v) because their masses (m) may differ. From the equation in the question, temperature is related to molecular momentum (mv) since it is related to average kinetic energy (choice A is a true statement and can be eliminated). The Boltzmann constant, with units of J/K, relates energy per unit temperature. As a constant, it should therefore be independent of the absolute quantity of temperature (choice C is a true statement and can be eliminated). Finally, Figure 1 shows that Z and T (average kinetic energy) are inversely related at high pressures (choice D is true and can be eliminated)

2. **D** Looking at Equation 1, a value of $Z = 1$ results in the Ideal Gas Law, implying that a compressibility factor equal to this represents an ideal gas. Choice D shows a gas with a constant value of $Z = 1$.

3. **A** The passage states that the van der Waals equation corrects for real pressures and volumes. Looking at Equation 2, a is associated with the pressure term, while b is associated with the volume term. At high pressures and low temperatures, real gas molecules experience attractive forces and the gas is more compressible. The real gas pressure is therefore lower than ideal pressure and requires an additive correction ($P_{ideal} = P_{real} + an^2/V^2$). At high pressures, real gas molecular volume becomes significant and the gas is less compressible. The real gas volume is therefore higher than ideal volume and requires a subtractive correction ($V_{ideal} = V_{real} - nb$).

4. **C** Compressibility of $Z = 0.8$ is relatively close to the ideal value of $Z = 1$. The table shows that the small, prototypically inert gases H_2 and N_2 each have Z values near 1 under the studied conditions. Molecules which best exhibit ideal gas behavior have low molecular weights and weak intermolecular forces. Ammonia and water undergo hydrogen bonding, a strong intermolecular force, eliminating choices B and D. Bromine, which is nonpolar like methane, is nonetheless heavier than methane with a larger molecular volume, eliminating choice A and leaving choice C as the best answer.

5. **A**   A calculation of the pressure of UF_6 acting ideally (below) reveals a theoretical pressure equal to the measured pressure.

$$PV = nRT$$

$$P \approx ((0.5\ \text{mol})(0.1\ \text{L·atm·mol}^{-1}\text{·K}^{-1})(500\ \text{K}))/(50\ \text{L}))$$

$$P \approx 0.5\ \text{atm}$$

If UF_6 acts ideally at a specific temperature and pressure, it is safe to assume He does as well. Equal molar amounts of the two gases would result in identical pressures, and by Dalton's Law of Partial Pressures, the total pressure is the sum of the two.

6. **D**   Whereas compressibility does change with changes in temperature, the most important difference in the answer choices is that the equilibrium phase of water at three of the listed temperatures (choices A, B, and C) is gas, while the last (choice D) is liquid. As a rule, liquids are substantially less compressible than gases.

Chapter 26
Kinetics

FREESTANDING QUESTIONS: KINETICS

1. A chemist wishes to measure the rate of the reaction described below. What best describes the rate of the reaction?

$$2 S_2O_3^{2-}(aq) + I_2(aq) \rightarrow S_4O_6^{2-}(aq) + 2 I^-(aq)$$

A) Two times the rate of disappearance of $S_2O_3^{2-}$
B) Rate of disappearance of I_2
C) One-half the rate of formation of $S_4O_6^{2-}$
D) Two times the rate of formation of I^-

2. What is the rate law for the mechanism shown?

$$H_2(g) + ICl(g) \rightarrow HI(g) + HCl(g) \text{ (slow)}$$
$$HI(g) + ICl(g) \rightarrow I_2(g) + HCl(g) \text{ (fast)}$$

A) rate = $k[ICl]$
B) rate = $k[H_2][ICl]$
C) rate = $k[H][ICl]^2$
D) rate = $k[HI][ICl]$

3. The rate law for the first step in the thermal decomposition of acetaldehyde was determined to be rate = $k[CH_3CHO]^{3/2}$. What are the units of k?

A) s^{-1}
B) Ms^{-1}
C) $M^{-1/2}s^{-1}$
D) $M^{-3/2}s^{-1}$

4. Addition of a catalyst to the second step in the following mechanism will have what impact on the overall reaction rate?

$$2 NO(g) \rightarrow N_2O_2(g) \text{ (slow)}$$
$$N_2O_2(g) + O_2(g) \rightarrow 2 NO_2(g) \text{ (fast)}$$

A) Increase the overall reaction rate by lowering activation energy
B) Increase the overall reaction rate by stabilizing the transition state
C) Increase the overall reaction rate by increasing reactant concentrations
D) Have no effect on the overall reaction rate

5. A research team studying the oxidation of bromide by hypochlorite has proposed a three-step reaction mechanism. Which of the following, if true, would lend support to the mechanism as shown below?

$$OCl^- + H_2O \rightarrow HOCl + OH^- \text{ (fast)}$$
$$HOCl + Br^- \rightarrow HOBr + Cl^- \text{ (slow)}$$
$$HOBr + OH^- \rightarrow OBr^- + H_2O \text{ (fast)}$$

A) Catalyzing the first step of the mechanism will increase the overall reaction rate.
B) The addition of KBr increases the overall reaction rate.
C) The overall rate law is zero order for HOCl.
D) Doubling both [HOCl] and [Br$^-$] causes the reaction rate to double.

6. Given the experimental results below, what is the rate law for the reaction in question?

Experiment	$[NH_4^+]$	$[NO_2^-]$	Rate (M/s)
1	1.2×10^{-3}	3.2×10^{-4}	1.9×10^{-7}
2	4.6×10^{-3}	3.4×10^{-4}	7.8×10^{-7}
3	1.2×10^{-3}	6.4×10^{-4}	3.8×10^{-7}
4	1.4×10^{-2}	3.4×10^{-4}	2.5×10^{-6}

A) rate $= k[NH_4^+]$
B) rate $= k[NH_4^+][NO_2^-]$
C) rate $= k[NH_4^+]^2[NO_2^-]$
D) rate $= k[NH_4^+][NO_2^-]^2$

7. What can be concluded about the reaction diagrammed below?

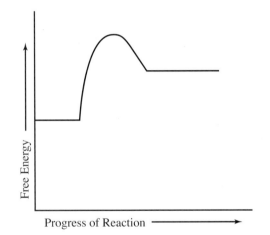

A) The reaction absorbs heat.
B) The reaction is spontaneous.
C) Increasing temperature decreases E_a.
D) $E_a > \Delta G$

8. A chemist is studying the following reaction mechanism and notes that when he adds IO^- to the reaction mixture, the rate of the overall reaction increases. What best describes IO^- in this reaction?

$$H_2O_2(aq) + I^-(aq) \rightarrow H_2O(l) + IO^-(aq) \text{ (fast)}$$
$$H_2O_2(aq) + IO^-(aq) \rightarrow H_2O(l) + O_2(g) + I^-(aq) \text{ (slow)}$$

A) An intermediate
B) A homogeneous catalyst
C) A heterogeneous catalyst
D) An uncompetitive inhibitor

9. Monitoring the reaction $2\,NO + 2\,H_2 \rightarrow 2\,H_2O + N_2$ by infrared spectroscopy indicated the quick production and accumulation of a species believed to be N_2O_2, followed by its gradual consumption. From this observation, a mechanism involving the following three steps was postulated:

Step 1: $NO + NO \rightarrow N_2O_2$
Step 2: $N_2O_2 + H_2 \rightarrow N_2O + H_2O$
Step 3: $N_2O + H_2 \rightarrow N_2 + H_2O$

Which of the following rate laws is consistent with the experimental observations, and the proposed mechanism?

A) Rate $= k[N_2O_2][H_2]$
B) Rate $= k[NO]^2[H_2]^2$
C) Rate $= k[NO]^2[H_2]$
D) Rate $= k[NO][H_2][N_2O_2]$

10. Given the rate law constant (k), activation energy (E_a), temperature in Kelvin (T), and gas law constant (R), a plot of $\ln(k)$ vs. $1/T$ will result in which of the following functions?

A) An exponential increase equal to $e^{(E_a/RT)}$
B) An exponential decrease equal to $e^{(-E_a/RT)}$
C) A linear increase with slope equal to E_a/R
D) A linear decrease with slope equal to $-E_a/R$

KINETICS PRACTICE PASSAGE

Legionnaires' disease is a serious type of pneumonia with symptoms including cough, shortness of breath, and fever. The responsible pathogen is *Legionella* bacteria, which is found naturally in freshwater environments. It may pose a serious health concern in communities with water that is not properly treated. Industrial water treatment can be achieved using various methods such as the application of biocides. One biocide used is bromine monochloride, which can be produced using the following reaction:

$$Cl(g) + Br_2(g) \rightarrow BrCl(g) + Br(g)$$

Reaction 1

This reaction is an example of a bimolecular reaction where two reactants collide to form one activated complex. The rate of a bimolecular reaction depends in part on the frequency of collisions between two molecules that occur with sufficient energy to create a reactive complex. The change in concentration of the reactants and products can be monitored over time, as depicted in Figure 1, and can be used to approximate the rate of a reaction. A tangential line to the initial portion of the slope can approximate the initial rate of the reaction. From the data presented in Figure 1, the rate law for Reaction 1 was determined to follow second-order kinetics, being first order in both [Cl] and [Br$_2$].

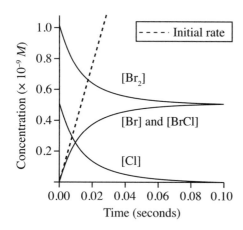

Figure 1   Reaction between Br$_2$ and Cl at 304 K

Although the rate constant is determined experimentally, for a bimolecular reaction in the gas phase, it can be estimated using Equation 1:

$$k_T = Z\rho e^{\left(\frac{-E_a}{RT}\right)}$$

Equation 1

where ρ is the steric factor, E_a is the activation energy, R is the gas constant, T is the temperature, and Z is the collision frequency. The steric factor is the ratio between the experimental and predicted rate constants, and takes into consideration that the probability of a reaction occurring depends on the orientation of the reactant molecules. The collision frequency is the average collisions per unit time, and is determined using Equation 2:

$$Z = N_A^2 \sigma_{AB} \sqrt{\frac{8k_B T}{\pi \mu_{AB}}}$$

Equation 2

where N_A is Avogadro's number (6.02×10^{23} mol^{-1}), σ_{AB} is the reaction cross-section, k_B is Boltzmann's constant (1.38×10^{-23} J·K^{-1}), and μ_{AB} is the reduced mass.

1. What is the rate constant of Reaction 1 at 304 K?

A) 8×10^1 $M^{-1}s^{-1}$
B) 8×10^1 s^{-1}
C) 8×10^{10} s^{-1}
D) 8×10^{10} $M^{-1}s^{-1}$

2. An increase in temperature by a factor of 4 would:

A)   increase Z by a factor of 2 and increase k_T overall.
B)   increase Z by a factor of 2 and decrease k_T overall.
C)   increase Z by a factor of 4 and decrease k_T overall.
D)   increase Z by a factor of 4 and increase k_T overall.

3. Which of the following statements regarding reaction kinetics is most accurate?

A) The activated complex can be measured in solution, although it is not a net product of the reaction.
B) The steric factor for more complex reactions is smaller than for simpler reactions.
C) The rate constant depends on the initial concentration of the reactants.
D) The rate law of a one-step bimolecular reaction cannot be determined using stoichiometry, but rather can only be calculated experimentally.

4. If the initial amount of Br_2 used in Reaction 1 were doubled and the volume of the reaction vessel decreased by a factor of two, how would the rate of the reaction be affected?

A) The rate of the reaction will increase by a factor of $2^{1/2}$.
B) The rate of the reaction will increase by a factor of 4.
C) The rate of the reaction will increase by a factor of 8.
D) The rate change cannot be determined from the given information.

5. A chamber of adjustable volume is loaded with $Cl(g)$ and $Br_2(g)$. At a time shortly after the beginning of the reaction, the chamber volume of the container is non-adiabatically halved. What is the correct rate expression for the resultant system immediately after the volume reduction?

A) rate = $k[Cl]^2[Br_2]^2$
B) rate = $k[Cl]^{(0.5)}[Br]^{(0.5)}$
C) rate = $k[Cl][Br_2]$
D) The rate law cannot be determined from the given information.

SOLUTIONS TO FREESTANDING QUESTIONS: KINETICS

1. **B** Reaction rate can be measured by the rate of disappearance of reactants or the rate of formation of products. This must, however, be adjusted for the various molar ratios in a reaction. The rate of disappearance or formation of each reactant or product, respectively, is therefore divided by its coefficient to give the reaction rate. For this reaction, this would mean the rate = $-\frac{1}{2}(\Delta[S_2O_3^{2-}]/\Delta t) = -(\Delta[I_2]/\Delta t) = (\Delta[S_4O_6^{2-}]/\Delta t) = \frac{1}{2}(\Delta[I^-]/\Delta t)$. The reaction rate can therefore be determined by the rate of disappearance of I_2 (choice B is correct).

2. **B** In a mechanism, the slowest step serves as the rate-determining step, which dictates the rate of the overall reaction. Rate laws for a given reaction can be determined by multiplying the rate constant by the concentration of the reactants raised to the power of their coefficient in the rate-limiting elementary step. The rate law for the overall reaction therefore is rate = $k[H_2][ICl]$ (choice B is correct).

3. **C** The units for a rate constant depend upon the order of reactants in the rate law and following multiplication, must give the same units as reaction rate (M/s). If provided a rate law, simply solve for the rate constant and solve for units:

$$\text{rate} = k[CH_3CHO]^{3/2}$$

$$k = \text{rate}/[CH_3CHO]^{3/2}$$

$$k = (M/s)/M^{3/2}$$

$$k = M^1 s^{-1} \times M^{-3/2}$$

$$k = M^{-1/2} s^{-1}$$

4. **D** Addition of a catalyst increases the rate of a reaction by stabilizing the transition state and decreasing the activation energy for the reaction. Choices A and B can be eliminated, as they are effectively saying the same thing. Since the first step in this mechanism is the rate-determining step, catalyzing the second step will have no impact on the rate of the overall reaction (choice D is correct). While increasing reactant concentrations will increase a reaction rate, this does not occur due to the addition of a catalyst (choice C is wrong).

5. **B** The overall reaction rate is determined by the rate of the slow step, which in this case is the second step. This gives the rate law: rate = $k[HOCl][Br^-]$ (eliminate choice C). The addition of KBr, which will dissociate to form Br^- ions, will increase the rate of the second step and increase the overall reaction rate (choice B is correct). Adding a catalyst to increase the rate of the first elementary step will not affect the rate of the overall reaction since it is not the rate-limiting step. (eliminate choice A). Doubling the concentration of both reactants in the second step would increase the reaction rate by a factor of four, not two (eliminate choice D).

6. **B** This question requires use of the isolation method to find the rate law for a given reaction. First, identify two experiments where the concentration of only one reactant changes. To assess the order of NH_4^+, compare experiments 2 and 4. Given that the concentration of NO_2^- does not change, any change in rate must be due to the concentration change of NH_4^+. In these two experiments, the $[NH_4^+]$ triples, as does the reaction rate. The reaction is therefore first order for NH_4^+ (eliminate choice C). To determine the order of NO_2^-, compare experiments 1 and 3. Here the concentration doubles like the reaction rate, indicating the reaction is first order for NO_2^- (eliminate choices A and D). The rate law is therefore rate = $k[NH_4^+][NO_2^-]$.

7. **D** This reaction coordinate diagram illustrates a nonspontaneous ($\Delta G > 0$) reaction where the activation energy is greater than the change in free energy (eliminate choice B; choice D is correct). While you know the reaction is nonspontaneous, you cannot be certain that it absorbs heat (eliminate choice A). Given the equation $\Delta G = \Delta H - T\Delta S$, you cannot determine ΔH without knowing something about ΔS and potentially the temperature. Heating a reaction will increase its reaction rate by increasing the rate constant k, but it does so by providing more energy with which the activation energy (E_a) can be overcome (eliminate choice C).

8. **A** IO^- is generated and consumed during the reaction, meaning it is an intermediate. In the above mechanism, the second step serves as the rate-determining step and addition of reactants to that step (in this case IO^-) increases the overall reaction rate. Catalysts must always be regenerated in a mechanism and in this case IO^- does not appear in the products (eliminate choices B and C). If IO^- were an inhibitor, you would expect it to decrease reaction rate, not increase it (eliminate choice D).

9. **A** The observation of a build-up of N_2O_2 in the reaction mixture supports the assignment of Step 2 as the rate-limiting step. If the proposed mechanism is correct, the rate law will be first order in N_2O_2 and first order in H_2, since one of each of these species are present as reactants in the slowest step of the mechanism.

10. **D** The Arrhenius equation for the rate law constant k is $k = Ae^{(-E_a/RT)}$. Taking natural logs to eliminate the exponent, you get $\ln(k) = -(E_a/RT) + \ln(A) \rightarrow \ln(k) = -(E_a/R)(1/T) + \ln(A)$. This form correlates to the equation for a line, $y = mx + b$. If you plot $\ln(k)$ (y-axis) vs. $1/T$ (x-axis), the resulting slope is $-(E_a/R)$ while the y-intercept is $\ln(A)$.

SOLUTIONS TO KINETICS PRACTICE PASSAGE

1. **D** As both Figure 1 and the passage text indicate, the rate law for Reaction 1 must be rate = $k[Cl][Br_2]$. Using Figure 1, the initial concentration of Br_2 is 1×10^{-9} M and the initial concentration of Cl is 0.5×10^{-9} M. Since the initial rate tangent line passes through the origin, any point (such as $x = 0.02$, $y = 0.8$) along it can be used to solve for the slope and obtain the initial rate of the reaction:

$$\text{rate}_{\text{initial}} = \frac{\Delta \text{concentration}}{\Delta \text{time}} = \frac{0.8 \times 10^{-9} M}{2.0 \times 10^{-2} s} = 4 \times 10^{-8} M \cdot s^{-1}$$

Solving the rate equation for k, you get

$$k = \frac{\text{rate}_{\text{initial}}}{[\text{Cl}]_{\text{initial}}[\text{Br}_2]_{\text{initial}}}$$

$$k = \frac{4 \times 10^{-8}\, M \cdot s^{-1}}{(0.5 \times 10^{-9}\, M)(1.0 \times 10^{-9}\, M)} = 8 \times 10^{10}\, M^{-1}s^{-1}$$

Therefore, choices A and B can be eliminated because they report the wrong value, while choice C can be eliminated because it has the wrong units, leaving choice D as the correct answer.

2. **A**   This is a 2 × 2 question, and is best answered using Process of Elimination. Equations 1 and 2 can be used to answer this question. In Equation 2, $Z \propto T^{1/2}$, so increasing T by a factor of 4 would increase Z by a factor of 2. This eliminates choices C and D. If Z is increased, it causes k_T to increase according to Equation 1. Also, since k_T is proportional to $e^{-1/T}$ in that same equation, increased temperature directly increases k_T independent of Z. Therefore, choice B is eliminated, and choice A is correct.

3. **B**   Although intermediates can be detected, an activated complex is non-isolable and cannot be detected, eliminating choice A. As indicated by Equations 1 and 2, the rate constant is independent of reactant concentrations, eliminating choice C. For a one-step bimolecular reaction, the reaction order is 2 as indicated by the stoichiometry, eliminating choice D. The passage states the steric factor depends on reactants colliding with the correct orientation. In complex reactions, the reactants have a lower probability of colliding with correct orientation so the steric factor will be lower, making choice B the best answer.

4. **C**   According to the passage, the rate law for Reaction 1 was determined to follow second-order kinetics, being first order in both [Cl] and [Br₂]. This means the equation for the rate law is

$$\text{rate} = k[\text{Cl}][\text{Br}_2]$$

Decreasing the volume of the reaction vessel by a factor of two will double the initial concentrations of both Cl and Br₂. As the initial amount of Br₂ used is also doubled, the concentration of Br₂ is effectively quadrupled. This will lead to the rate of the reaction increasing by a factor of 8.

5. **C**   Changing the reaction volume of the chamber does increase the concentrations of the reactants in the reaction; however, it does not change the rate expression. The overall rate would increase by a factor of 4, but this is due to doubling both reactant concentrations, not changes in the rate expression.

Chapter 27
Equilibrium

FREESTANDING QUESTIONS: EQUILIBRIUM

1. Which of the following strategies would be effective in increasing the ratio of products to reactants in the following endothermic reaction at equilibrium?

$$FSO_3H(g) \rightleftharpoons SO_3(g) + HF(g)$$

A) Decreasing the reaction temperature
B) Increasing the reaction temperature
C) Increasing the initial amount of FSO_3H
D) Running the reaction in an HF atmosphere

2. Which of the following accurately describes the equilibrium constant for the following Pd-catalyzed hydrogenation equilibrium?

$$Cl_2TiH_2 \underset{}{\overset{Pd^o}{\rightleftharpoons}} TiCl_2 + H_2$$

A) $\dfrac{[Cl_2TiH_2]}{[TiCl_2][H_2]}$

B) $\dfrac{[Cl_2TiH_2][Pd]}{[TiCl_2][H_2]}$

C) $\dfrac{[TiCl_2][H_2]}{[Cl_2TiH_2]}$

D) $\dfrac{[TiCl_2][H_2]}{[Cl_2TiH_2][Pd]}$

3. The maximum solubility of sodium sulfide (Na_2S) in water at 0°C is 12.4 g per every 100 mL of water. What value most closely approximates the solubility product (K_{sp}) of Na_2S at 0°C in water?

A) 4.2×10^0
B) 1.8×10^{-1}
C) 1.8×10^1
D) 4.2×10^2

4. Which of the following salts is most likely to fully dissolve in a 5% saline solution?

A) $AgCl(s)$
B) $LiBr(s)$
C) $Na_2CO_3(s)$
D) $PbCl_2(s)$

5. Given the equilibrium for the decomposition of dinitrogen tetroxide to nitrogen dioxide:

$$N_2O_4(g) \rightleftharpoons 2\,NO_2(g) \quad K_{eq} = 1.4 \times 10^{-1} \text{ at } 25°C$$

If both species have a partial pressure of 0.1 atm in a reaction vessel at 25°C, which way will the reaction proceed?

A) In a net forward direction
B) In a net reverse direction
C) In both directions at equal rates
D) Cannot be determined without the volume of the reaction vessels

6. A reaction at equilibrium has a K_{eq} of 154. All of the following are true for this reaction EXCEPT:

A) $\Delta G < 0$.
B) $\Delta G = 0$.
C) $Q = K_{eq}$.
D) $\Delta G° < 0$.

7. Which of the following systems is at equilibrium?

A) Combustion of propane in a propane fire
B) Bubbles forming in a freshly poured glass of soda
C) A saturated solution of NaCl sitting over solid NaCl
D) Rust forming on an exposed metal surface

8. Dissolved carbon monoxide can be quantified in solution through a distinctive peak in the solution's infrared (IR) absorbance spectrum at ~1800 cm^{-1}, which increases in intensity with increasing [CO]. If ethanol was subjected to an applied CO pressure, which combination of pressure and temperature would yield the most intense CO peak in the IR spectrum of the solution?

A) 1 atm CO at 373 K
B) 2 atm CO at 273 K
C) 1 atm CO at 273 K
D) 2 atm CO at 373 K

9. Nitrogen is a relatively inert species; therefore, high temperatures and pressures are required to produce appreciable amounts of ammonia in the gas phase by the following reaction:

$$N_2 + 3 H_2 \rightleftharpoons 2 NH_3$$

In a reactor of fixed volume containing only the gases in equilibrium and temperature fixed with external controls, which of the following relationships explains the enhancement in the production of ammonia at higher pressures?

A) $n \propto T$
B) $V \propto 1/P$
C) $P \propto R$
D) $P \propto n$

10. When 50 mL of a 0.10 M MgCl$_2$ solution is added to 50 mL of a 0.20 M LiCl solution, the final concentration of chloride ions will be:

A) 0.15 M.
B) 0.20 M.
C) 0.30 M.
D) 0.40 M.

EQUILIBRIUM PRACTICE PASSAGE

Creatine is a naturally occurring biomolecule, produced in the kidney and liver, which is used by the body to help store energy for use in muscle tissues. Once creatine is biosynthesized, it is transformed by creatine kinase to creatine phosphate. The phosphorylated molecule is stored in muscle tissue as an easily metabolized form of quick energy. It is broken down in body tissues to form the cyclic urea creatinine.

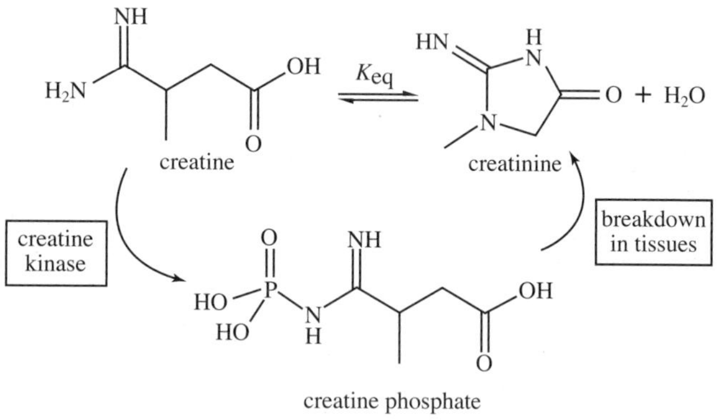

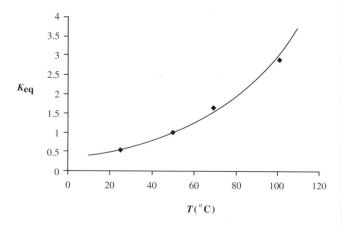

Figure 1   Conversion of creatine to creatinine

Synthetic creatine is known to exist in equilibrium with creatinine in aqueous solution, as depicted in Figure 1 above. The equilibrium constant (K_{eq}) for this conversion is known to be temperature dependent, as shown in Figure 2.

K_{eq}

$T(^{\circ}C)$

Figure 2 K_{eq} of creatinine formation at pH = 7

1. The ΔH° for the equilibrium in Figure 1 was determined to be +4.3 kcal/mol. Which of the following must also be true?

A) ΔG°_{363K} has a positive value.
B) ΔS°_{363K} has a negative value.
C) ΔS°_{363K} has a positive value.
D) ΔG°_{293K} has a negative value.

2. A pH-neutral creatine solution is brought to reflux in water (100°C) and found to have a creatinine concentration of 0.45 M. At this temperature, what is the expected concentration of creatine?

A) 0.45 M
B) 0.23 M
C) 0.15 M
D) 0.10 M

3. A test solution at 50°C was found to have a creatinine concentration of 1 M. When the temperature was raised to 85°C, what was the value determined for the equilibrium concentration of creatinine?

A) 0.66 M
B) 0.50 M
C) 1.50 M
D) 1.33 M

4. In the active site of creatine kinase, a number of amino acids are responsible for holding and directing the phosphate and nitrogen-bearing terminus of creatine in the facilitation of bond formation. Which of the following amino acid residues is most likely found active in this role?

A) Histidine
B) Valine
C) Glycine
D) Phenylalanine

5. When 0.5 M of creatine is dissolved in acetonitrile (CH_3CN), a near complete conversion to creatinine was observed. Which of the following is a plausible explanation for this observation?

A) Acetonitrile cannot hydrogen bond with creatine.
B) Removal of the excess of water allows the equilibrium to shift heavily to the products.
C) Creatine is easily deprotonated by acetonitrile, halting equilibrium.
D) The formation of water is extremely thermodynamically unfavorable in acetonitrile.

SOLUTIONS TO FREESTANDING QUESTIONS: EQUILIBRIUM

1. **B** Choices C and D can be eliminated, as equilibrium constants (ratios of the concentrations of products to reactants) are not altered with changes in initial concentrations of starting materials or products. Both choices A and B will change the equilibrium constant of the reaction, but only increasing the temperature (choice B) will change it in favor of the products. In endothermic reactions, heat can be treated as a reactant. Therefore, increasing temperature will shift the reaction to the right, using up reactants to make products, and as a result, increasing the ratio of products to reactants (K_{eq}).

2. **C** The equilibrium constant for the following generic reaction

    $$aA + bB \rightleftharpoons cC + dD$$

    is $([C]^c[D]^d)/[A]^a[B]^b)$. Choices B and D may be eliminated, as they both include the concentration of the Pd catalyst in the equilibrium constant. Catalysts play no role in the thermodynamics of the system. Choice C has the correct form (products/reactants), while choice A has the terms reversed.

3. **C** 12.4 g of Na_2S (78 g/mol) in 100 mL of water translates to 124 g in 1 L, allowing the following calculation:

    $$(124 \text{ g/L})/(78 \text{ g/mol}) \approx 125/75 \text{ mol/L} = 5/3 \ M = 1.66 \ M$$

    This result implies that at saturation there are 1.66 mol of S^{2-} in solution, and two times this amount (3.33 mol) of Na^+. The expression for K_{sp} for Na_2S may be written as follows:

    $$K_{sp} = [Na^+]^2[S^{2-}]$$
    $$K_{sp} = [3.33]^2[1.66]$$

    To estimate the math, round 3.33 to 4 and 1.66 to 2. This leads to an answer of $16 \times 2 = 32$, representing the upper limit of the correct answer to seek. Now assume 3.33 = 3 and 1.66 = 1, leading to a lower limit of 9. With these two boundaries in place, choice C is the only appropriate answer.

4. **B** According to the common-ion effect, only LiBr(s) dissolution will remain unaffected by the Na^+ and Cl^- ions present in a 5% saline solution. These ions will shift the equilibria of the remaining choices to the left, making them less likely to completely dissolve. In addition, LiBr is the most soluble of all the species listed.

5. **A** First, calculate the reaction quotient, Q:

    $$Q = \frac{P_{NO_2}^2}{P_{N_2O_4}} = \frac{0.1^2}{0.1} = 0.1$$

    Under these conditions, $Q < K_{eq}$. The reaction will proceed forward until $Q = K_{eq}$. If moles were given instead of partial pressures, then either the total pressure or volume of the vessel would be required to solve the problem.

6. **A**   Any reaction at equilibrium has no net change in free energy. Therefore, $\Delta G = 0$ at present for this reaction, and choice B can be eliminated. When a reaction is at equilibrium, $Q = K_{eq}$, eliminating choice C. Regarding the standard state free energy change for this reaction, because $K_{eq} > 1$, the products are favored at equilibrium and $\Delta G° < 0$ according to the following equation:

$$\Delta G° = -2.3RT \log K_{eq}$$

7. **C**   When propane burns, no propane is reformed, and if the reverse reaction doesn't occur, the system can't be at equilibrium. In a freshly poured glass of soda, the amount of carbon dioxide leaving the solution far exceeds the amount of carbon dioxide reentering the soda, so the system is not at equilibrium. In a saturated solution, the amount of solid precipitating from the solution is exactly equal to the amount re-dissolving, so choice C is correct. If rust is forming on an exposed metal surface, the amount of rust being created must be greater than the amount reverting back to metal.

8. **B**   The peak at ~1800 cm^{-1} becomes more intense with increasing CO concentration in solution. Keeping in mind the dissolution equilibrium expression

$$CO(g) \rightleftharpoons CO(sol)$$

it is clear that larger values of $CO(g)$ will lead to larger values of $CO(sol)$. Choices A and C may be eliminated as the applied CO pressure is 1 atm, rather than 2 atm. As gases have higher solubility in solution at low temperatures, choice B is the correct answer.

9. **D**   As temperature and volume are held constant, the only relationship valid in the system is that between P and n, and the only way to increase P is to increase n. Therefore, you know that elevated pressures means greater numbers of moles present. In the reaction

$$N_2 + 3\,H_2 \rightleftharpoons 2\,NH_3$$

the reactants comprise four moles of gas, while the products only two. At high pressures, and hence high molarity (large n at fixed volume), the reaction will be driven toward the products. For this reason, choice D is correct. Volume is held constant, and hence not proportional to 1/pressure in the system described, eliminating choice B. Choice A is incorrect for the same reason; T is explicitly held constant while n is not. R is the universal gas constant and is not proportional to a changeable quantity like P.

10. **B**   To calculate the final [Cl⁻] in terms of molarity (mol/L, or mmol/mL), find the total number of moles of Cl⁻ ions in each solution and divide by the total volume of the resulting mixture. You cannot simply add the concentrations of the solutions together, as choice C might suggest. In addition, the formulas of each compound must be taken into consideration. $MgCl_2$ will dissociate in solution to produce twice as many chloride ions as magnesium ions, so while the concentration of $MgCl_2$ is 0.10 M, the concentration of Cl⁻ in the same solution is 0.20 M. Ignoring the formula in this way may lead to choosing the wrong answer, choice A. To calculate the final concentration:

$$\frac{[(2)(0.10\ M\ \text{Cl}^-)(50\ \text{mL})] + [(0.20\ M\ \text{Cl}^-)(50\ \text{mL})]}{50\ \text{mL} + 50\ \text{mL}} = \frac{20\ \text{mmol Cl}^-}{100\ \text{mL}} = 0.20\ M\ \text{Cl}^-$$

SOLUTIONS TO EQUILIBRIUM PRACTICE PASSAGE

1. **C**   At 363 K (90°C), K_{eq} for the reaction is greater than 1, while at 293 K (20°C) the value is less than 1. The relation between $\Delta G°$ and K_{eq} is as follows:

   $$\Delta G° = -RT \ln K_{eq}$$

   When $K_{eq} > 1$, the value of $\Delta G° < 0$, and conversely, when $K_{eq} < 1$, the value of $\Delta G° > 0$. These two statements eliminate choices A and D, respectively. Since it is established that $\Delta G°_{363K}$ must be negative, $\Delta S°_{363K}$ must be positive, as there is no way to achieve a negative $\Delta G°$ value with a positive $\Delta H°_{363K}$ and negative $\Delta S°_{363K}$ according to the relationship $\Delta G° = \Delta H° - T\Delta S°$ (eliminate choice B).

2. **C**   According to Figure 2, at 100°C the value of K_{eq} is ~3. The following calculation can be written to arrive at the answer:

   $$K_{eq} = [\text{creatinine}]/[\text{creatine}]$$

   $$3 = 0.45/[\text{creatine}]$$

   $$[\text{creatine}] = 0.45/3 = 0.15$$

3. **D**   According to Figure 2, at 50°C K_{eq} is ~1. This means that [creatine] = [creatinine] = 1 M. At 85°C K_{eq} is ~2. As the change in creatinine must be equal and opposite to the change in creatine as temperature changes, the following equation can be written:

   $$K_{eq} = [1 + x]/[1 - x] = 2$$

   $$1 + x = 2 - 2x$$

   $$3x = 1$$

   $$x = 1/3 = 0.33$$

   The total final value for creatinine at 85°C is [1 + x], or 1.33 M.

4. **A**   The presence of numerous hydrogen-bonding moieties on both the active end of creatine and on the phosphate suggests that hydrogen bonding will be responsible for the orientation of the reactants in the active site. Of the four amino acids listed, only histidine (below) is capable of hydrogen bonding, making choice A the correct answer.

5. **B** In aqueous solution, water is available in vast excess and is not expressed as part of the equilibrium constant, since its value does not appreciably change during the reaction. If the reaction is run in a non-aqueous solvent, water is scarce. If the equilibrium constant of the reaction was in the range of 1–3 in a vast excess of water, in the absence of water the reaction will likely be converted almost wholly to products. Acetonitrile is capable of accepting hydrogen bonds with any one of the many H-bond donors on creatine (eliminate choice A). Choice C may be eliminated both because acetonitrile is very weakly basic and cannot deprotonate a carboxylic acid, and because such a deprotonation of the reactant would shift the equilibrium to the left, decreasing the amount of product. Choice D may be eliminated due to the fact that there is no reason to think that water is unstable in acetonitrile (it is not), but also because if water were unstable, and high energy in acetonitrile, the equilibrium would lie predominantly with the reactants.

Chapter 28
Acids and Bases

FREESTANDING QUESTIONS: ACIDS AND BASES

1. The label "strong" versus "weak" when referring to an acid indicates which of the following?

   A) Whether the pH of the acid solution will be ~7 or significantly less than 7
   B) How likely it is for the acid to react with a base
   C) Whether the ratio of [acid] to [conjugate base] is < 1 or > 1
   D) The likelihood of a color change occurring when a proton is lost

2. Given a pK_a of 10.3 for bicarbonate, which of the following is FALSE?

   A) The conjugate base of bicarbonate will increase the pH of water.
   B) The pK_b of carbonic acid is 3.7.
   C) At equilibrium, more bicarbonate is present in solution than carbonate upon dissociation.
   D) Bicarbonate can function as an acid or a base.

3. Addition of what volume of 0.5 M NaOH to 100 mL of 1.0 M malonic acid (pK_{a1} = 2.8, pK_{a2} = 5.7) will generate a solution best able to resist pH change at 5.7?

   A) 100 mL
   B) 200 mL
   C) 300 mL
   D) 400 mL

4. A scientist wishes to select an indicator to demonstrate a color change upon neutralization of a solution of acetic acid with a strong base. Which of the following would be the best choice?

   A) Crystal violet (pK_a = 1.1)
   B) Bromocresol green (pK_a = 4.9)
   C) Bromocresol purple (pK_a = 6.3)
   D) Phenol red (pK_a = 7.9)

5. Ba(NO$_2$)$_2$ is a basic salt due to the interaction of the nitrite ion with water according to the following reaction:

   $$NO_2^- + H_2O \rightleftharpoons HNO_2 + OH^-$$

   Why does the equilibrium shown favor the left side of the reaction?

   A) H_2O is a weaker base than OH^-.
   B) NO_2^- is a weaker base than OH^-.
   C) H_2O is a stronger acid than HNO_2.
   D) NO_2^- is a stronger base than OH^-.

6. Which of the following statements is true about a solution of propanoic acid in equilibrium?

   $$CH_3CH_2COOH(aq) \rightleftharpoons H^+(aq) + CH_3CH_2COO^-(aq)$$

   A) When NaOH is added, CH_3CH_2COOH acts as a Lewis acid.
   B) When HCl is added, $CH_3CH_2COO^-$ acts as a Brønsted-Lowry base.
   C) When HI is added, CH_3CH_2COOH acts as a Brønsted-Lowry acid.
   D) When HF is added, CH_3CH_2COOH acts as an Arrhenius base.

7. Pure water will react with itself to form hydronium and hydroxide ions in a process called autoionization, represented by the following reaction:

   $$2 H_2O \rightleftharpoons H_3O^+ + OH^-$$

   In this reaction, which of the following can be considered a Brønsted-Lowry base?

   A) H_2O
   B) H_3O^+
   C) OH^-
   D) Both A and C

8. If 50 mL of each of the following solutions are combined as indicated, which of the following will create an acidic final solution?

   A) 0.3 M HCl with 0.1 M Fe(OH)$_3$
   B) 0.1 M HClO$_3$ with 0.1 M Ca(OH)$_2$
   C) 0.2 M HF with 0.2 M LiOH
   D) 0.2 M NH$_3$ with 0.1 M HI

9. The K_a values for HF and HCN are 6.3×10^{-4} and 6.2×10^{-10}, respectively. Compared to the conjugate base F$^-$, CN$^-$ is a:

   A) weak conjugate base that is weaker than F$^-$.
   B) strong conjugate base that is weaker than F$^-$.
   C) weak conjugate base that is stronger than F$^-$.
   D) strong conjugate base that is stronger than F$^-$.

10. Compare the two weak Brønsted-Lowry acids HBrO$_3$ and HIO$_3$. Which acid is stronger, and why?

    A) HBrO$_3$ is stronger because bromine is more electronegative than iodine.
    B) HIO$_3$ is stronger because iodine is more electronegative than bromine.
    C) HIO$_3$ is stronger because iodine is a larger atom than bromine.
    D) HBrO$_3$ is stronger because bromine forms shorter, stronger bonds with oxygen than iodine.

ACIDS AND BASES PRACTICE PASSAGE

Ocean acidification is a consequence of ocean waters absorbing atmospheric CO_2 at the air-water interface to form carbonic acid. This acid ultimately dissociates to form bicarbonate and carbonate ions:

$$CO_2(g) + H_2O(l) \rightarrow H_2CO_3 \, (aq)$$
Reaction 1

$$H_2CO_3(aq) \rightleftharpoons H^+ \, (aq) + HCO_3^- \, (aq) \quad K_2 = 2.5 \times 10^{-4} \text{ (at 25°C)}$$
Reaction 2

$$HCO_3^-(aq) \rightleftharpoons H^+ \, (aq) + CO_3^{2-} \, (aq) \quad K_2 = 5.6 \times 10^{-11} \text{ (at 25°C)}$$
Reaction 3

The complex equilibria are summarized in Figure 1 below, which describes the relationship between seawater pH and the concentrations of carbon dioxide, bicarbonate ions, and carbonate ions.

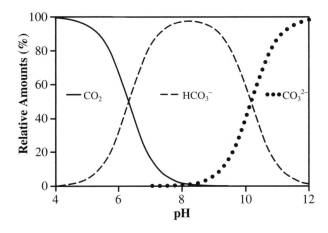

Figure 1 Concentration of CO_2, HCO_3^-, and CO_3^{2-} with varying seawater pH

Ocean acidification is of great interest for marine biologists because of its effects on the calcium carbonate exoskeletons of mollusks and corals. The equilibrium governing the mineralization and dissolution of calcium carbonate exoskeletons is described by the following equation:

$$CaCO_3(s) \rightleftharpoons Ca^{2+} \, (aq) + CO_3^{2-} \, (aq) \quad K_{sp} = 8.7 \times 10^{-9} \text{ (at 25°C)}$$
Reaction 4

In the marine environment, the solubility of calcium carbonate decreases with increasing temperature. Organisms that need to generate calcium carbonate for their exoskeletons are usually found in shallow waters due to the relative saturation of calcium and carbonate ions at this depth. However, it is hypothesized that ocean acidification and its effects on calcium carbonate availability may lead to mass migrations of these organisms.

1. Which of the following is a consequence of increased CO_2 absorption in ocean water?

A) A decrease in seawater pOH
B) A decrease in the K_a of Reaction 2
C) A decrease in the thickness of mollusk shells
D) A decrease in calcium ions in seawater

2. According to the passage, which of the following is true regarding the K_{sp} of $CaCO_3$ in seawater?

A) K_{sp} does not change with changes in temperature.
B) K_{sp} (23°C) > K_{sp} (50°C)
C) K_{sp} (23°C) < K_{sp} (50°C)
D) The change in K_{sp} is not predictable without further data.

3. Titration of a 1.0 M solution of H_2CO_3 with 2.5 M NaOH will result in a titration curve with two plateaus close to which pH values?

A) 2.5 and 4.0
B) 2.5 and 5.6
C) 3.6 and 10.2
D) 5.6 and 11.0

4. Groundwater, often found with dissolved calcium and carbonate ions, may contain high levels of carbon dioxide while underground. Which of the following will occur when this water surfaces and expels the excess carbon dioxide?

A) Water acidity decreases and calcium carbonate may precipitate.
B) Water acidity decreases and calcium carbonate will remain in solution.
C) Water acidity increases and calcium carbonate will remain in solution.
D) Water acidity increases and calcium carbonate may precipitate.

5. A scientist samples a liter of seawater and notices a calcium carbonate precipitate settle to the bottom of the flask when placed in a 25°C water bath. Roughly how many moles of calcium carbonate will be dissolved in this solution?

A) 3×10^{-3}
B) 9×10^{-5}
C) 9×10^{-9}
D) 9×10^{-18}

SOLUTIONS TO FREESTANDING QUESTIONS:
ACIDS AND BASES

1. **C** The term "strong" versus "weak" with respect to acids and bases refers to their degree of dissociation, and therefore how much of the acid is present compared to the amount of its conjugate base (choice C is correct). While it is tempting to conclude that a strong acid necessarily has a very low pH when in solution, this is concentration dependent (eliminate choice A). For instance, a 10^{-6} M solution of the strong acid HCl has a pH of 6. All acids will react to completion with a base (eliminate choice B). The color of an acid (or its conjugate base)—if it has one as indicators do—is a function of the structure of the molecule, not how readily it loses a proton (eliminate choice D).

2. **B** The relation $pK_a + pK_b = 14$ only applies when comparing the pK_a of an acid with the pK_b of its conjugate base (or when comparing the pK_b of a base with the pK_a of its conjugate acid). Here you are given the pK_a of bicarbonate, so while the pK_b of carbonate is 3.7, you do not know the pK_b of carbonic acid (choice B is a false statement and the correct answer). The conjugate base of a weak acid is basic (choice A is a true statement and not the correct answer) and weak acids only dissociate to a limited extent (choice C is a true statement and not the correct answer). While independent of the given pK_a value in the question, bicarbonate is an amphoteric species, meaning it can function as either an acid or a base (choice D is a true statement and not the correct answer).

3. **C** Solutions of weak acids and their conjugate bases best serve as buffers (or resist pH change upon the addition of acid or base) when the concentrations of the conjugate pair are roughly equal. When they are exactly equal, the pH of the solution is equal to the acid pK_a. On a titration curve, these are commonly known as half-equivalence points. Given there are 0.1 moles of malonic acid (1.0 M × 0.1 L), addition of 100 mL of 0.5 M NaOH (0.05 moles) would generate a buffer capable of resisting changes in pH nearest pH 2.8 (choice A is wrong). Addition of 200 mL of NaOH (0.1 moles) would bring the solution to the equivalence point and would not function as a buffer (choice B is wrong). Addition of 300 mL of NaOH (0.15 moles) would reach the second half-equivalence point, which is then able to resist pH change nearest a pH of 5.7 (choice C is correct). Adding 400 mL of NaOH (0.2 moles) reaches the second equivalence point, which cannot serve as a buffer (choice D is wrong).

4. **D** Neutralization of a weak acid with a strong base will result in a basic solution, and our indicator should therefore change color at a pH greater than 7 (choice D is correct). Note that without the specific concentration of acetic acid and the base you begin with, it is not possible to determine the precise final pH upon complete neutralization (adding an equal molar quantity of strong base to the acetic acid).

5. **B** Acid/base equilibria always favor the weaker acid/base pair. Since NO_2^- has a negative charge and no proton to donate, it must be the base, making water the acid. Therefore, NO_2^- and H_2O are the weakest base and acid, respectively, eliminating choices C and D. While water is a weaker base than OH^-, making choice A a true statement, water is not acting as a base in this particular reaction (eliminate choice A).

6. **B** In the presence of a strong acid, $CH_3CH_2COO^-$ will behave as a Brønsted-Lowry base by accepting a proton, and the equilibrium will shift to the left. This eliminates choice C and makes choice B the correct answer. In the presence of a strong base, H^+ and not CH_3CH_2COOH will behave as a Lewis acid and accept electrons from OH^-, eliminating choice A. CH_3CH_2COOH does not contain the hydroxide ion, even though the formula for a carboxylic acid (COOH) might suggest that. Therefore, it cannot behave as an Arrhenius base, so choice D can be eliminated.

7. **D** Recall that a Brønsted-Lowry base is a proton acceptor. On the left side of the equation, one H_2O will act as an acid and the other as a base in the forward reaction. On the right side of the equation, OH^- will also accept a proton in the reverse reaction (choice D is correct). It is important to note here that we are concerned with *both directions* of the reaction for the purposes of answering this question correctly.

8. **A** When equimolar amounts of acid and base are neutralized, the salt composed of their respective conjugates determines whether the resultant solution is acidic or basic. In choice A, the only significant species left in solution after neutralization is Fe^{3+}, which is the conjugate acid of the weak base $Fe(OH)_3$. The resulting solution is therefore acidic, so choice A is the correct answer. In choice B, only half of the initial base is neutralized by the acid, so the resulting solution is basic (eliminate choice B). In choice C, the neutralization is complete and the significant species left in solution is F^- (the conjugate base of the weak acid HF), yielding a basic solution (eliminate choice C). In choice D, exactly half the base is neutralized, yielding another basic solution (eliminate choice D).

9. **C** This is a 2×2 question, which is best answered by first addressing one of the assertions. Any conjugate base of a weak acid is a weak base. HCN is a weak acid, so CN^- must be a weak conjugate base (eliminate choices B and D). Since HCN has a lower K_a than HF, HCN is a weaker acid. This means that HCN has a stronger conjugate base than F^- because the weaker an acid is, the *stronger* its conjugate base (eliminate choice A).

10. **A** The conjugate base that is better able to stabilize its negative charge has the stronger conjugate acid. Br is more electronegative than I and will better stabilize the negative charge on the adjacent oxygen atom in the conjugate base (eliminate choice B; choice A is correct). Although iodine is a larger atom than bromine, the negative charge in question is delocalized via resonance over the three oxygen atoms in each ion so size does not come into play (eliminate choice C). While Br—O bonds will be shorter and stronger than I—O bonds due to the smaller size of Br, the bond strength of the O—H bonds are the important ones to consider when comparing acidities (eliminate choice D).

SOLUTIONS TO ACIDS AND BASES PRACTICE PASSAGE

1. **C** Looking at Figure 1, as more carbon dioxide is absorbed, the pH of ocean water decreases, causing the pOH to increase (eliminate choice A). An increase in CO_2 concentration will not cause the K_a to change, since equilibrium constants change only with temperature (eliminate choice B). Choice D is incorrect because Figure 1 shows that as CO_2 concentration in seawater increases, CO_3^{2-} ion concentration decreases. Consequently, the equilibrium in Reaction 4 will shift to the right, resulting in increased calcium ion concentration. For the same reason, more calcium carbonate dissolves and the thickness of the shells would be expected to decrease.

2. **B** The passage states, "In the marine environment, the solubility of calcium carbonate decreases with increasing temperature." This statement eliminates choice D. Decreased solubility of $CaCO_3$ indicates a smaller solubility product (K_{sp}), rather than a larger one (eliminate choice C), or one of the same size (eliminate choice A).

3. **C** Plateaus in a titration curve indicate the buffer region when a weak acid, like H_2CO_3, is titrated with a strong base, like NaOH. These regions are the half-equivalence points where pH equals pK_a of the acid, and it will occur at these pH values regardless of the concentrations of the acid and base. Since H_2CO_3 is diprotic, there will be two buffering regions at pH values that correspond to the pK_a values of H_2CO_3 and HCO_3^-. Based on the K_a values given in Reactions 2 and 3, the pK_a values should be between 3 and 4 (3.6) for H_2CO_3 and between 10 and 11 (10.2) for HCO_3^-.

4. **A** The general theme of this passage is that as carbon dioxide levels increase, water acidity increases and CO_3^{2-} ion concentration decreases. Thus, if carbon dioxide is removed, the acidity decreases (eliminate choices C and D) and the CO_3^{2-} ion concentration increases. Since this is the case, the equilibrium shown in Reaction 4 will shift to the left indicating that calcium carbonate may precipitate out of solution if the saturation point of the solution is reached.

5. **B** Since a precipitate forms, the solution above it must be saturated. Given the stoichiometry of the solubility equilibrium: $CaCO_3(s) \rightleftharpoons Ca^{2+}(aq) + CO_3^{2-}(aq)$, x moles of calcium carbonate will dissociate into x moles of calcium ions and x moles of carbonate ions. Writing out the K_{sp} expression for this reaction and substituting, you get

$$K_{sp} = [Ca^{2+}][CO_3^{2-}] = [x][x]$$
$$K_{sp} = x^2$$
$$8.7 \times 10^{-9} = x^2 \approx 9 \times 10^{-9}$$
$$\text{so } x \approx 3 \times 10^{-4.5} \ M$$

This is closest to choice B, in which the order of magnitude given is 10^{-5}. This will correspond to 9×10^{-5} moles of solute in the 1 L solution given.

Chapter 29
Electrochemistry

FREESTANDING QUESTIONS: ELECTROCHEMISTRY

1. Gold can be spontaneously electrodeposited on an iron surface if clean iron is immersed in a solution of Au^{3+} ions. The reaction is described by the following equation:

$$3\ Fe^0 + 2\ Au^{3+} \rightarrow 2\ Au^0 + 3\ Fe^{2+}$$

The reducing agent in this reaction is which of the following?

A) Fe^0
B) Fe^{2+}
C) Au^0
D) Au^{3+}

2. In a lead acid battery, a Pb^0 electrode and a PbO_2 electrode (depicted below) are oxidized and reduced, respectively, to $PbSO_4$. Reactions with sulfates to form sulfur-containing products are known to occur in many such cells. Which of the following sulfur side reactions is most likely to occur at the anode in the concentrated H_2SO_4 environment under discharge conditions?

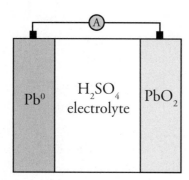

A) $8\ H^+ + PbSO_4 \rightarrow PbS + 4\ H_2O$
B) $2\ H^+ + H_2SO_4 \rightarrow SO_2 + 2\ H_2O$
C) $H_2O + SO_2 \rightarrow SO_3 + 2\ H^+$
D) $SO_3 + 6\ H^+ \rightarrow S^0 + 3\ H_2O$

3. A small toy car is driven by a hydrogen fuel cell for 2 minutes at 2 amps of current. What mass of hydrogen gas is consumed in this operation? Hydrogen is consumed by the fuel fell in the following half reaction: $H_2 \rightarrow 2\ H^+ + 2e^-$. (Faraday's constant is 96,500 C/mol e^-)

A) 26.0 mg H_2
B) 2.5 mg H_2
C) 50.0 mg H_2
D) 12.5 mg H_2

4. A cell is constructed with two iron electrodes, one of which is placed in a 1.0 M aqueous solution of $FeCl_2$, while the other is submerged in 1.0 $M\ FeCl_3$. Given the following reduction potentials, which best approximates the initial voltage of this galvanic cell?

$$Fe^{3+} + e^- \rightarrow Fe^{2+} \qquad E^\circ = 0.77\ V$$

$$Fe^{2+} + 2e^- \rightarrow Fe^0 \qquad E^\circ = -0.44\ V$$

$$Fe^{3+} + 3e^- \rightarrow Fe^0 \qquad E^\circ = -0.04\ V$$

A) 0.48 V
B) 1.21 V
C) 0.33 V
D) −0.73 V

5. Heavy main group elements are frequently capable of more oxidation states than the lighter members of the group. Below is a table of reduction potentials for half reactions involving Pb and Sn:

$Pb^{2+} + 2e^- \rightarrow Pb(s)$	$E^\circ = -0.13\ V$
$Pb^{4+} + 2e^- \rightarrow Pb^{2+}$	$E^\circ = +1.69\ V$
$Sn^{4+} + 2e^- \rightarrow Sn^{2+}$	$E^\circ = +0.15\ V$
$Sn^{2+} + 2e^- \rightarrow Sn(s)$	$E^\circ = -0.14\ V$

Which of the following mono-elemental reactions is the most electrochemically favorable?

A) $Sn^{4+} + Sn(s) \rightarrow 2\ Sn^{2+}$
B) $Pb^{4+} + Pb(s) \rightarrow 2\ Pb^{2+}$
C) $2\ Sn^{2+} \rightarrow Sn(s) + Sn^{4+}$
D) $2\ Pb^{2+} \rightarrow Pb(s) + Pb^{4+}$

6. In the cell below, a voltage is externally applied to enable the oxidation of Pt^0 and its re-deposition on the surface of an FeO electrode. Which reaction occurs at the negatively charged (−) electrode?

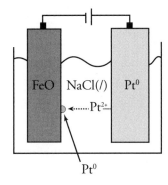

A) $Pt^0(s) \rightarrow Pt^{2+} + 2e^-$
B) $Pt^{2+} + 2e^- \rightarrow Pt^0(s)$
C) $FeO(s) + Pt^{2+} \rightarrow Fe^{2+} + PtO(s)$
D) $Pt^0(s) + NaCl \rightarrow PtCl(s) + Na^+ + e^-$

7. Transition metals in very high oxidation states (large and positive) tend to be very good oxidizing agents. Based on this criterion, which of the following species is likely the best oxidizing agent?

A) OsO_2
B) $MnO_2(NH_3)_2$
C) WCl_3
D) $KMnO_4$

8. The voltage of a galvanic cell composed of one Zn and one Fe electrode, in 1 M aqueous solutions of their respective ions, is measured to be 0.33 V, confirming the tabulated half-reaction values below, referenced against the standard hydrogen electrode.

$$Fe^{2+} + 2e^- \rightarrow Fe^0 \qquad E° = -0.44 \text{ V}$$
$$Zn^0 \rightarrow 2e^- + Zn^{2+} \qquad E° = +0.77 \text{ V}$$

If enough H_2SO_4 is added to each chamber of the cell to make the solution 1 M in H^+, how will the cell's $\Delta G°$ change? ($\Delta G° = -nFE°$, F = 96,500 C/mol e^-, 1 J = 1 C·V)

A) $\Delta G°_2 - \Delta G°_1 = -85$ kJ/mol
B) $\Delta G°_2 - \Delta G°_1 = -148$ kJ/mol
C) $\Delta G°_2 - \Delta G°_1 = +85$ kJ/mol
D) $\Delta G°_2 - \Delta G°_1 = +148$ kJ/mol

9. A galvanic cell is constructed using platinum and iron electrodes in 1 M solutions of their respective salts. The half reactions for these two elements are provided as follows:

$$Pt^{2+}(aq) + 2e^- \rightarrow Pt(s) \qquad E° = +1.2 \text{ V}$$
$$Fe^{3+}(aq) + 3e^- \rightarrow Fe(s) \qquad E° = -0.036 \text{ V}$$

Which of the following statements is correct regarding this cell?

A) $E°$ = 1.164 V, and Pt^{2+} is the reducing agent.
B) $E°$ = 1.164 V, and Fe^{3+} is the reducing agent.
C) $E°$ = 1.236 V, and Pt^{2+} is the oxidizing agent.
D) $E°$ = 1.236 V, and Fe^{3+} is the oxidizing agent.

10. Pennies are fabricated by the electrodeposition of copper on zinc. If this is a non-spontaneous reaction, which of the following is true with respect to zinc?

A) It is connected to the positive terminal of the battery where copper is oxidized.
B) It is connected to the positive terminal of the battery where copper is reduced.
C) It is connected to the negative terminal of the battery where copper is oxidized.
D) It is connected to the negative terminal of the battery where copper is reduced.

ELECTROCHEMISTRY PRACTICE PASSAGE

Research into the electrolysis of water has taken on increasing importance with hopes that molecular hydrogen might fuel the future world energy economy. Unfortunately, conversion of H_2O into O_2 and H_2 is thermodynamically unfavorable, and requires the input of energy. The electrical energy required for this conversion can be monitored through the design and testing of water-electrolysis cells, such as described by Figure 1.

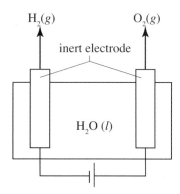

Figure 1 A water-electrolysis cell

In any cell design, a voltage is supplied across the inert electrodes submerged in water, resulting in a flow of current. The overall reaction is below.

$$H_2O(l) \rightarrow H_2(g) + \tfrac{1}{2} O_2(g)$$

$$(\Delta H = 286 \text{ kJ and } \Delta S = 0.16 \text{ kJ K}^{-1})$$

Efficiency is an important factor in cell design and is affected by changes in temperature. Real-world cells are designed for performance under non-standard conditions; therefore, adjustments of reaction conditions must be made according to the Nernst equation (below) in conjunction with the data in Table 1.

$$E_{cell} = E_{cell}^{\circ} - \frac{RT}{nF} \ln Q$$

In this relation, E_{cell} is the standard cell potential, $R = 8.31$ J K^{-1} mol^{-1}, n is the number of electrons transferred per mole of reactant consumed, $F = 96{,}500$ C mol^{-1}, and Q is the reaction quotient.

Half-reaction	E (V)
$Na^+(aq) + e^- \rightarrow Na(s)$	−2.71
$2\,H_2O(l) + 2\,e^- \rightarrow H_2(g) + 2\,OH^-\,(aq)$	−0.83
$2\,H^+(aq) + 2\,e^- \rightarrow H_2(g)$	0.00
$O_2(g) + 2\,H_2O(l) + 4\,e^- \rightarrow 4\,OH^-\,(aq)$	0.40
$O_2(g) + 4\,H^+(aq) + 4\,e^- \rightarrow 2\,H_2O(l)$	1.23
$Cl_2(g) + 2\,e^- \rightarrow 2\,Cl^-\,(aq)$	1.36

Table 1

1. The standard cell potential for electrolysis of water is:

A) −1.23 V.
B) −0.83 V.
C) 0.40 V.
D) 1.23 V.

2. In the electrolysis of pure water, $E_{cell} = 0$ when $T = 400$ K. This is consistent with which of the following?

A) The reaction is no longer at equilibrium.
B) The K_{eq} at 400 K is greater than the K_{eq} at 298 K.
C) More free energy is required from the circuit at 400 K compared to 298 K.
D) E° cell is greater at 400 K compared to 298 K.

3. $NaCl(s)$ is added to pure water in an electrolysis unit with the goal of increasing the rate of oxygen production. Will this be effective?

A) No, because the standard reduction potential of $Na^+(aq)$ is less than that of $H^+(aq)$.
B) No, because $Cl^-(aq)$ will be preferentially oxidized at the anode to produce chlorine gas.
C) Yes, because $Na^+(aq)$ will migrate to the cathode and alleviate the buildup of negative charge.
D) Yes, because the overall conductivity of water will be decreased with the addition of solute.

4. Which of the following is true about the electrolysis of water?

    I.   Oxygen gas is formed at the cathode.
    II.   Electrons flow from anode to cathode.
    III. The anode is positively charged.

A) I only
B) II only
C) I and II only
D) II and III only

5. When adding an electrolyte to water during the production of hydrogen gas, it is important to choose one that contains:

A) a cation with a higher reduction potential than hydroxide.
B) a cation with a higher reduction potential than hydronium.
C) an anion with a higher reduction potential than hydronium.
D) an anion with a higher reduction potential than hydroxide.

SOLUTIONS TO FREESTANDING QUESTIONS: ELECTROCHEMISTRY

1. **A**   The reducing agent in this reaction will be the species supplying the electrons for the forward reaction, and which is in turn oxidized. Choices B and C list product species in the reaction as it is written, and can therefore be eliminated. The electrons taken from Fe^0 are responsible for the reduction of Au^{3+}, therefore Fe^0 (choice A) is correct. Au^{3+} is the oxidizing agent in this reaction.

2. **C**   The anode of an electrochemical cell is the site of oxidation. In order to determine the correct answer, start by assessing which of the listed reactions are reductions and which are oxidations. In choice A, S goes from S^{6+} to S^{2-}. In choice B, the transformation is S^{6+} to S^{4+}. In choice D, S^{6+} becomes S^0. All of these reactions are reduction reactions, and are likely the source of reducing electrons (the cathode!). In choice C, S^{4+} is oxidized to S^{6+}, which is the most likely of the four reactions to occur at the oxidizing anode.

3. **B**   The following calculation can be used to determine the mass of consumed hydrogen:

    $$2 \text{ min} \times 60 \text{ sec/min} = 120 \text{ sec}$$

    $$2 \text{ C/sec} \times 120 \text{ sec} = 240 \text{ C}$$

    $$240 \text{ C} \times (1 \text{ mol } e^-/96{,}500 \text{ C}) \approx 25/10{,}000$$

    $$= 25/(100 \times 10^2) = 0.25 \times 10^{-2} = 0.0025 \text{ mol } e^-$$

    $$(1 \text{ mol } H_2/2 \text{ mol } e^-) \times 0.0025 \text{ mol } e^- = 0.00125 \text{ mol } H_2$$

    $$0.00125 \text{ mol } H_2 \times (2 \text{ g}/1 \text{ mol } H_2) = 0.0025 \text{ g } H_2$$

4. **B**   Galvanic cells should have a positive voltage (eliminate choice D). By comparison of the equations, the most energetically favorable reaction is $Fe^0 + 2 \ Fe^{3+} \rightarrow 3 \ Fe^{2+}$. The summation of the first equation in the forward direction and the middle equation in the reverse direction gives a total of 1.21 V.

5. **B**   In order to compute the voltage for the overall reaction, the two constitutive half reactions must be summed. The reactions in choices C and D result in negative cell potentials, and can therefore be eliminated. The overall size of the potential for the reaction $Pb^{4+} \rightarrow Pb^{2+}$ is much larger than any of the other reduction potentials. This points to the fact that the best overall equation is going to include this half-reaction in the forward (reducing) direction. Choice B includes the reduction of Pb^{4+}, and in conjunction with the oxidation of Pb(*s*), has an overall cell potential of +1.82 V. This is far larger than possible for the Sn reaction in choice A.

6. **B**   Since the question states that the reaction must be driven by an external voltage, the cell can be classified as electrolytic. This means that the cathode is negatively charged, and the anode is positively charged. Reduction reactions occur at the cathode, so oxidation reactions in the choices may be eliminated (choices A and D). The reaction in choice C is not a redox

reaction, as no oxidation states change. It can likewise be eliminated by the fact that no PtO is noted in the cell. Choice B is the reductive electrodeposition of Pt^{2+}, which occurs at the negatively charged cathode.

7. **D** The largest positive oxidation state among these choices is the +7 of Mn in $KMnO_4$ ($4 \times O = -8$, $K = +1$, $Mn = +7$). The two ammonia ligands in $MnO_2(NH_3)_2$ carry no charge, so Mn in this compound is only +4. Os in OsO_2 is also +4, and W in WCl_3 is +3.

8. **A** The reduction potential of H^+ is the standard for the standard hydrogen electrode ($E° = 0.00$ V). This makes H^+ a better cathode-reactant than Fe^{2+}, which it will replace in the cell's chemistry. The overall voltage of the cell will become more positive, so by the equation $\Delta G° = -nFE°$, choices C and D may be eliminated. If reaction 1 includes the reduction of Fe, and reaction 2 includes the reduction of H^+, two equations may be written for their respective free energies:

$$\Delta G°_1 = -nFE°_1 = -nF(0.33)$$

$$\Delta G°_2 = -nFE°_2 = -nF(0.77)$$

The difference in these two values of $\Delta G°$ can thereby be written as follows:

$$\Delta G°_2 - \Delta G°_1 = -nF(0.77 - 0.33) = -nF(0.44)$$

$$= -2 \text{ mol} \times 96{,}500 \text{ C/mol} \times 0.44 \text{ V} \approx -2 \text{ mol} \times 96{,}500 \text{ C/mol} \times 0.5 \text{ V}$$

$$\approx -96{,}500 \text{ C·V} = -96.5 \text{ kJ}$$

As we've rounded 0.44 to 0.5, this number represents an upper limit on the magnitude of the absolute value of the overall answer. The only answer that fits is choice A.

9. **C** The reduction potential of Pt^{2+} is large and positive, indicating a propensity to be reduced, or act as an oxidizing agent. The reduction potential of Fe^{3+} is small and negative, which points to the employment of this equation in reverse, with Fe(s) acting as the reducing agent. The full reaction is therefore $3 Pt^{2+}(aq) + 2 Fe(s) \rightarrow 2 Fe^{3+}(aq) + 3 Pt(s)$. This equation eliminates choices B and D, since Fe^{3+} is a product, and neither an oxidizing nor reducing agent. Correct calculation of the reduction potential for the cell yields $E° = 1.2$ V $+ 0.036$ V $= 1.236$ V, eliminating choice A.

10. **D** This is a 2 × 2 question, which is best answered by first addressing one of the assertions. Since copper solid is produced, the reaction occurring on the zinc surface must be

$$Cu^{2+}(aq) + 2e^- \rightarrow Cu(s)$$

This is a reduction reaction since copper ions from solution are gaining electrons to form metallic copper (eliminate choices A and C). Reduction always occurs at the cathode, which is connected to the negative terminal of a battery in applications requiring an external power supply such as an electrolytic cell (choice D is correct).

SOLUTIONS TO ELECTROCHEMISTRY PRACTICE PASSAGE

1. **A** Choices C and D can be eliminated since positive potentials only occur for spontaneous reactions (which we do not have here since an external battery is required to drive the reaction). The problem can be solved using two different sets of half reactions from Table 1, whose addition will give the reaction for hydrolysis in the passage. In the first option, the reduction reaction of oxygen gas to water under acidic conditions is reversed (changing the sign), and the stoichiometry is divided by 2 (no effect on the magnitude of potential):

   Cathode: $H^+(aq) + 2e^- \rightarrow H_2(g)$ $E° = 0.00$

   Anode: $H_2O(l) \rightarrow \frac{1}{2}O_2(g) + 2H^+(aq) + 2e^-$ $E° = -1.23$

   Cell: $H_2O(l) \rightarrow H_2(g) + \frac{1}{2}O_2(g)$ $E° = -1.23$

   In the second option, the reduction of oxygen gas to hydroxide is again reversed (changing the sign), and the stoichiometry is divided by 2 (no effect on the magnitude of potential):

   Cathode: $H_2O(l) + 2e^- \rightarrow H_2(g) + 2OH^-(aq)$ $E° = -0.83$

   Anode: $OH^-(aq) \rightarrow \frac{1}{2}O_2(g) + H_2O(l) + 2e^-$ $E° = -0.40$

   Cell: $H_2O(l) \rightarrow H_2(g) + \frac{1}{2}O_2(g)$ $E° = -1.23$

2. **B** When $E_{cell} = 0$, the reaction is at equilibrium (eliminate choice A). At equilibrium, $Q = K_{eq}$ and the Nernst equation can be solved as follows:

$$E_{cell} = E°_{cell} - \frac{RT}{nF}\ln Q$$

$$0 = E°_{cell} - \frac{RT}{nF}\ln K_{eq}$$

$$\ln K_{eq} = \frac{E°_{cell}\,nF}{RT}$$

   $E°_{cell} = -1.23$ V is a constant (eliminate choice D), and the only factors that are changing are K_{eq} and T:

$$\ln K_{eq} \propto \frac{-1.23}{T}$$

   Because the standard cell potential is negative, as T increases from 298 to 400 K, $\ln K_{eq}$ also increases (becomes less negative). This makes sense because you can expect K_{eq} to increase with increasing temperature for an endothermic reaction. Since the environment is contributing more energy at higher temperatures, the battery does not have to contribute as much free energy (eliminate choice C).

3. **C**   During hydrolysis, a negative charge accumulates in the fluid around the cathode, and a positive charge accumulates in the fluid around the anode:

$$2\,H^+(aq) + 2e^- \rightarrow H_2(g) \qquad \text{(reduction at cathode)}$$

$$H_2O(l) \rightarrow \frac{1}{2}\,O_2\,(g) + 2\,H^+\,(aq) + 2e^- \quad \text{(oxidation at anode)}$$

This imbalance inhibits the flow of electrons, and it is the reason why the hydrolysis of pure water is very slow. Electrolytes in solution function as a salt bridge in that they neutralize this charge buildup. Cations migrate to the surface of the cathode, while anions migrate to the anode. Adding an electrolyte increases conductivity (eliminate choice D) and increases the rate of hydrolysis (eliminate choices A and B). The fact that $Na^+(aq)$ has a lower reduction potential than $H^+(aq)$ and $Cl^-(aq)$ has a lower oxidation potential than hydroxide ensures no alteration of the reaction products.

4. **D**   Start by analyzing Item I, since it appears in exactly two of the answer choices; whether it is true or false, you can eliminate half the answers. Item I is false: oxidation always occurs at the anode and reduction always occurs at the cathode of all cells. Oxygen gas is produced from the oxidation of water (or hydroxide ion) at the anode (choices A and C can be eliminated). Since both remaining answer choices include Item II, it must be true and you can focus on Item III. Item III is true: electrolysis is not spontaneous, so electrons are forced toward a charge they would not go toward spontaneously; therefore, the cathode is considered negative and the anode is considered positive in electrolytic cells (choice B can be eliminated, and choice D is correct). Note that Item II is in fact true: since oxidation is the loss of electrons and always occurs at the anode, electrons must flow from anode to cathode in all electrolytic cells.

5. **D**   Adding an electrolyte minimizes charge buildup and increases conductivity in electrolysis. However, it is important that the electrolyte is not preferentially oxidized or reduced instead of water. Therefore, the cation should be less likely to be reduced than hydronium (eliminate choice B), and the anion should be less likely to be oxidized (more likely to be reduced) than hydroxide (choice D is correct). The important comparisons are between the two cations in solution competing for reduction (eliminate choice A) or between the two anions in solution competing for oxidation (eliminate choice C).

Part 6

MCAT
Organic Chemistry

Chapter 30
Structure and Stability

FREESTANDING QUESTIONS: STRUCTURE AND STABILITY

1. Aluminum chloride (AlCl$_3$) is known to efficiently extract Cl$^-$ from both organic and inorganic species, forming [AlCl$_4^-$] and a de-chlorinated cation. If 3,5,6,7-tetrachloro-1,4-cyclooctadiene were treated with an equimolar amount of AlCl$_3$, which of the Cl atoms will be extracted?

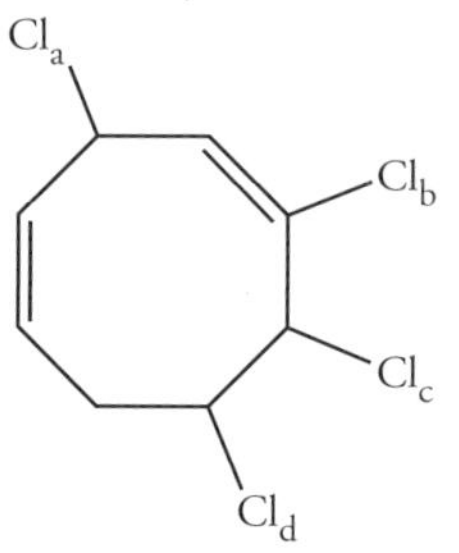

A) Cl$_a$
B) Cl$_b$
C) Cl$_c$
D) Cl$_d$

2. Which of the following stereochemical descriptions most accurately describes the products in the reaction shown below?

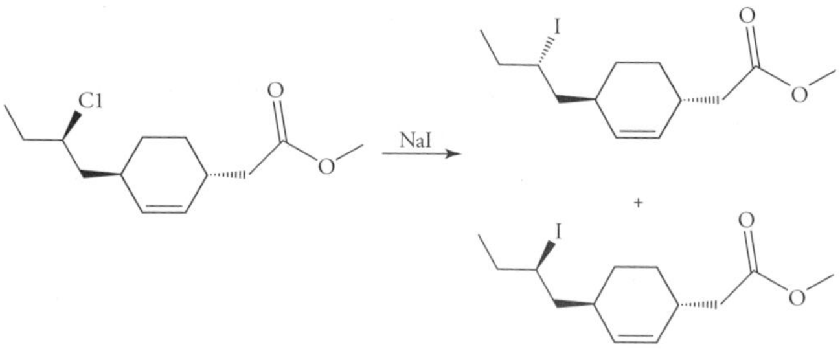

A) The product is a mixture of diastereomers.
B) The product is a mixture of enantiomers.
C) The product has meso stereochemistry.
D) The product is a racemic mixture.

3. When natural fatty acids are heated at high temperatures, the natural Z-double bonds may be isomerized to E-double bonds. Which of the following fatty acids is most prone to such isomerization?

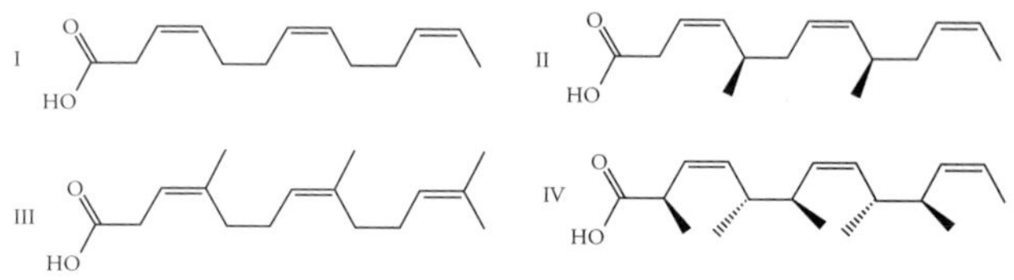

A) I
B) II
C) III
D) IV

4. Rank the following in terms of increasing acidity:

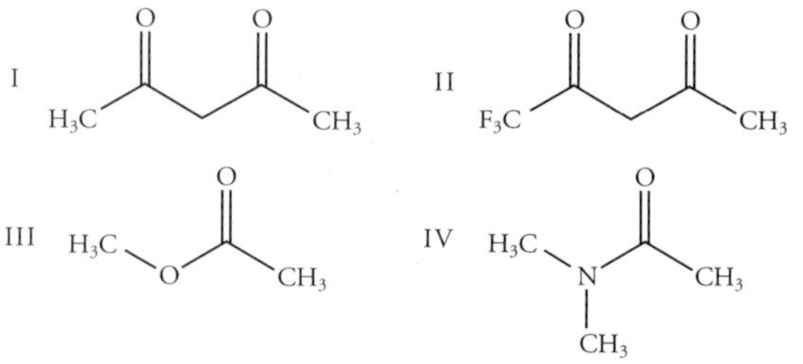

A) III < I < IV < II
B) IV < III < II < I
C) IV < III < I < II
D) II < I < III < IV

5. When compared to γ-butyrolactone, the increased susceptibility to nucleophilic attack of α-acetolactone is due to which of the following factors?

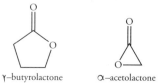

γ–butyrolactone   α–acetolactone

I.   There is more ring strain in γ-butyrolactone than in α-acetolactone.

II. The bond angles deviate more from ideality in α-acetolactone than in γ-butyrolactone.

III. There is greater freedom of rotation about the C—C bond at the carbonyl carbon in γ-butyrolactone than in α-acetolactone.

A) II only
B) III only
C) I and III only
D) II and III only

6. Which of the following is true based on the structure shown below?

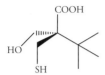

A) The highest priority group is $-C(CH_3)_3$, and the chiral center has an *R* configuration.
B) The highest priority group is $-CH_2SH$, and the chiral center has an *S* configuration.
C) The highest priority group is $-COOH$, and the chiral center has an *S* configuration.
D) The highest priority group is $-CH_2SH$, and the chiral center has an *R* configuration.

CHO
H———OH
HO———H
H———OH
H———OH
CH_2OH

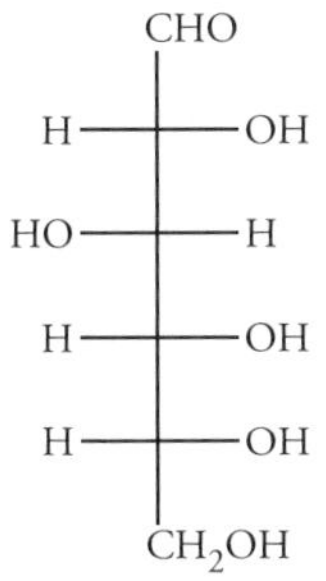

D–glucose

7. D-Galactose, a C-4 epimer of D-glucose (shown above), can be selectively oxidized at the primary carbons to produce galactaric acid. In aqueous solutions, galactaric acid exists in equilibrium with its cyclic form, galactaro-lactone. The linear structure of galactaric acid:

A) is a strong acid.
B) is water insoluble.
C) is optically inactive.
D) is a structural isomer of glucose.

8. Rank the following species in order of increasing nucleophilicity:

NH_3 HS^- H_2O CH_3O^-

A) $NH_3 < H_2O < HS^- < CH_3O^-$
B) $NH_3 < CH_3O^- < H_2O < HS^-$
C) $H_2O < NH_3 < CH_3O^- < HS^-$
D) $H_2O < CH_3O^- < HS^- < NH_3$

9. In the reaction below, what is the expected specific rotation of the product?

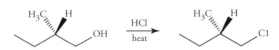

(*S*)-2-methyl-1-butanol
$[\alpha] = -5.76°$

A) $-5.76°$
B) $+5.76°$
C) $0.00°$
D) Unable to predict

10. The *cis* isomer of the aldehyde shown is less susceptible to nucleophilic addition than the *trans* isomer because:

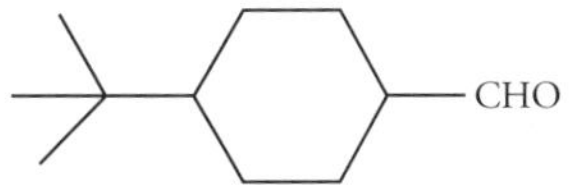

I. the axial *tert*-butyl group sterically hinders the aldehyde from nucleophilic attack.
II. the intermediate formed from addition to its equatorial aldehyde has increased steric interactions.
III. the intermediate formed from addition to its axial aldehyde has increased steric interactions.

A) II only
B) III only
C) I and II only
D) I and III only

11. Reactions of esters with nucleophiles potentially can proceed via either acyl-oxygen cleavage or alkyl-oxygen cleavage. These two processes are illustrated below for thermal reaction of a phthalate ester, Compound I, with ammonia.

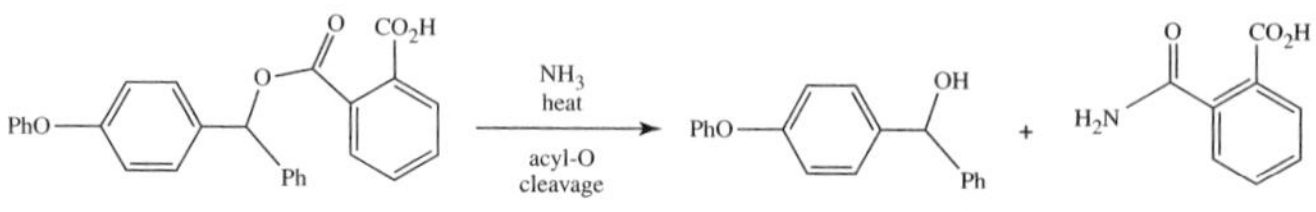

Compound I → (NH₃, heat, acyl-O cleavage) → Compound II + Compound III

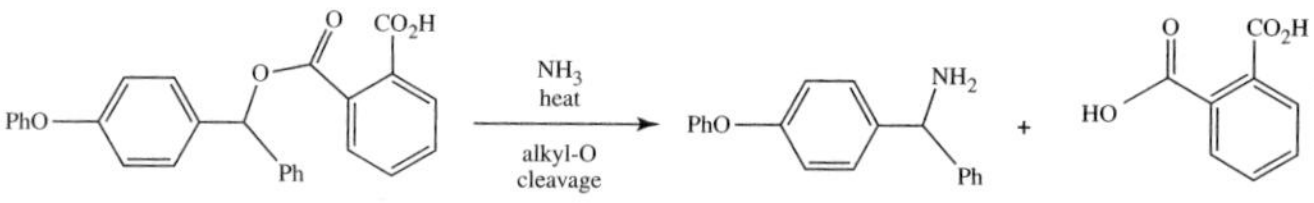

Compound I → (NH₃, heat, alkyl-O cleavage) → Compound IV + Compound V

Reaction of optically active Compound I with ammonia has been reported to afford racemic products. Which one of the following statements is most consistent with this observation?

A) Reaction of Compound I with ammonia affords Compounds IV and V.
B) Reaction of Compound I with ammonia proceeds via acyl-oxygen cleavage.
C) Compound II is formed with inversion of configuration at the original chiral center in Compound I.
D) Compound IV is formed with inversion of configuration at the original chiral center in Compound I.

12. Consider the proton NMR spectra of Compounds I, II, and III below in $CDCl_3$ solution:

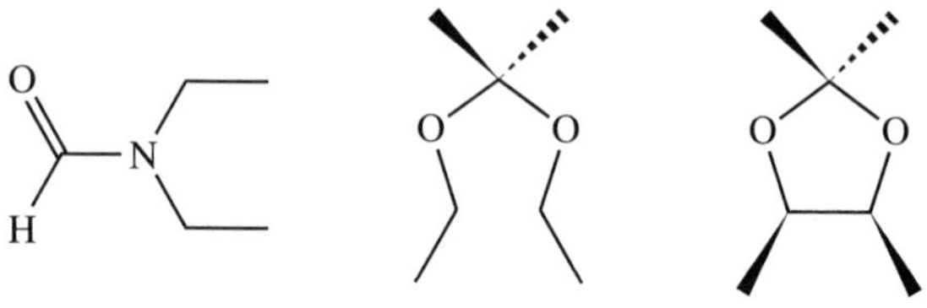

I   **II**   **III**

Which of these compounds is/are expected to produce an NMR spectrum that consists exclusively of one singlet, one triplet, and one quartet?

A) I only
B) II only
C) I and III only
D) II and III only

13. Neurotrophins belong to a family of proteins that control neurogenesis in mammalian brains. Jiadifenolide, a sesquiterpenoid natural product isolated from the fruit of *Illicium jiadifengpi*, has been reported to exhibit neurotrophic activity on human neuronal precursor cells. The structure of (–)-jiadifenolide, $C_{15}H_{18}O_7$, is shown below.

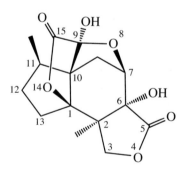

How many chiral centers are found in (–)-jiadifenolide, and what is the absolute configuration at the hemiacetal carbon atom?

A) 6 chiral centers, and the hemiacetal carbon atom possesses the *R*-configuration
B) 7 chiral centers, and the hemiacetal carbon atom possesses the *R*-configuration
C) 6 chiral centers, and the hemiacetal carbon atom possesses the *S*-configuration
D) 7 chiral centers, and the hemiacetal carbon atom possesses the *S*-configuration

14. 2,4-Dibromo-3-methylpentane contains three chiral centers for which a maximum of $2^3 = 8$ stereoisomers can be drawn, as shown below.

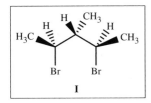

I

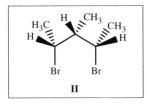

II

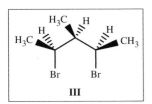

III

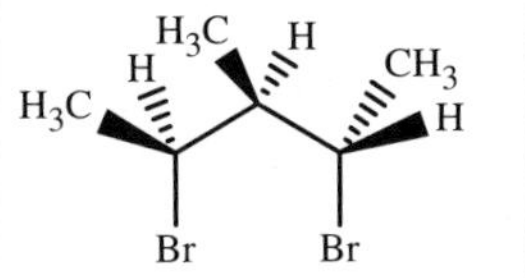

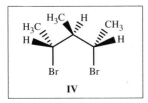

IV

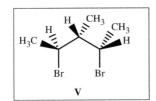

V

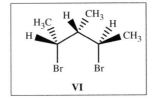

VI

VII

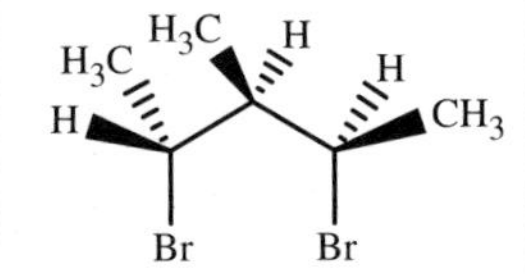

VIII

A mixture of all possible stereoisomers of 2,4-dibromo-3-methylpentane is spotted on a silica gel TLC plate, and the spot is eluted with 5% chloroform in hexane. By assuming that the components of this mixture can be separated under the experimental conditions employed, what is the *maximum number* of spots that can appear on the TLC plate after elution has been completed?

A) 4
B) 5
C) 6
D) 7

STRUCTURE AND STABILITY PRACTICE PASSAGE

Chlorosulpholipids are a class of organic toxin found in shell-fish that are responsible for some illnesses associated with the consumption of tainted seafood. Much like conventional lipids, these molecules bear both hydrophobic and hydrophilic regions, but differ from normal human lipids in that their backbones contain a number of chlorine atoms and one or more sulfonyl groups. A representative, stereochemically defined chlorosul-pholipid is shown in Figure 1.

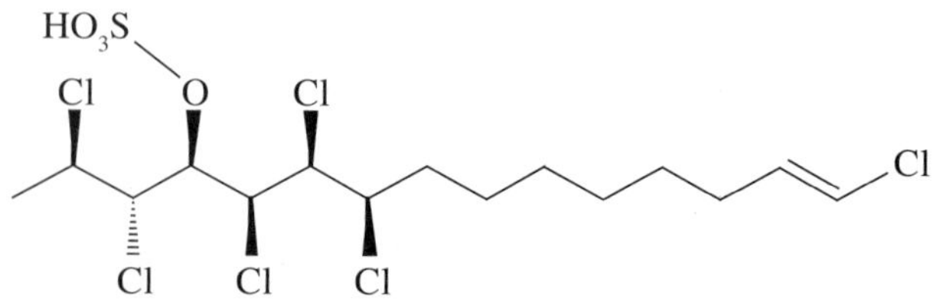

Figure 1   Chlorosulpholipid

Some chlorosulpholipids, however, play more beneficial roles, such as malhamensilipin A (Figure 2), which is employed as a protein kinase inhibitor. This molecule is derived from algae, but due to its stereochemical complexity its structure is not well defined.

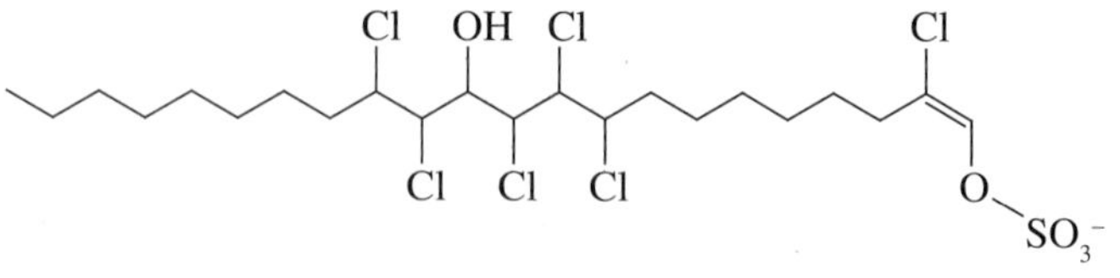

Figure 2   Malhamensilipin A

Since these molecules can only be isolated from their aquatic sources in small quantities, finding a method to synthesize them is important to allow for further study of their biological effects. Multiple chlorine atoms can be introduced through ad-dition reactions to the double bonds in the carbon backbone of unsaturated lipids. Addition across double bonds can happen in one of two ways: *syn* addition, where both chlorine atoms are added to the same side of a planar double bond, or *anti* addition, where the chlorine atoms are added to opposite sides of the planar double bond (Figure 3).

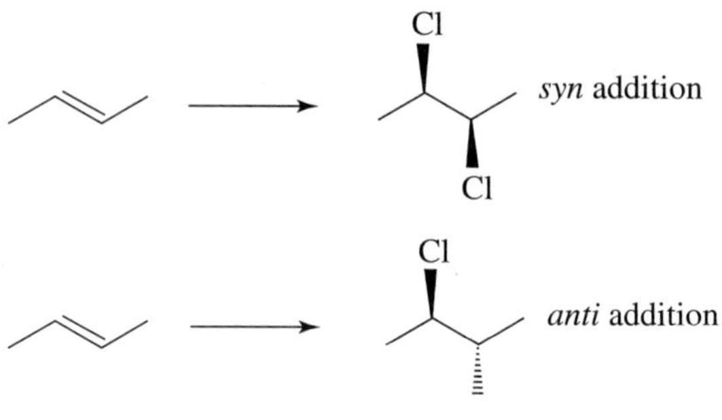

Figure 3   *Syn* vs. *anti* addition to alkenes

1. If malhamensilipin A is known to contain an *E* alkene but the rest of the stereochemistry in the molecule is unknown, what is the maximum number of stereoisomers possible for the molecule?

A) 2
B) 8
C) 32
D) 64

2. The ^{1}H NMR spectrum of the chlorosulpholipid in Figure 1 exhibits one doublet upfield and one doublet downfield. What is the ratio of their respective integration?

A) 3:1
B) 1:1
C) 1:2
D) 1:3

3. The chlorosulpholipid in Figure 1 can act as a:

A) strong Lewis base.
B) Brønsted acid
C) reducing agent.
D) Brønsted base.

4. A chemist treats the following *Z*-alkene with a reagent intending to add two chlorine atoms across the double bond in a *syn* fashion:

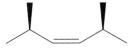

Assuming the reagent is effective and selective in the *syn* addition, which of the following best describes the product(s) of the reaction?

A) A pair of enantiomers
B) A mix of four diastereomers
C) A pair of diastereomers
D) A meso compound

5. Malhamensilipin A is treated with dimethyl sulfate, a strong methylating reagent, and purified by reverse phase HPLC. The retention time of the product, in relation to the starting material, would be:

A) longer, because the product is more polar than the starting material.
B) longer, because the product is less polar than the starting material.
C) shorter, because the product is more polar than the starting material.
D) shorter, because the product is less polar than the starting material.

6. What is the absolute configuration for C-13 and C-14, respectively, in the chlorosulpholipid in Figure 1?

A) *R, S*
B) *R, R*
C) *S, R*
D) *S, S*

SOLUTIONS TO FREESTANDING QUESTIONS: STRUCTURE AND STABILITY

1.   **A**   Extraction of Cl⁻ results in the formation of a carbocation at the carbon where the Cl was formerly bound. The Cl⁻ most likely to be extracted will be the one that leaves the most stable cation, which in this molecule means the one most efficiently stabilized by resonance. Extraction of Cl_a will result in the following highly-delocalized cation.

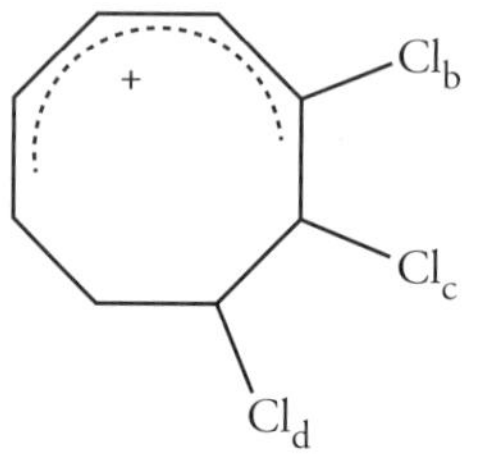

Neither the extraction of Cl_b nor Cl_d will allow delocalization into either of the two double bonds, and choices B and D can therefore be eliminated. Extraction of Cl_c only allows delocalization into one of the two double bonds (eliminate choice C).

2.   **A**   In the reaction shown, the two products differ at one stereocenter (the iodine), yet each has two other stereocenters that are unaltered in the reaction. As the product compounds are non-mirror-images, they are a pair of diastereomers. A racemic mixture is composed of an enantiomeric pair, making choices B and D equivalent, and both incorrect. Enantiomers have different stereochemistry at every chiral center and are mirror images. Meso compounds are achiral because they contain a plane of symmetry, which is absent in the products shown (eliminate choice C).

3.   **D**   The isomerization from Z to E is driven by the relaxation of the steric stress in the region shown below:

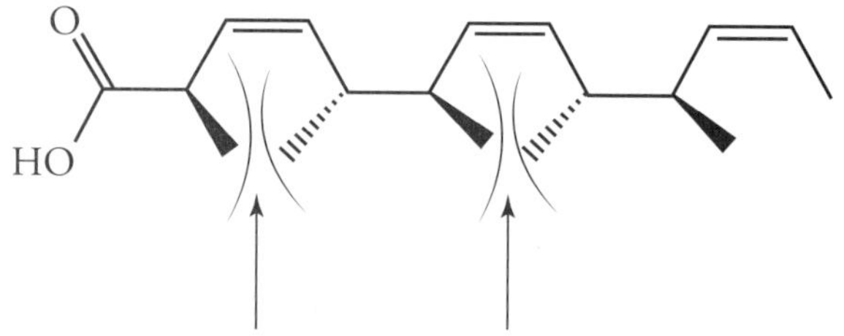

Acid IV has the greatest amount of steric strain and will benefit the most from isomerization.

4.   **C**   In a ranking question, an efficient POE strategy is to look for an extreme. Start by determining the most acidic hydrogen on the compounds. An α-proton located between two carbonyls is more acidic than a standard α-proton due to greater resonance stabilization over both carbonyl groups, therefore, compounds I and II are more acidic than compounds III and IV (eliminate choice D; choice A can also be eliminated if you're looking in the middle of the ranking). Compound II will be more acidic than compound I due to the nearby CF_3 group, which inductively withdraws electron density (eliminate choice B). Compounds

III and IV differ by an oxygen (ester) and nitrogen (amide) atom. Upon deprotonation, the enolate portion of the amide is less resonance stabilized because its nitrogen atom is more electron-donating by resonance compared to the ester oxygen. This grants the enolate portion of the ester greater relative ability to stabilize its carbanion, rendering it more acidic than the amide and making choice C correct.

5.   **A**   Ring strain is dependent on the bond angles associated with the cyclic structure and how much they deviate from the ideal angles, which are dependent on the hybridization of the atoms of the ring. α-Acetolactone is a three-member ring with a geometrically determined internal bond angle of ~60°, while γ-butyrolactone, a five-membered-ring, will have an internal geometrical angle of ~108°. Since the 108° angles of γ-butyrolactone are closer to the ideal angles of 109.5° for an sp^3 hybridized atom, Item II is correct (eliminate choice B) and Item I is incorrect (eliminate choice C). As part of a small (< 8 carbon) ring system, neither α-acetolactone nor γ-butyrolactone have any freedom of rotation around the C–CO–C bonds at their respective carbonyl carbons, making Item III false (eliminate choice D).

6.   **B**   To assign absolute configuration to a stereocenter, first prioritize the substituents based on the highest atomic number of the atoms at the first point of difference between each substituent. Since each substituent has a C attached to the chiral center, prioritize by the next atoms out on each chain. Sulfur has the highest atomic number, so the thiol is group 1 (eliminate choices A and C). The carboxylic acid has two oxygens compared to only one in the alcohol, so these groups are prioritized 2 and 3, respectively. Since the *t*-butyl group has only carbons attached, which has a smaller atomic number than oxygen, this is the last group. By rotating the molecule to put the number 4 group in the back, connecting groups 1 to 2 to 3 gives a counterclockwise arc, so this is an *S* configuration (eliminate choice D).

7.   **C**   Selective oxidation of D-galactose will convert the C-1 aldehyde and the C-6 primary alcohol to the carboxylic acids.

D–glucose   D–galactose   galactaric acid

Galactaric acid is a meso compound due to the plane of symmetry bisecting the bond between C-3 and C-4, and is therefore optically inactive. Carboxylic acids are relatively strong as organic acids go, but they still do not dissociate completely, making them weak (eliminate choice A). Galactaric acid contains four hydroxyl and two carboxylic acid groups. These hydrogen bonding groups will make it highly water soluble (eliminate choice B). Galactaric acid has a different chemical formula than glucose, and therefore the compounds cannot be isomers of any sort (eliminate choice D).

8. **C** For this ranking question, start by looking for extremes and eliminate answer choices. Nucleophilicity increases with greater charge, so the neutral compounds water and ammonia are worse nucleophiles than the methoxide or sulfide anions (eliminate choices B and D). When comparing elements in the same family like S and O, the larger, more polarizable element will be the better nucleophile (eliminate choice A). Similarly, looking at the other extreme for the ranking, choice A can be eliminated because when comparing elements in the same period like N and O, the less electronegative element will be the better nucleophile, making ammonia better than water.

9. **D** Since the reactant and product are completely different chiral compounds, they will NOT have the same optical rotation (eliminate choice A). The molecules are also not enantiomers, so the optical rotation will not be of equal magnitude but opposite sign (eliminate choice B). Since the reaction did not destroy or racemize the stereocenter, the product will retain some nonzero optical activity (eliminate choice C), though without measuring it directly, the optical rotation cannot be accurately predicted (choice D is correct).

10. **B** The *cis* and *trans* isomers of the compound are shown in their chair conformations below:

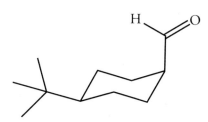 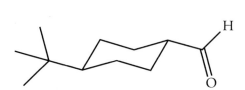

cis isomer, axial aldehyde   *trans* isomer, equatorial aldehyde

Since each of the Items appear in exactly two of the answer choices, it doesn't matter which Item you start analyzing, so start with Item I. Item I is false: the most stable conformation of a cyclohexane chair will put the largest substituent, in this case the *tert*-butyl group, in the equatorial position to avoid 1,3-diaxial interactions. With the orientation of the *tert*-butyl group assigned, the *cis* cyclohexane must have the aldehyde axial (both groups are on the top of the ring as shown) and the *trans* must have the aldehyde equatorial (one group is on the top, the other on the bottom of the ring). Item I is incorrect because it indicates the *tert*-butyl group is in the axial position (eliminate choices C and D). Item II says the *cis* cyclohexane has the aldehyde in the equatorial position, which is incorrect (eliminate choice A). Therefore, the correct answer has to be choice B. Upon nucleophilic addition to the aldehyde, the carbonyl carbon will become sp^3 hybridized and tetrahedral. This change in geometry gives the substituent increased 1,3-diaxial interactions with the hydrogens on the ring, making it less likely to change hybridization. Attack on the equatorial aldehyde, however, creates no such increase in steric strain, so addition to the *trans* isomer is more likely.

11. **A** Heterolytic alkyl-O cleavage in Compound I is expected to lead to the formation of a carbocation, thereby resulting in formation of racemic products. If Compound I were to react with ammonia with concomitant alkyl-O cleavage, racemic (optically inactive) Compound IV would be obtained. Note also that Compound V is achiral and thus is optically inactive (choice A is correct).

No bond to the chiral center in Compound I will be affected if the reaction were to proceed with concomitant acyl-oxygen cleavage. In this event, Compound II would be formed with *retention* of configuration at the original chiral center and thus would be optically active. This result is inconsistent with the statement included in the stem (choice B can be eliminated). Choices C and D indicate that products II and IV, respectively, are formed with concomitant inversion of configuration at the original chiral center in Compound I. In this event, both Compounds II and IV would be expected to be optically active (choices C and D can be eliminated).

12. **B** Since all Items appear in exactly two of the answer choices, it doesn't matter which Item you start analyzing, so start with Item I. Item I is false: compound I is *N,N*-dimethylformamide. Resonance interaction between the nitrogen lone pair of electrons and the adjacent carbonyl group is expected to confer partial double bond character upon the amide carbon-nitrogen bond. Consequently, these two ethyl groups are nonequivalent. As shown in the image below, the proton NMR spectrum of Compound I is expected to consist of two quartets (CH_2 groups spin-spin coupled to adjacent CH_3 groups), two triplets (CH_3 groups coupled to adjacent CH_2 groups) and one singlet (aldehyde **H**C=O proton).

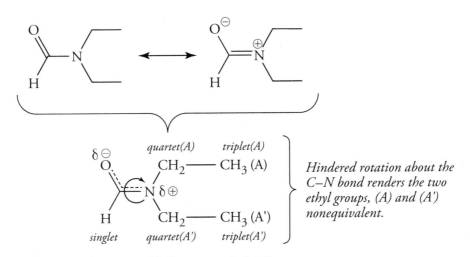

Compound I (Resonance hybrid)

Choices A and C can be eliminated. Note that both remaining choices include Item II, so it must be true, and you can focus on Item III. Item III is false: compound III contains two chiral centers but is optically inactive (*meso*). Accordingly, the *cis* C(4) and C(5) methyl groups are equivalent. Their signal is expected to be split into a doublet *via* spin-spin coupling to the adjacent proton. Similarly, protons H(4) and H(5) are equivalent, and their signal is expected to be split into a quartet *via* coupling to the adjacent methyl group.

Finally, the two geminal methyl groups are magnetically nonequivalent due to their *cis/trans* stereochemical relationship to the *cis* C(4) and C(5) methyl groups. Thus, the geminal CH_3 groups are expected to give rise to two singlets in the proton NMR spectrum of Compound III (choice D can be eliminated, and choice B is correct).

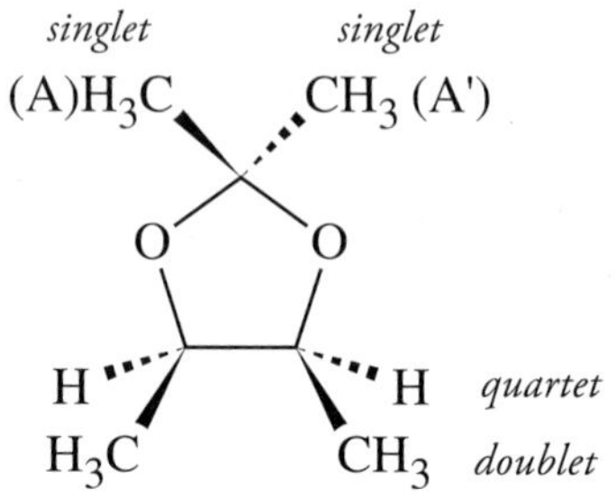

Compound III

Item II is in fact true: the proton NMR spectrum of Compound II is expected to consist of one singlet (due to the geminal methyl groups) along with one triplet and one quartet (due to the two equivalent CH_2CH_3 groups).

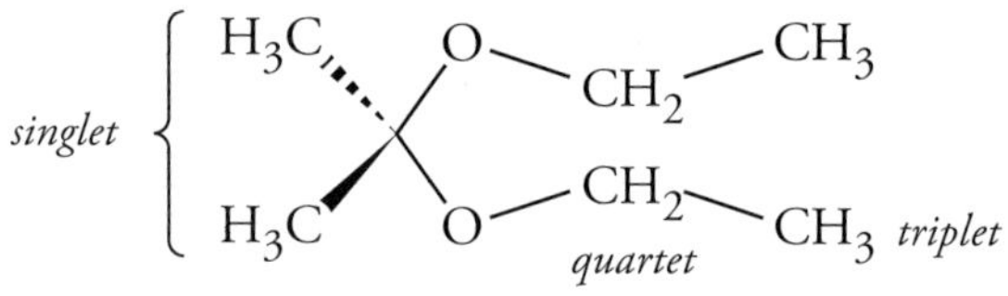

Compound II

Note: You are likely to recognize the characteristic absorption signal pattern associated with an isolated X-CH_2CH_3 group, i.e., one CH_3 triplet and one CH_2 quartet. In addition, you are expected to recognize that the proton NMR spectrum of Compound II meets the criteria stated in the question stem. A higher level of understanding is required to recognize that the expected appearance of the corresponding spectrum of Compound I is inconsistent with these criteria; however, since "I and II only" is not offered as one of the four answer choices, it is possible to arrive at the correct response (choice B) without necessarily understanding why the expected appearance of the spectrum of Compound I does not meet the criteria stated in the stem.

13. **D** Jiadifenolide contains seven chiral centers (choices A and C can be eliminated), which are located at C(1), C(2), C(6), C(7), C(9), C(10), and C(11). Each of these centers is marked by an asterisk in the structure shown below:

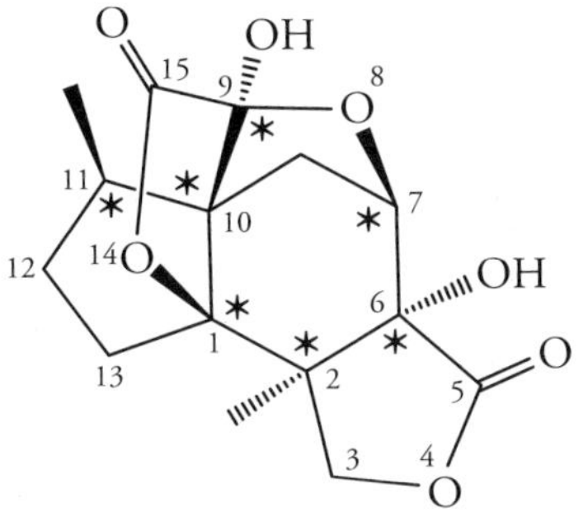

Hemiacetals possess the general structure RCH(OH)OR′. Jiadifenolide contains one hemiacetal functionality at C(9). Cahn-Ingold-Prelog (CIP) rules must be applied in order to establish the R,S absolute configuration at this chiral center. Priorities at C(9) are seen to decrease in the order O(8) > OH > O=C(15) > C(10). When the molecule is viewed correctly down the C(9)-C(10) bond [i.e., viewed down the bond of lowest priority with C(10) positioned away from the viewer], the remaining three bonds decrease in priority along a counterclockwise direction as indicated below:

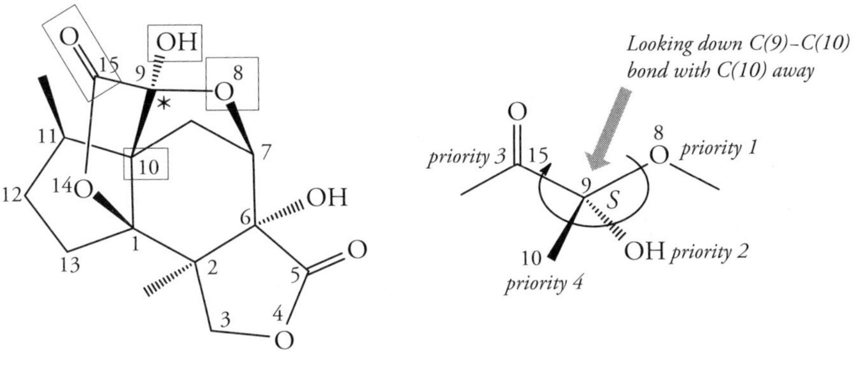

This shows that C(9), the central carbon atom in the hemiacetal moiety in (–)-jiadifenolide, possesses the S-configuration (choice B can be eliminated, and choice D is correct).

14. **A** It is necessary first to evaluate the eight structures shown in the stem by determining which are enantiomeric pairs and which are achiral (*meso*). It can be seen that the given set of structures consists of two enantiomeric pairs (V-VIII and VI-VII) and two diastereoisomeric *meso* structures (I and III). It should be noted that the remaining structures, II and IV, are identical to III and I, respectively. Hence, 2,4-dibromo-3-methylpentane consists of six stereoisomers, i.e., two enantiomeric pairs and two *meso* structures.

Note that separation of enantiomers by TLC would require either the use of a chiral solvent and/or a chiral stationary phase. Since the conditions indicated in the stem lack any chiral element, V cannot be separated from VIII nor can VI be separated from VII on a silica gel TLC plate by eluting with 5% chloroform in hexane. Thus, separation of a total of four diastereoisomeric compounds can be carried out under the indicated TLC conditions.

> Spot 1 contains racemic V and VIII.
> Spot 2 contains racemic VI and VII.
> Spot 3 contains *meso* structure I (same as IV).
> Spot 4 contains *meso* structure III (same as II).

Choice A indicates that a maximum of four spots are expected to appear on the TLC plate after elution has been completed, and it is the correct answer.

SOLUTIONS TO STRUCTURE AND STABILITY PRACTICE PASSAGE

1. **D**   The maximum number of stereoisomers will be 2^n, where, in this case n (the number of chiral centers) is 6. Therefore, $2^6 = 64$.

2. **A**   According to the $n + 1$ splitting rule, where n = # of non-equivalent neighboring hydrogens, doublets in the NMR spectrum represent hydrogens with one hydrogen neighbor. The C-15 methyl group and the single vinyl hydrogen on C-1 fit this requirement. The methyl group is shifted slightly downfield by the Cl atom on C-14, but should appear between 2–3 ppm. Vinyl hydrogens typically appear around 5–6 ppm, but this one will be shifted even farther downfield by the Cl atom on C-1. The ratio of upfield to downfield is therefore 3:1.

3. **B**   The $-SO_3^-$ group shown on malhamensilipin A suggests that the $-SO_3H$ group can act as a Brønsted acid and donate a proton. This leaves a stable product (due to resonance). In fact, the $-SO_3H$ group on the molecule is reminiscent of H_2SO_4, a strong Brønsted acid. Choice B is the correct answer. The molecule doesn't have any easily donated electron pairs, and therefore isn't a strong Lewis base or Brønsted base (eliminate choices A and D). Also, it has no groups that are easily oxidized, so it cannot be a reducing agent (eliminate choice C).

4. **D**   The reactant contains no stereocenters, but two new ones are introduced in the reaction. The maximum number of stereoisomers any compound with two stereocenters can have is four (2^2). All four options are not created, however, due to the nature of the reaction and the symmetry of the reactant. The *syn* addition of two Cl atoms to the double bond in the reactant will lead to the following meso product, regardless of the face of the double bond that reacts:

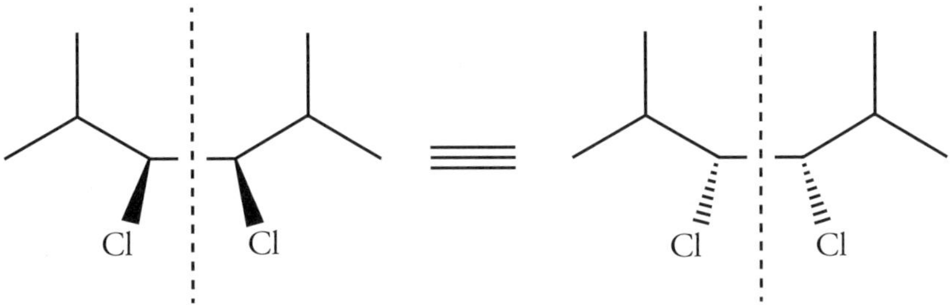

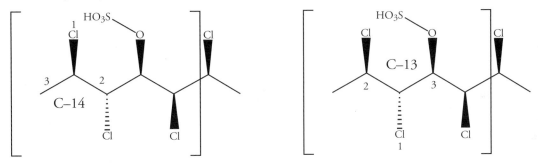

Since the product is meso, it has no enantiomer, and therefore we expect only one compound from the reaction.

5. **B** In the alkylation reaction, both the hydroxyl and the sulfoxide anion will be methylated. This will decrease the polarity of the compound (eliminate choices A and C). In reverse phase HPLC, the stationary phase is nonpolar, and opposite flash column chromatography in which the stationary phase is polar. Since the stationary phase is nonpolar, less polar compounds will interact more with the stationary phase thus having a longer retention time (eliminate choice D).

6. **C** C-13 and C-14 are the two leftmost chiral carbons in Figure 1. Numbering starts at the double-bond end of the molecule. Shown below are the individual stereocenters in question with the priority of each substituent labeled.

For each stereocenter, the Cl atom gets first priority because it has the highest atomic number. For C-14, the bulk of the molecule gets second priority due to more substitution compared to the methyl group of C-15. The #4 priority hydrogen, not drawn, is already in the back, and connecting 1, 2, and 3 makes a clockwise circle. As such, C-14 is *R* (eliminate choices A and D). For assigning the second priority for C-13, the first point of difference in the substituents occurs with the Cl on C-14 and the O on C-12. Because Cl has a higher atomic number, the shorter end of the molecule gets second priority. The #4 priority hydrogen for C-14 comes out of the page. Therefore, connecting the ordered substituents will give the opposite configuration. Connecting 1, 2, and 3 shown gives a clockwise rotation, so the actual rotation is counterclockwise, and as such, C-13 is *S* (eliminate choice B).

Chapter 31
Organic Chemistry
Reactions: Nucleophilic
Substitution and
Addition

FREESTANDING QUESTIONS: ORGANIC CHEMISTRY REACTIONS, NUCLEOPHILIC SUBSTITUTION AND ADDITION

1. Which of the following enolates would be expected from the reaction of the dione below with the bulky base lithium hexamethyldisilazane at –78°C?

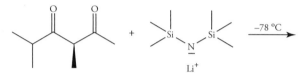

A)

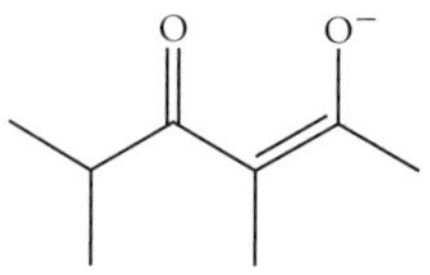

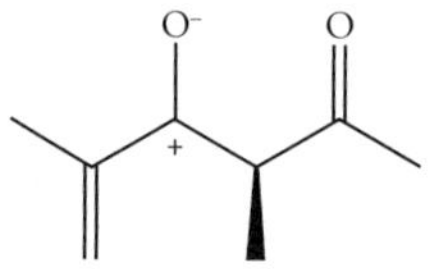

B)

C)

D)

2. The acid-catalyzed reaction between l benzoate and propanol is a(n):

A) reversible reaction, producing propyl benzoate and methanol.
B) reversible reaction, producing methyl propanoate and benzyl alcohol.
C) irreversible reaction, producing propyl benzoate and methanol.
D) irreversible reaction, producing methyl propanoate and benzyl alcohol.

3. Testosterone cypionate is an injectable slow release steroid formulation. The prodrug can be converted to testosterone and cypionic acid in the muscle tissue by which of the following reaction types?

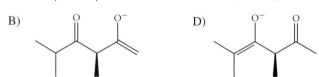

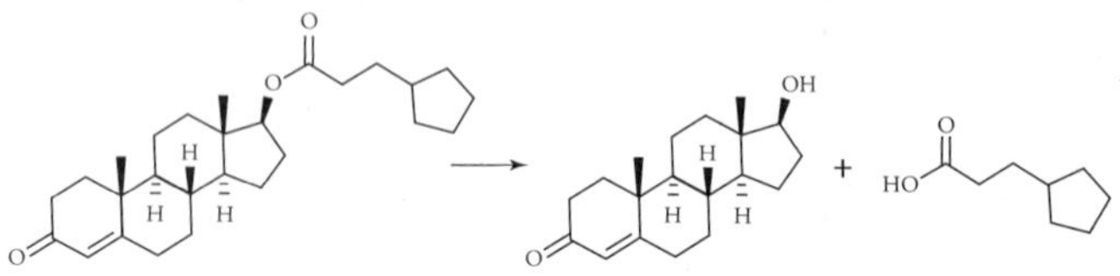

A) Reduction
B) Retro aldol
C) Decarboxylation
D) Hydrolysis

4. Which of the following reagents could be used to synthesize the compound below?

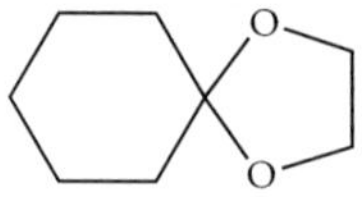

A)

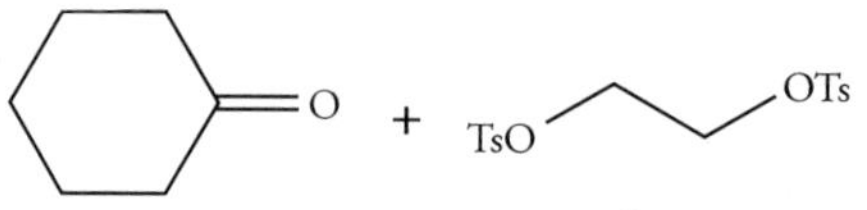

B)

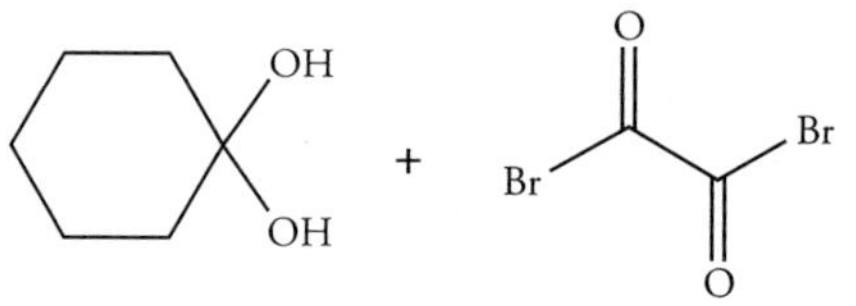

C)

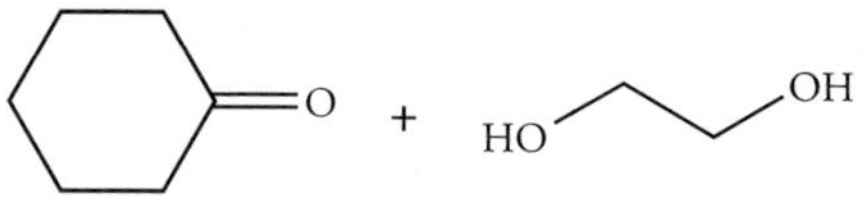

D)

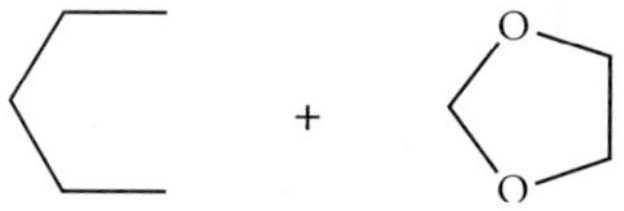

5. In which of the following reactions will the equilibrium lie toward the reactants?

I.

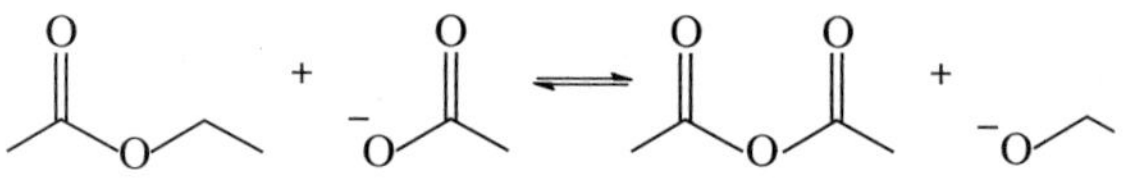

II.

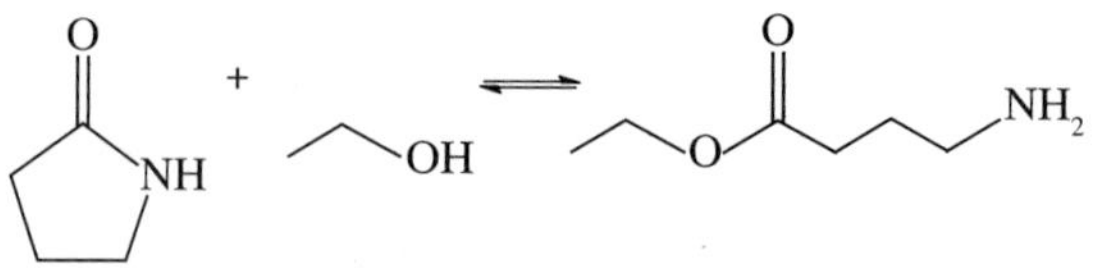

III.

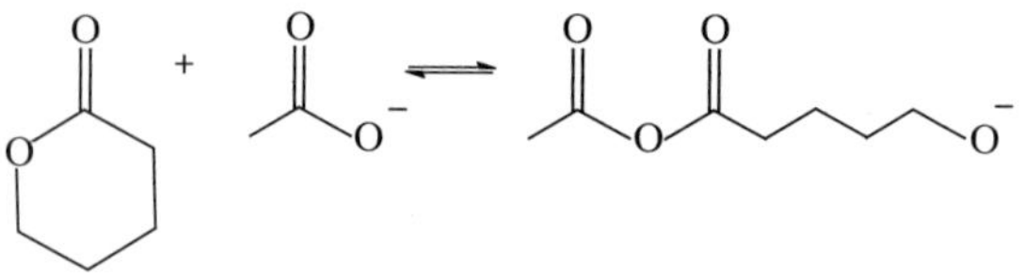

A) I only
B) II only
C) II and III only
D) I, II, and III

6. The reaction between cyclohex-3-ene-1-carboxylic acid and dimethylamine does not form the desired amide. Which of the following best explains this observation?

O
OH
+
H
N
O
N

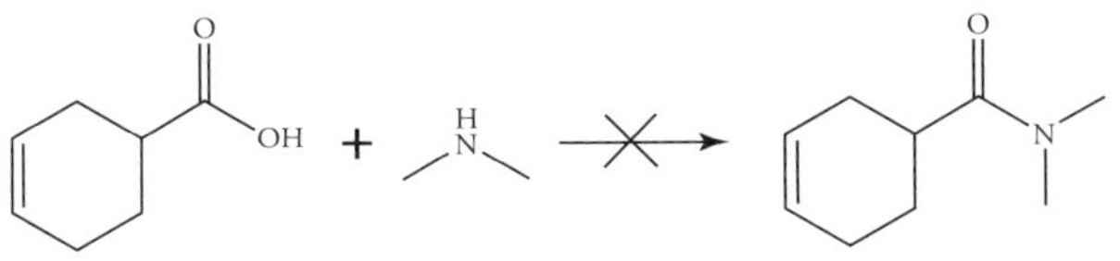

A) The intermediate formed in the reaction preferentially loses $N(CH_3)_2$ to regenerate starting materials.
B) Proton transfer reactions are very fast.
C) Dimethylamine is a gas at standard temperature and pressure.
D) Amides can be synthesized from acid chlorides and amines.

7. The first step in the reaction of pyrrolidine with cyclohexanone shown below is:

O
+
H
N
H₂SO₄
Δ
N
+ H₂O

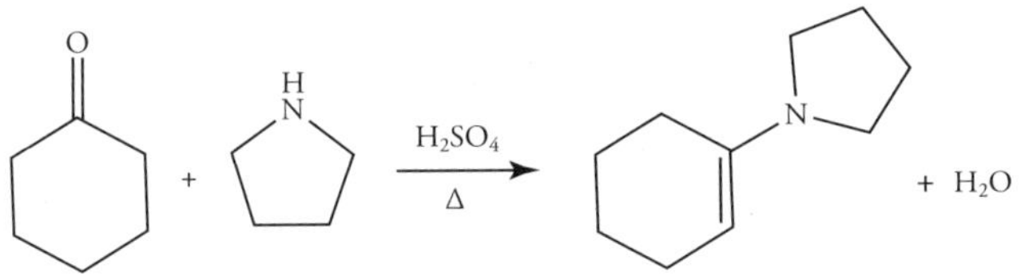

A) protonation of the carbonyl oxygen.
B) attack by the amine nitrogen on the carbonyl carbon.
C) deprotonation of an α-hydrogen in cyclohexanone.
D) dehydration of a reaction intermediate.

8. Which of the following reactions could be used to prepare 2-butanol?

A)
O
H
1. EtMgBr/Et₂O
2. H⁺

B)
O
H
1. CH₃CH₂Li/MeOH
2. H⁺

C)
O
O
H⁺/H₂O

D)
O
NaBH₄/DMF

9. Which of the following reactions is capable of yielding the compound shown?

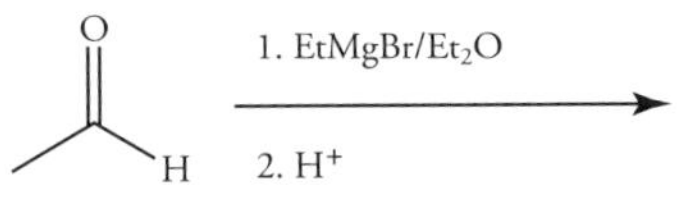

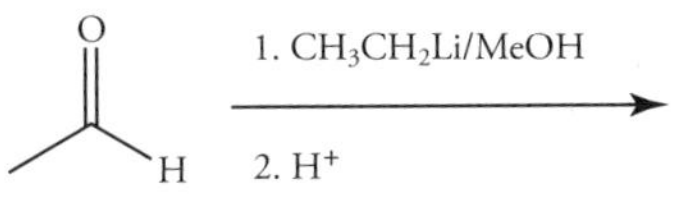

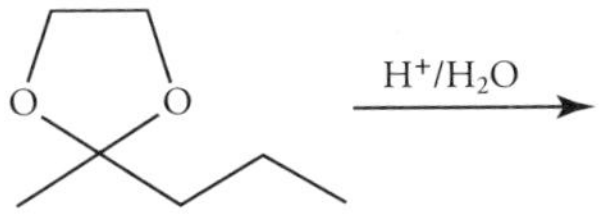

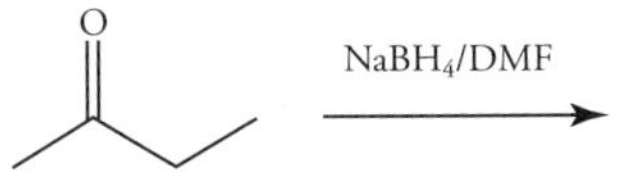

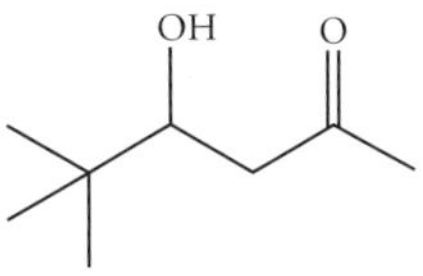

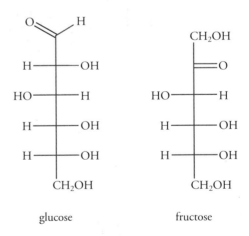

OH
O

A)
O
OH
H⁺/H₂O
heat

B)
O
O
NaBH₄

C)
O
H
+
O
catalytic H⁺

D)
O
+
H
O
catalytic H⁺

O
H
H
OH
HO
H
H
OH
H
OH
CH₂OH

glucose

CH₂OH
O
HO
H
H
OH
H
OH
CH₂OH

fructose

10. Glucose and fructose share metabolic pathways and can each be interconverted. Under which conditions could glucose be converted to fructose?

A) An oxidizing environment
B) A reducing environment
C) An aqueous basic environment
D) An aqueous acidic environment

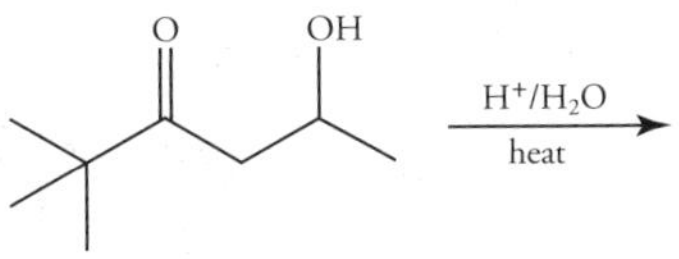

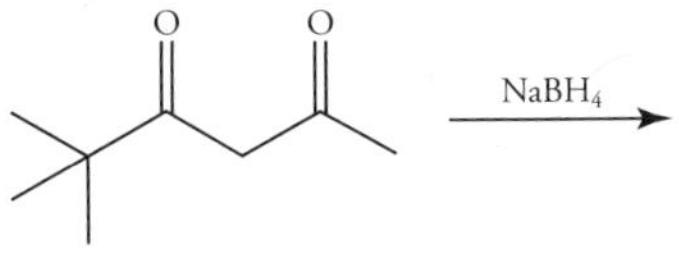

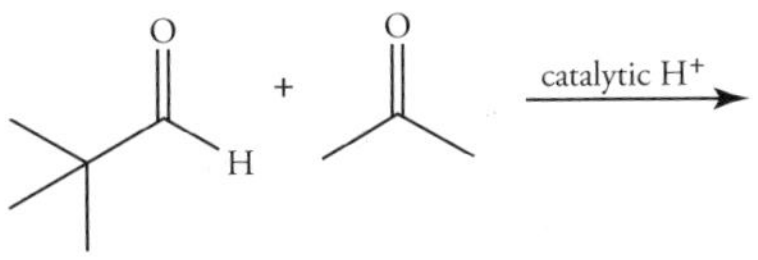

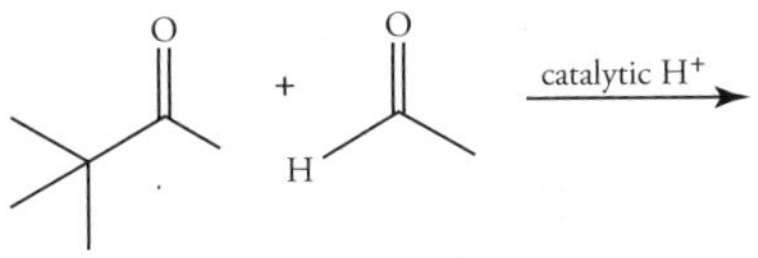

Questions 11 and 12 refer to the reaction mechanism shown below:

Pantothenic acid (Vitamin B$_5$) functions in living organisms as a precursor to Coenzyme A and thus is essential to sustain all forms of life. The sequence of reactions shown below parallels an early total synthesis of pantothenic acid.

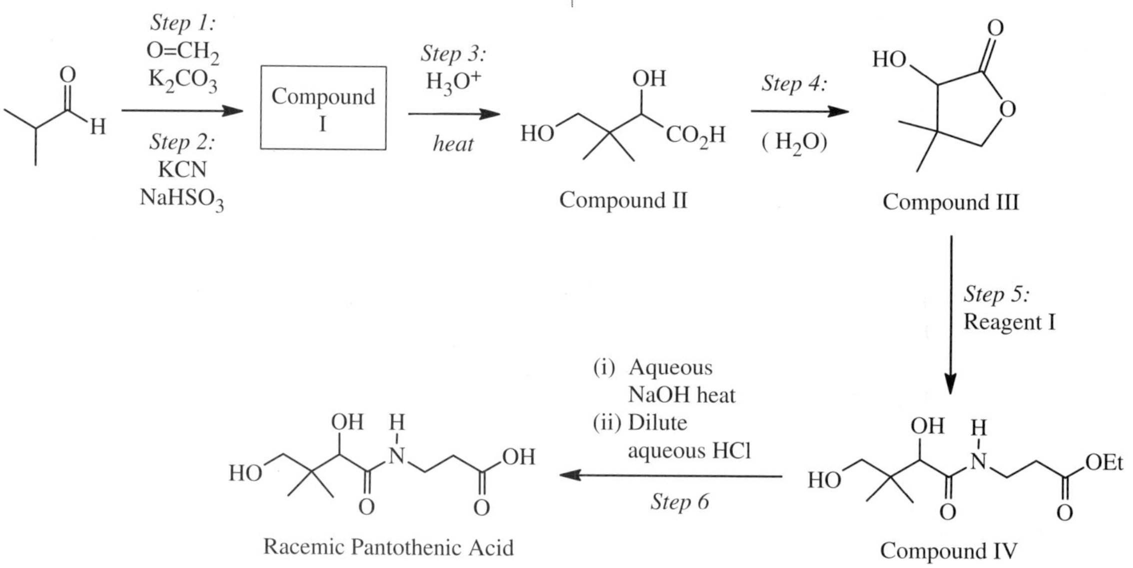

11. Compound I, the product formed via Steps 1 and 2, is a member of which class of compounds?

A) Nitrile
B) Cyanohydrin
C) Isocyanide
D) Amide

12. Which compound could best be employed as Reagent I in Step 5 in the reaction sequence?

A) Ethyl 3-aminopropanoate
B) Ethyl 4-aminopropanoate
C) Ethyl 3-aminobutanoate
D) Ethyl 4-aminobutanoate

13. A solution of CH_3CH_2MgBr (0.09 mol) in diethyl ether was added dropwise with vigorous stirring to a solution of methyl benzoate (0.1 mol) in diethyl ether. The reaction mixture was quenched with cold aqueous HCl, the layers were separated, and the organic layer was dried, filtered, and concentrated. Which of the following statements most accurately describes the contents of the crude reaction product obtained?

A) 1-Phenyl-1-propanol along with a small amount of unreacted methyl benzoate
B) 2-Phenyl-2-butanol, ethyl phenyl ketone, and unreacted methyl benzoate
C) 1-Phenyl-1-propanol and ethyl phenyl ketone
D) 3-Phenyl-3-pentanol and unreacted methyl benzoate

14. Compound J reacts with Compound K at 20°C to form a mixture of two products, L (20%) and M (80%). When the reaction is performed at 60°C, Compounds L and M are formed in 80% and 20% yields, respectively. When the reaction mixture obtained at 20°C is heated to 60°C and allowed to stand overnight, the composition of the mixture slowly changes to 80% L/20% M and remains invariant at longer reaction times. Which of the following statements is most consistent with the information given above?

A) An equilibrium mixture of L and M is obtained at 60°C.
B) The activation energy for formation of L is lower than that for M.
C) M is more stable than L.
D) L is formed faster than M.

15. Which of the following procedures could best be used to convert Compound X into Compound Y?

Compound X   Compound Y

A) (i) $NaBH_4$, CH_3OH; (ii) H_3O^+, heat
B) (ii) $LiAlH_4$, Et_2O; (ii) H_2O
C) (i) $HO-CH_2CH_2-OH$, TsOH, benzene; (ii) $LiAlH_4$, Et_2O; (iii) H_2O
D) (i) $HO-CH_2CH_2-OH$, TsOH, benzene; (ii) $NaBH_4$, CH_3OH; (iii) H_2O

ORGANIC CHEMISTRY REACTIONS: NUCLEOPHILIC SUBSTITUTION AND ADDITION PRACTICE PASSAGE 1

Gelsemine (Figure 1) has been widely studied due to its complex structure that includes a total of six rings, and several attempts have been made at its stereoselective synthesis.

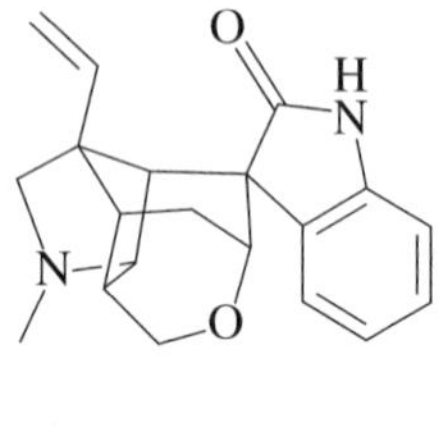

Figure 1   Gelsemine

Part of one synthesis is shown in Figure 2, illustrating the successful addition of the fourth and fifth rings of the compound.

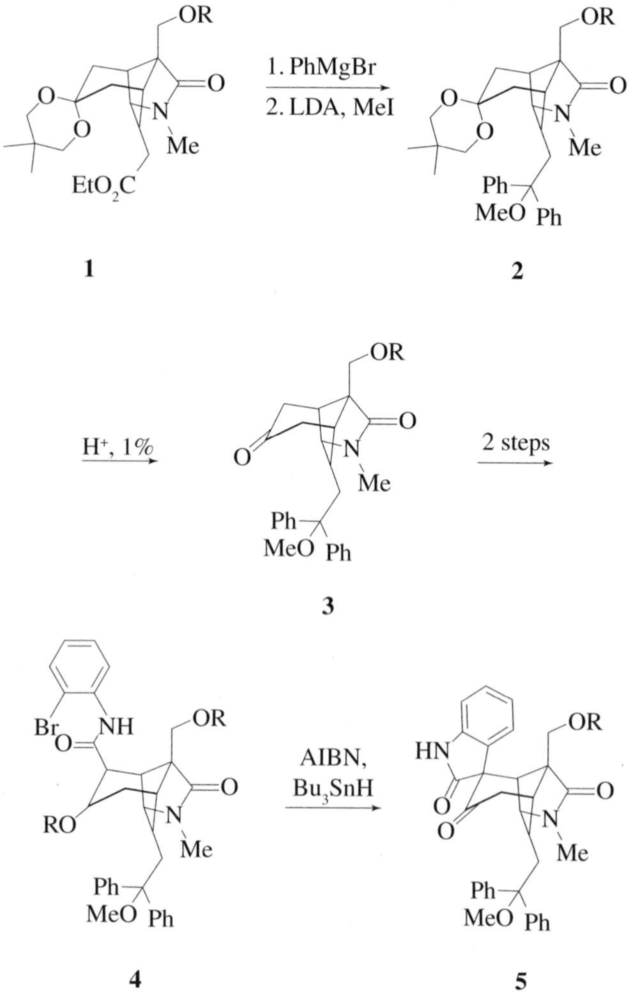

Figure 2   Partial synthesis of gelsemine

(Atarashi, S.; et. al., *J. Am. Chem. Soc.*, 1997, *119*, 6226-6241.)

Two key steps along the synthetic route to the tetracyclic Compound 1 are shown below in Figure 3.

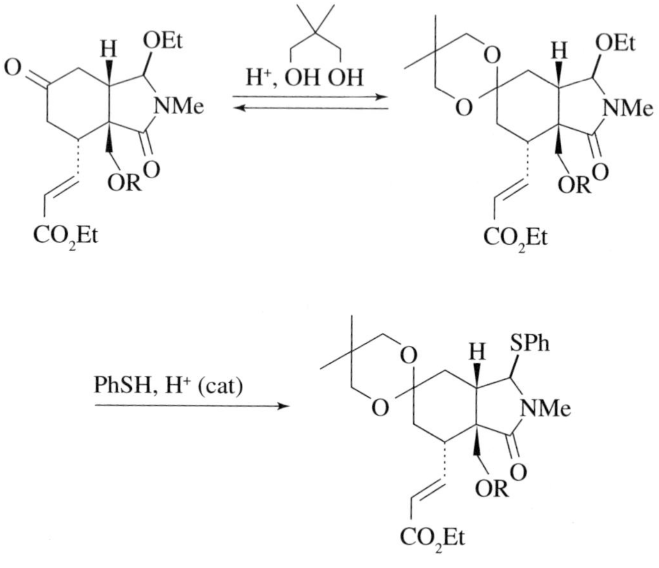

Figure 3   Early steps of gelsemine synthesis

1. Why is the ketone in Compound 3 protected during the first two steps of the synthesis?

A) The hemiacetal prevents the less reactive ketone from being deprotonated.
B) The acetal prevents Grignard addition to the ketone.
C) The acetal, being equatorial, provides extra stability.
D) The hemiacetal prevents the ketone from forming a tertiary alcohol during the Grignard addition.

2. If the conversion of Compound 1 to Compound 2 was monitored by IR spectroscopy, what would be observed as the reaction progressed?

A) The disappearance of all peaks in the region between 1650 cm^{-1} and 1750 cm^{-1}.
B) The appearance of a moderately strong band near 2100 cm^{-1}.
C) The elimination of one of the two strong peaks between 1650 cm^{-1} and 1750 cm^{-1}.
D) The disappearance of a set of three moderately strong peaks between 1450 cm^{-1} and 1580 cm^{-1}.

3. Why is no Grignard addition to the carbonyl of the amide observed in Step 1 of Figure 1?

A) The carbonyl carbon in the amide is less electrophilic than that of the ester.
B) The carbonyl carbon in the amide is more electrophilic than that of the ester, but the leaving group ($-NR_2$) is not as stable.
C) The carbonyl carbon of the ester is less electrophilic than that of the amide, but its leaving group ($-OEt$) is less stable.
D) Addition to the ester results in a release of steric strain.

4. The equilibrium depicted in the first step in Figure 3, in which a carbonyl is protected as an acetal, can be pushed in the forward direction via which of the following strategies?

A) Protecting the amido-carbonyl prior to treatment with the diol
B) Using a 1,3-propanediol with large, bulky substituents at the 2-position
C) The use of an alcohol solvent
D) Rigorously removing water from the system

5. How many chiral centers does gelsemine have?

A) 5
B) 6
C) 7
D) 8

ORGANIC CHEMISTRY REACTIONS: NUCLEOPHILIC SUBSTITUTION AND ADDITION PRACTICE PASSAGE 2

A number of enzyme-catalyzed Claisen-type condensations are involved in the synthesis and degradation of fatty acids. Fatty acids are degraded by β-oxidation, the final step of which involves enzyme-catalyzed removal of an acetyl group from a β-ketoacyl-CoA moiety.

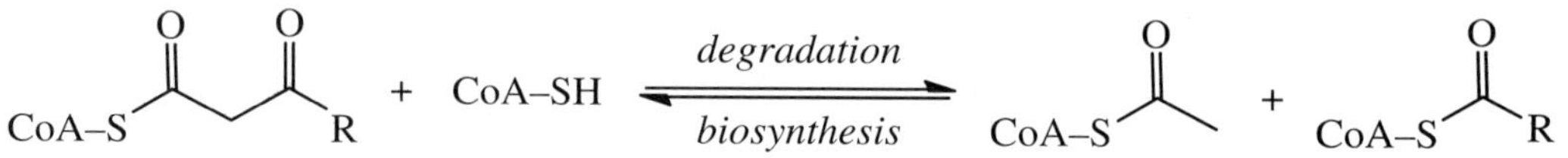

Two potential reaction mechanisms for base-promoted self-Claisen condensation of ethyl acetate are shown below. Mechanism I proceeds via a rapid, reversible first step followed by a second, rate-determining step, rate constant k_2. In Mechanism II, the first step is slow and irreversible, rate constant k_4.

Mechanism I

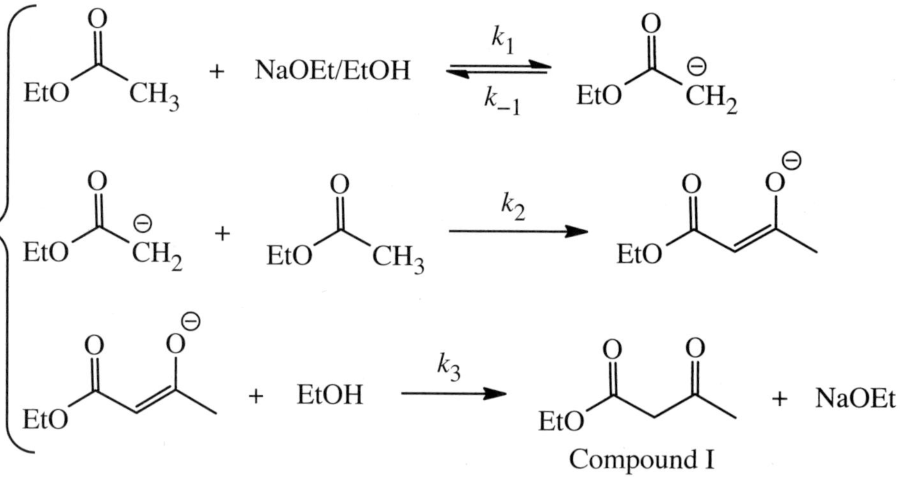

Mechanism II

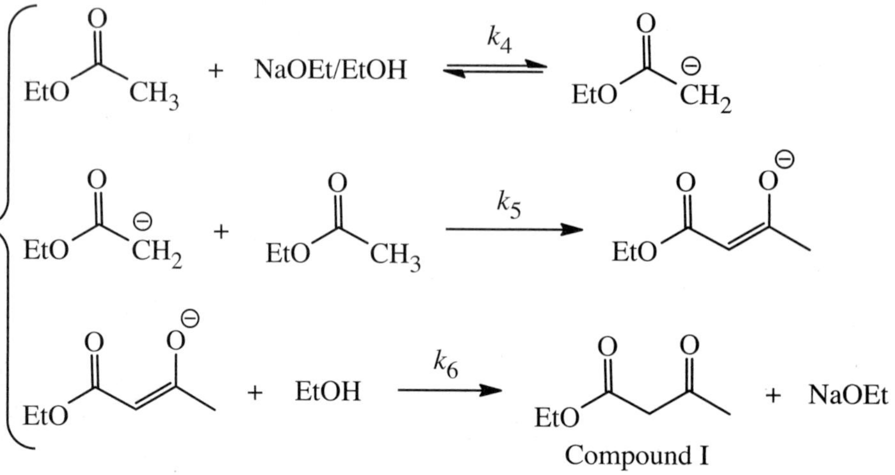

1. The reaction shown in the passage is performed in the presence of deuterium labeled CH_3CH_2OD. The reaction is run to 50% completion and then is quenched immediately. Unreacted starting material (ethyl acetate) is recovered from the reaction mixture and subsequently is subjected to mass spectrometric analysis. Which one of the following statements is correct?

A) If Mechanism I is operative, recovered ethyl acetate will be found to contain only $CH_3CH_2O\text{-}C(=O)\text{-}CH_3$.
B) If Mechanism I is operative, recovered ethyl acetate will be found to contain $CH_3CH_2O\text{-}C(=O)\text{-}CH_2D$.
C) If Mechanism II is operative, recovered ethyl acetate will be found to contain $CH_3CHD\text{-}O\text{-}C(=O)\text{-}CH_3$.
D) If Mechanism II is operative, recovered ethyl acetate will be found to contain $CH_3CH_2O\text{-}C(=O)\text{-}CH_2D$.

2. Which one of the following structures is expected to be the major product formed *via* the three-step reaction sequence shown below?

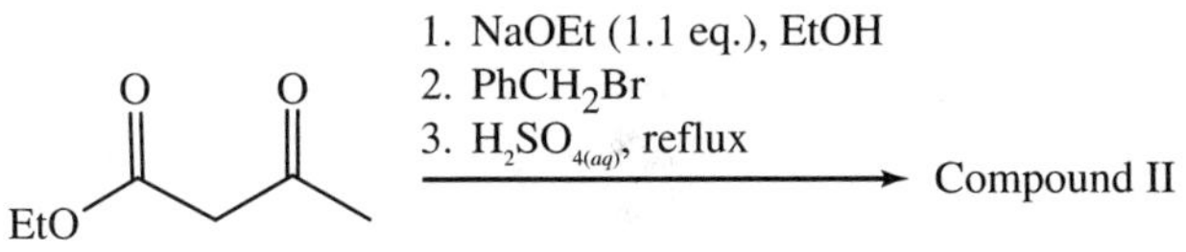

Compound I

1. NaOEt (1.1 eq.), EtOH
2. PhCH₂Br
3. $H_2SO_{4(aq)}$, reflux
→ Compound II

A)

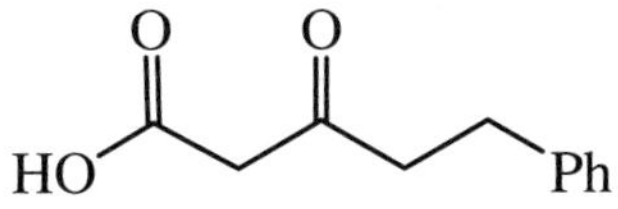

B)

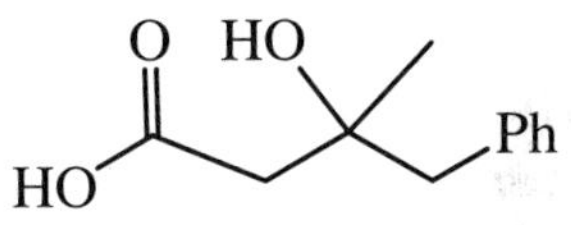

C)

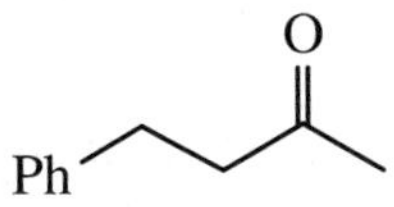

D)

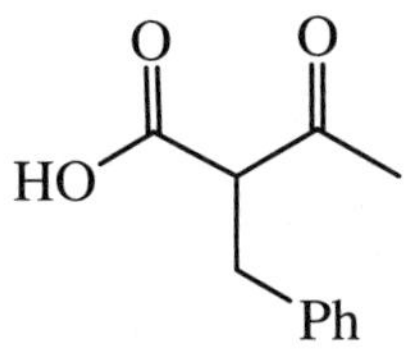

3. Which of the following spectral regions would be expected to display absorption peaks in the infrared spectrum of Compound I but are *not* present in the corresponding IR spectrum of ethyl acetate?

I. 3300–3500 cm^{-1}
II. 1700–1750 cm^{-1}
III. 1630–1650 cm^{-1}

A) I only
B) I and III only
C) II and III only
D) I, II, and III

4. Base-promoted self-Claisen condensation is performed by using optically active Compound III as starting material.

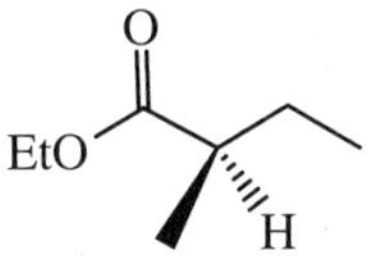

Compound III

The reaction is run to 50% completion and then is quenched immediately. Which one of the following statements is most consistent with information presented in the passage?

A) If the reaction proceeds via Mechanism I, recovered Compound III will be optically inactive.
B) If the reaction proceeds via Mechanism I, the chiral center in recovered Compound III will have undergone inversion of configuration.
C) If the reaction proceeds via Mechanism I, the product formed via self-Claisen condensation of Compound III will be optically active.
D) If the reaction proceeds via Mechanism II, the chiral center in recovered Compound III will have undergone inversion of configuration.

5. Which one of the four proton NMR spectra shown below is most likely to correspond to that of Compound I?

A)

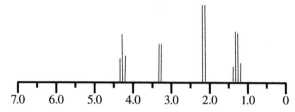

B)

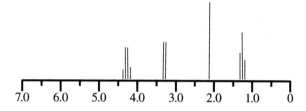

C)

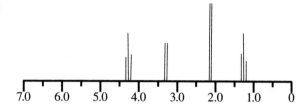

D)

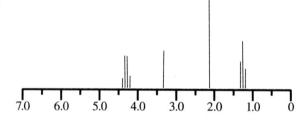

6. Decarboxylation is mechanistically similar to a reverse (retro) Claisen reaction. One process involved in the citric acid cycle involves a two-step enzyme-mediated conversion of isocitrate to α-ketoglutarate and carbon dioxide.

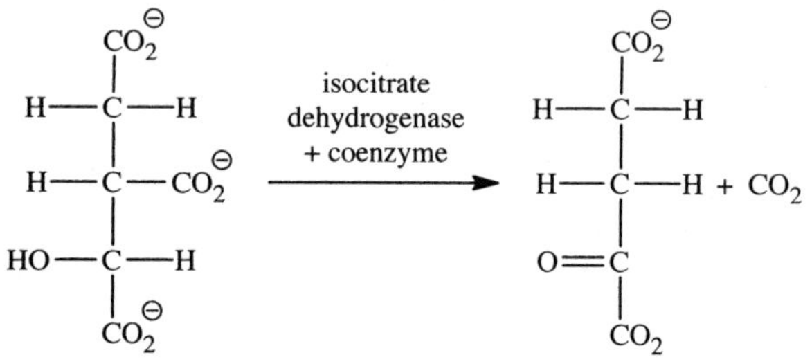

Which statement offers the most accurate description of this process?

A) Decarboxylation followed by reaction with NADH (coenzyme)
B) Decarboxylation followed by reaction with NAD⁺ (coenzyme)
C) Reaction with NADH (coenzyme) followed by decarboxylation
D) Reaction with NAD⁺ (coenzyme) followed by decarboxylation

SOLUTIONS TO FREESTANDING QUESTIONS: ORGANIC CHEMISTRY REACTIONS, NUCLEOPHILIC SUBSTITUTION AND ADDITION

1. **B** The combination of a bulky base and extremely low reaction temperature point to the formation of the kinetic enolate, through the deprotonation of the most easily accessible α-proton. There are 3 different α-proton environments on the initial substrate, as shown below:

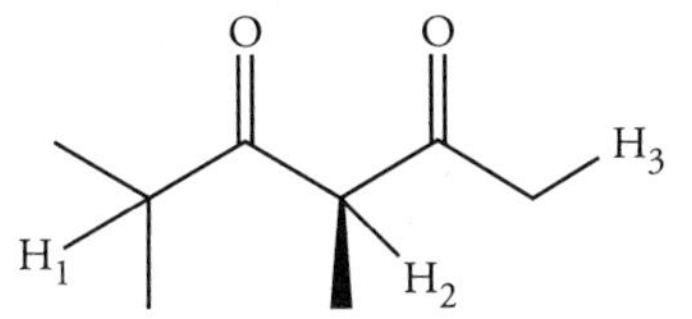

   H_2 is the most acidic of the three, but not the most accessible. Its deprotonation would yield the thermodynamic enolate (choice A). The protons at H_3 have minimal steric bulk in their vicinity, and hence are easily removed by the strong, bulky base, even at very low temperatures. Deprotonation of H_3 will yield the enolate in choice B. Choice C is not an enolate at all, and it cannot be produced from the simple deprotonation of the initial substrate. Choice D is the product of the deprotonation of H_1, which is a valid α-proton, but not as acidic as H_2, or as accessible as H_3.

2. **A** As a reminder of ester nomenclature (important in this question), the first group mentioned in the name of the ester is the group on the oxygen side of the ester. In this acid-catalyzed transesterification reaction, propanol attacks the acid-protonated methyl benzoate at the carbonyl carbon. The overall transesterification reaction is given below.

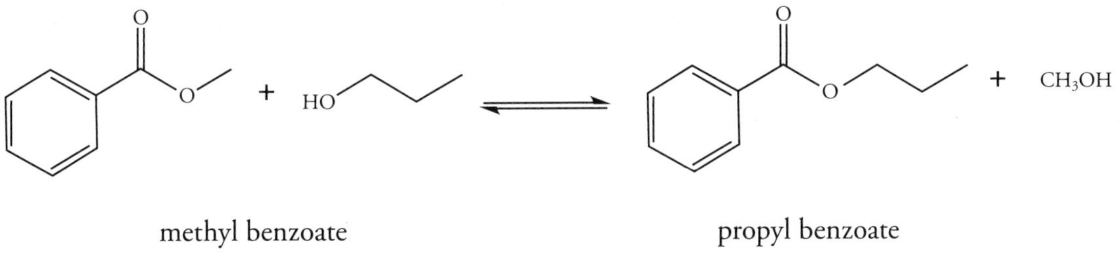

   methyl benzoate   propyl benzoate

   After proton exchange, methanol leaves, creating propyl benzoate (eliminate choices B and D). This reaction is reversible, as nothing prevents methanol from undertaking a similar attack and regenerating the starting materials (eliminate choice C).

3. **D** The reaction is an ester hydrolysis resulting in an alcohol (testosterone) and cypionic acid. Reduction involves the addition of hydrogen to a molecule, or the loss of oxygen. While this is tempting—in this case, looking at the steroid molecule product—the cleavage of the ester bond is achieved by insertion of water, not H_2. Therefore, this is not a reduction (eliminate choice A). Retro aldol reactions require β-hydroxy carbonyl compounds as starting materials and yield two carbonyl compounds with the cleavage of a carbon-carbon bond (eliminate choice B). Decarboxylation is the removal of carbon dioxide from a molecule. Decarboxylation occurs with a β-ketoacid, which is not present here (eliminate choice C).

4. **C**   The compound in question is a cyclic acetal, which can be synthesized from a carbonyl compound and a diol (choice C) in an equivalent fashion to acetal formation with two independent alcohols. Choice A is incorrect, since ketones are only very slightly nucleophilic, and do not react with electrophiles, even when they have good leaving groups attached like tosylates. Choice B can be eliminated, as the attack of the hydroxyls on the acid bromide would leave behind ester groups, which are not present in the desired products. Choice D has the right number of carbons, but it requires forming new carbon-carbon bonds and functionalization of a linear alkane, which would be impossible in the absence of specialized, aggressive reagents.

5. **D**   To approach this question, compare the relative reactivities of the carboxylic acid derivatives on either side of the reaction arrow. Each reaction will be favored toward the less reactive derivative. In Item I, the ester in the reactants is less reactive than the anhydride in the products because the anhydride has a resonance-stabilized leaving group. Since Item I favors reactants, eliminate choices B and C. To get to the right answer, you only need to evaluate Item II or Item III. Item II is true: amides are less reactive than esters because an alcohol is a better leaving group than an amine. Therefore, the reactants are again favored (choice A can be eliminated, and choice D is correct). Note that in Item III, you again see the comparison of an ester (in this case a cyclic one, or a lactone) and an anhydride. Item III will therefore also favor the reactants.

6. **B**   Carboxylic acids protonate amines to form salts because proton transfer reactions are much faster than nucleophilic additions. Protonated amines are not nucleophilic and therefore do not react with carbonyl compounds, so no tetrahedral intermediate is formed (eliminate choice A). Choices C and D are both true but irrelevant to the question.

7. **A**   The first step in the reaction mechanism for the condensation of a ketone with a secondary amine to form an enamine involves the protonation of the carbonyl oxygen. Protonation increases the electrophilicity of the carbonyl carbon, permitting subsequent attack by the amine nitrogen at the electrophilic site (eliminate choice B). Choice D is a later step in the reaction mechanism, so is incorrect. Choice C does not occur at all in this reaction.

8. **A**   Grignard reagents react with aldehydes in polar aprotic solvents to yield secondary alcohols. Adding ethyl Grignard to acetaldehyde results in the four carbon chain of 2-butanol. Alkyl lithium reagents are strong bases and strong nucleophiles, and add to carbonyl compounds in aprotic solvents as well, but choice B uses the polar protic solvent methanol. Choice C depicts the hydrolysis of an acetal, which would give rise to 2-butanone. The reagent in choice D is sodium tetrafluoroborate, which is not to be confused with the reducing agent $NaBH_4$, which could achieve the desired product by reducing the ketone.

9. **C**   The reaction in choice A requires the oxidation of one hydroxyl and the reduction of a ketone, which will not be driven by an acidic aqueous solution. The reaction in choice B can be eliminated, as the addition of $NaBH_4$ would either lead to a diol, if $NaBH_4$ was used in excess, or in the reduction of the less sterically hindered ketone if one equivalent was used. Choice C is an aldol condensation between acetone and an aldehyde with no α-hydrogens, leading to the desired product. The reaction in choice D can yield multiple products as each reactant bears acidic α-hydrogens, but none of the end products are the desired molecule.

10. **C** In order for glucose to be converted into fructose, an isomerization must occur. Keto-enol tautomerism will allow for this. An oxidizing environment will oxidize the aldehyde to a carboxylic acid (eliminate choice A). A reducing environment will reduce the aldehyde to an alcohol (eliminate choice B). In an aqueous acidic environment, the carbonyl oxygen of the aldehyde will be protonated, promoting hemiacetal formation and cyclization into a ring (eliminate choice D). In an aqueous basic environment, the α-hydrogen on the aldehyde can be deprotonated, allowing for keto-enol tautomerism. This transformation can permit isomerization of the aldehyde into a ketone as shown below. Note the location of the bolded hydrogen atom shown in the carbohydrate molecules.

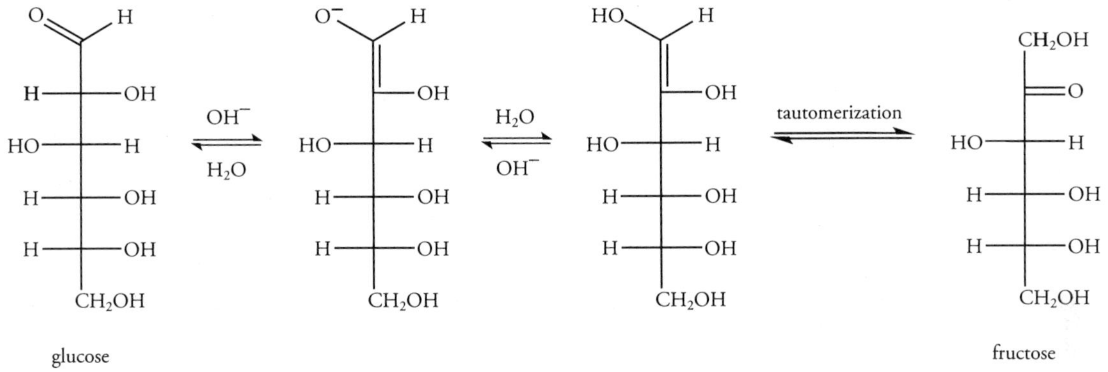

glucose   fructose

11. **B** Outside of the CO_2H group, Compound II differs from the starting material (2-methyl-propanal) by the addition of one carbon atom. Thus, 2-methylpropanal can serve as substrate in a crossed aldol addition reaction with formaldehyde to increase its chain length by one carbon atom. The intermediate product obtained from this addition is expected to be 2,2-dimethyl-3-hydroxypropanal. Subsequent reaction of this aldehyde with KCN is expected to result in the formation of the corresponding cyanohydrin (Compound I) which undergoes subsequent hydrolysis in *Step 3* to afford Compound II.

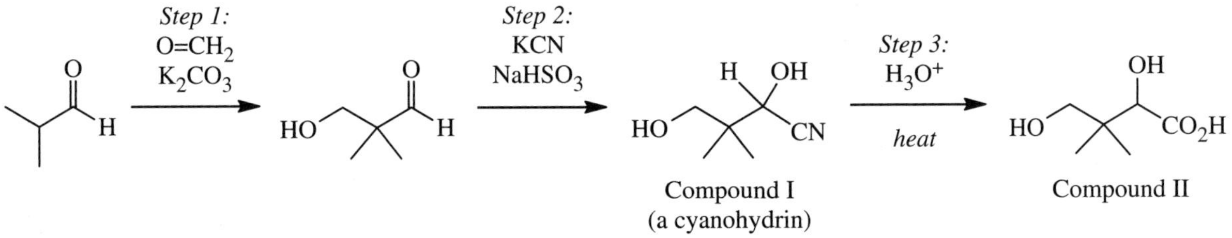

Compound I
(a cyanohydrin)

Compound II

12. **A** It is necessary to recognize that Compound IV is formed by converting Compound III (a lactone) into the corresponding amide. As illustrated below, ethyl 3-aminopropanoate serves as an appropriately-functionalized amine, which will undergo an addition-elimination reaction with Compound III.

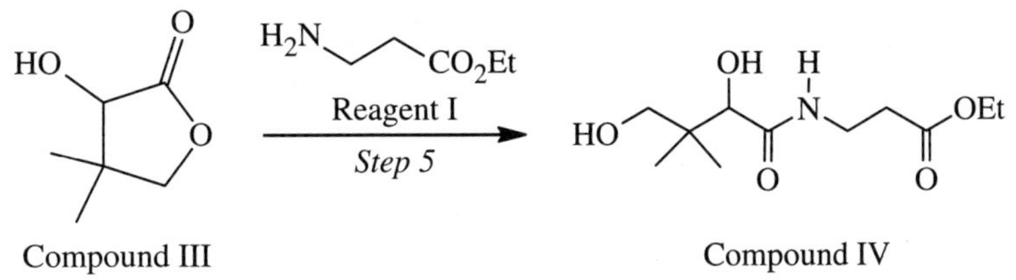

Compound III   Compound IV

13. **D** The reaction described in the stem employs an insufficient quantity of CH_3CH_2MgBr (0.9 equivalents). Hence, it is important to recognize that CH_3CH_2MgBr is the limiting reagent in this reaction. For this reason, roughly half of the methyl benzoate is expected to remain unreacted and the portion of ester that does react with CH_3CH_2MgBr is expected to follow the reaction sequence shown below:

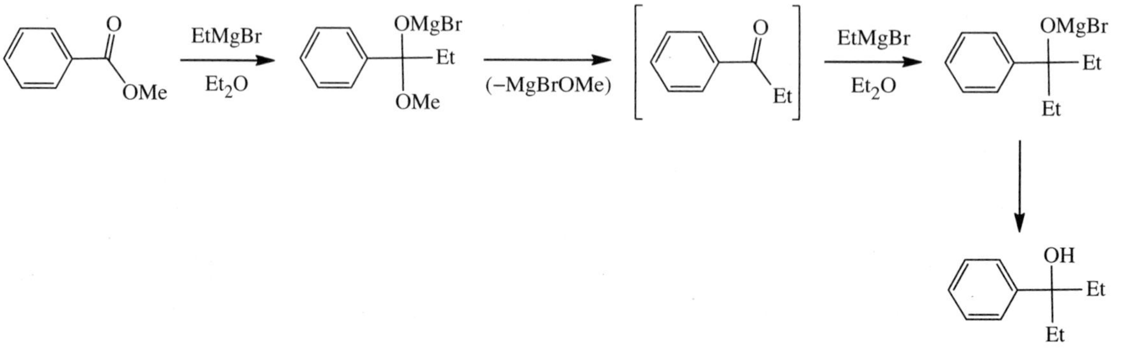

Note that propiophenone (i.e., ethyl phenyl ketone) is formed as a reaction intermediate. Once formed, a competition exists between this ketone and methyl benzoate in the ensuing reaction with CH_3CH_2MgBr. As nucleophiles react more rapidly with ketone C=O groups than with ester C=O groups, ethyl phenyl ketone is expected to be consumed preferentially, thereby ensuring that this compound will not be found among the crude reaction products (choices B and C can be eliminated). Upon preferential reaction with CH_3CH_2MgBr, ethyl phenyl ketone is converted to 3-phenyl-3-pentanol. This alcohol and unreacted methyl benzoate therefore are expected to be found among the crude reaction products (choice D is correct, and choice A is wrong).

14. **A** The observation that the composition of the reaction mixture remains constant at 80% L/20% M when the reaction mixture is maintained at 60°C over a long period of time indicates that this product ratio represents the equilibrium product composition at that temperature (choice A is correct), thereby demonstrating that L is more stable than M (choice C is wrong). The fact that M is the major product when the reaction of K with L is performed at 20°C suggests that the activation energy for formation of M is lower than that for L, thus M is formed faster than L (choices B and D are wrong).

15. **C** Sodium borohydride in choice A is expected to reduce the ketone carbonyl group in Compound X. However, this metal hydride is not sufficiently reactive to reduce the ester carbonyl group in the corresponding lactone moiety, as shown below (choice A can be eliminated):

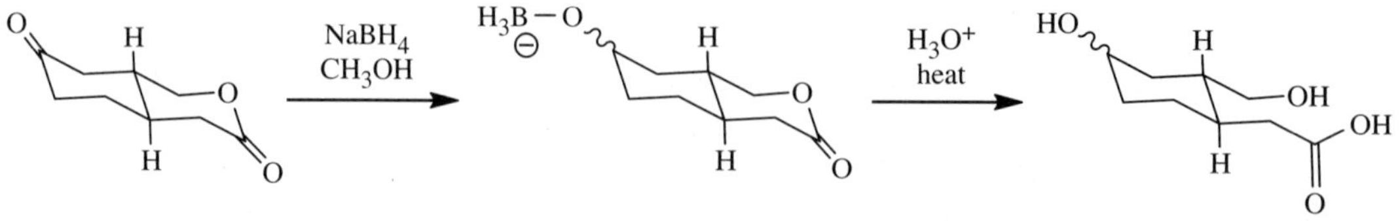

In contrast, lithium aluminum hydride in choice B, a more powerful reducing agent than sodium borohydride, is expected to reduce both the ketone and ester carbonyl groups, as shown below (choice B can be eliminated):

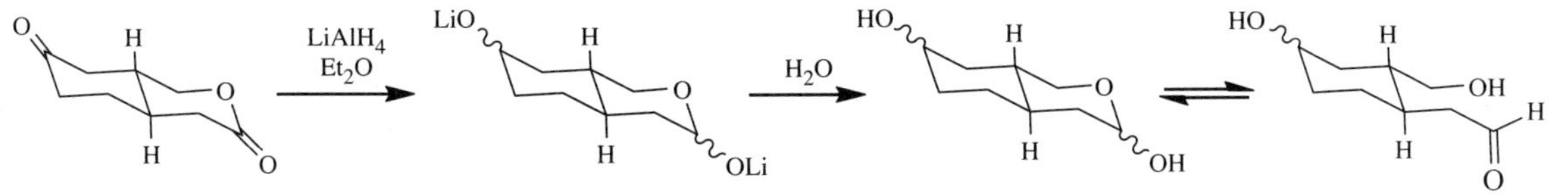

It is important to recognize the need to protect the ketone carbonyl group prior to reducing the lactone carbonyl group in Compound X. In choice C, acid-catalyzed reaction of Compound X with 1,2-ethanediol is employed for this purpose to yield a cyclic acetal protecting group. Subsequent reaction with aqueous acid regenerates the ketone C=O group and also results in hydrolysis of the hemiacetal moiety formed *via* reduction of the lactone carbonyl group (choice C is correct).

SOLUTIONS TO ORGANIC CHEMISTRY REACTIONS: NUCLEOPHILIC SUBSTITUTION AND ADDITION PRACTICE PASSAGE 1

1. **B** Hemiacetals and acetals have the general structures shown below. These structures illustrate that the functional group in the molecule is an acetal (eliminate choices A and D).

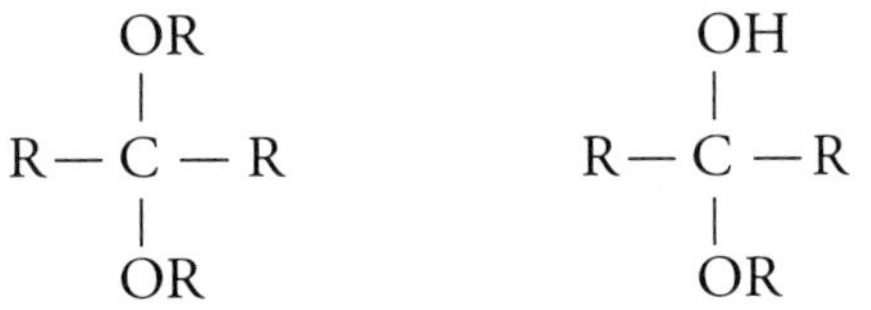

$$
\begin{array}{cc}
\text{OR} & \text{OH} \\
| & | \\
\text{R}-\text{C}-\text{R} & \text{R}-\text{C}-\text{R} \\
| & | \\
\text{OR} & \text{OR} \\
\textbf{acetal} & \textbf{hemiacetal}
\end{array}
$$

The acetal has two bonds to the six-membered ring, one of which is axial and the other equatorial (eliminate choice C). Ketones are more reactive than esters; therefore, if the ketone had been present during the Grignard addition, the Grignard reagent would have added there instead.

2. **C** As Compound 1 is converted to Compound 2, one of the two carbonyl moieties is converted into an ether as a result of the addition of two phenyl rings. The C=O stretches of carbonyl compounds appear in the same area, but do not necessarily appear at the same exact wavenumbers. Seeing one of the two initial stretches in the carbonyl region between 1650 cm^{-1} and 1750 cm^{-1} disappear would be a clear indication that the reaction had progressed as shown. Elimination of all the stretches in this region would indicate the reaction

of all C=O units in the molecule, which does not fit the reaction scheme (eliminate choice A). Stretches near 2100 cm^{-1} generally derive from carbon-carbon triple bonds, which play no role in the chemistry presented (eliminate choice B). Sets of multiple peaks in the region between 1450 cm^{-1} and 1580 cm^{-1} usually come from aromatic C=C bonds; therefore, the appearance of these peaks would be expected, not their disappearance (eliminate choice D).

3.　**A**　Amides are less electrophilic at the carbonyl carbon because the two oxygen atoms of the ester inductively withdraw more electron density from the carbon than the nitrogen and oxygen atoms of the amide (choice A is correct; eliminate choice B). When comparing the possible leaving groups (NR_2 or –OR), –OR is the better leaving group because oxygen is more electronegative than nitrogen, and it can better stabilize a negative charge (eliminate choice C). Addition to the amide might result in a release of strain from breaking the ring; however, there is no such strain present in the ester (eliminate choice D).

4.　**D**　The formation of the acetal in the presence of H^+ results in the elimination of water. This water can re-attack the acetal, causing a reversion to the carbonyl, giving rise to the equilibrium in the equation. If this water is removed from the system by a drying agent, the equilibrium will be pushed in the forward direction. The amido-carbonyl does not need protection, as the amide is already of sufficient stability for the following steps, and its protection has no bearing on the ease of protection of the ketone in the equation (eliminate choice A). A bulky substituent at the 2-position of the 1,3-propanediol will, if anything, inhibit the attack of the diol, pushing the equilibrium to the reactants side of the equations (eliminate choice B). The use of an alcohol solvent would greatly complicate the equilibrium, as there would be competing reactions involving the addition of solvent molecules, rather than the desired diol (eliminate choice C).

5.　**C**　Carbons with four different substituents are chiral. The chiral centers of gelsemine are marked in the structure below.

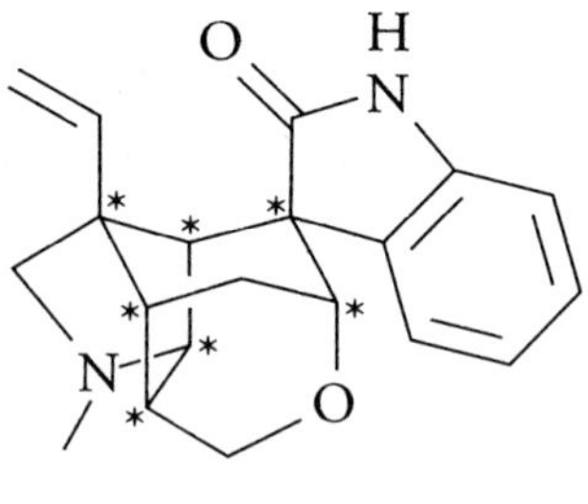

SOLUTIONS TO ORGANIC CHEMISTRY REACTIONS: NUCLEOPHILIC SUBSTITUTION AND ADDITION PRACTICE PASSAGE 2

1. **B** As indicated in the passage, the initial step in Mechanism I is rapid and reversible. Since the second step is rate-determining, it follows that $k_{-1} > k_2$. By the time that the reaction has been quenched after 50% completion, rapid H-D exchange will have occurred at the α-carbon atom. Hence, recovered starting material is expected to contain CH_3CH_2O-$C(=O)$-CH_2D (choice B). Choice A, which neglects base-promoted H-D exchange at the α-position in ethyl acetate, can be eliminated.

The initial step in Mechanism II is stated in the passage to be both rate-determining and irreversible. Under these conditions, the intermediate enolate ion cannot revert to starting material *via* reaction with EtOD (choice D can be eliminated). Choice C indicates incorrectly that H-D exchange would occur in the (unactivated) ethoxy CH_2 group in the starting material.

2. **C** As indicated in the passage, the initial step in both Mechanisms I and II involves base-promoted abstraction of an α-hydrogen in ethyl acetate to afford the corresponding enolate anion. Recall that in Compound I the C(2) α-hydrogens are considerably more acidic than the C(4) α-hydrogens. The use of NaOEt in a hydroxylic solvent (EtOH) suggests that the thermodynamic (rather than kinetic) enolate will be formed. The three-step reaction sequence shown in the stem is expected to proceed in the manner outlined below.

Choice A is expected to result via kinetically controlled base-promoted alkylation of Compound I and can be eliminated. Choice B suggests incorrectly that the ketone C=O group in Compound I undergoes nucleophilic addition by benzyl anion; this species is not produced in the reaction sequence shown in the stem (choice B can be eliminated). Although the β-keto acid shown in choice D is formed during *Step 3*, this compound is not expected to survive the stated experimental conditions (i.e., reflux in acid solution) and thus will spontaneously decarboxylate to afford the structure shown in choice C, along with CO_2 and H^+.

3. **B** Whereas ethyl acetate exists almost completely in the keto form, the enol form of Compound I receives stabilization *via* intramolecular hydrogen bonding and thus is expected to be present to a significant extent in the tautomeric equilibrium shown below.

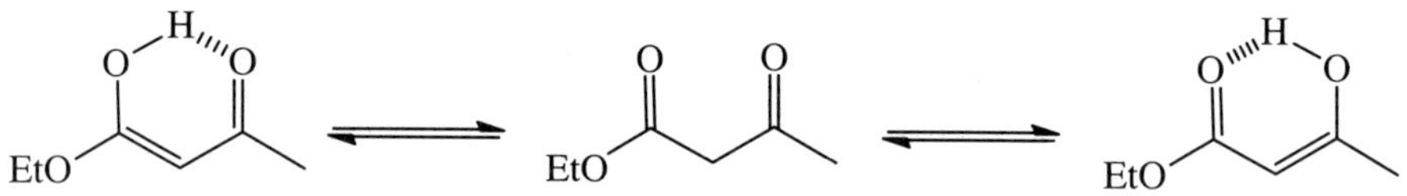

As a result, the IR spectrum of Compound I, but not that of ethyl acetate, is expected to display absorption in the region 3300–3500 cm^{-1} (I, enol O–H stretching vibration) and the region 1630–1650 cm^{-1} (IV, enol C=C double bond stretch). Both Compound I and ethyl acetate are expected to display intense absorption in the region 1700–1750 cm^{-1} (C=O stretch). Only the response given in choice B is consistent with the foregoing conclusions.

4. **A** As indicated in the passage, Mechanism I proceeds via a rapid, reversible deprotonation at the α-carbon in in the first step followed by a second, rate-determining step. When the reaction is quenched after 50% completion, Compound III (the starting material) is expected to be recovered. This compound is expected to be optically inactive due to racemization, which occurred during protonation of the achiral enolate intermediate, as indicated below:

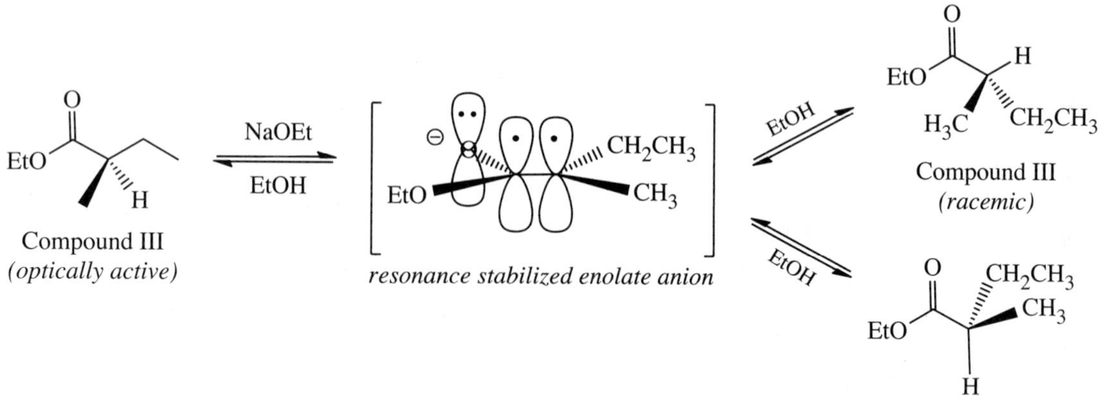

Eliminate choice B, as Mechanism I is expected to afford recovered Compound III in which the chiral center is 50% retained, 50% inverted. Eliminate choice C, since racemic Compound III is formed more rapidly via Mechanism I than its corresponding self-Claisen condensation product, from which it follows that the reaction product also is expected to be optically inactive. Eliminate choice D, since the first step in Mechanism II is stated to be irreversible, thus recovered Compound III will be the original optically active molecule.

5. **D** Compound I contains four types of mutually nonequivalent protons: ester CH_3, ester CH_2, ketone CH_3, and $O=C-CH_2-C=O$. The chemical shifts of the four types of protons show negligible differences in each of the four answer choices. Hence, only the spin-spin coupling patterns should be considered. The ester CH_3 and CH_2 groups are mutually coupled and afford a triplet and quartet, respectively. Choice B can be eliminated, as it does not display a quartet. Both the ketone $O=C-C\underline{\textbf{H}}_3$ and $O=C-C\underline{\textbf{H}}_2-C=O$ groups are expected to appear as singlets. Thus, the NMR spectrum of Compound I is expected to consist of one quartet, one triplet, and two singlets. Only choice D meets this criterion and is the correct answer.

6. **D** Recall that the presence of a β-carbonyl group serves to activate decarboxylation in a β-keto acid. Thus, an oxidation step necessarily must precede decarboxylation of isocitrate in order to produce α-ketoglutarate under biological conditions. Eliminate choices A and B, each of which indicates incorrectly that the decarboxylation step precedes oxidation during conversion of isocitrate to α-ketoglutarate. The first step of this reaction sequence requires a coenzyme that can function as an oxidizing agent in a redox reaction by acting as a hydride ion acceptor. Note that NAD^+ serves this function in a variety of metabolic processes, e.g., citric acid cycle, glycolysis, and fatty acid β-oxidation. The resulting two-step reaction sequence is summarized below.

Isocitrate → Oxalosuccinate → α–Ketoglutarate

Note that choices A and C indicate incorrectly that a *reducing agent*, NADH (rather than NAD^+), functions as coenzyme to promote the oxidation step. Choice D indicates correctly that NAD^+-mediated oxidation occurs first followed by decarboxylation.

Chapter 32
Biologically Important Molecules

FREESTANDING QUESTIONS: BIOLOGICALLY IMPORTANT MOLECULES

1. At what pH would the net charge on a 0.3 M solution of the amino acid asparagine (pK_a α-COOH = 2.0, pK_a α-NH$_3^+$ = 8.8) be minimized?

A) 2.0
B) 5.4
C) 8.8
D) 12.0

2. Predict the products of the following reaction:

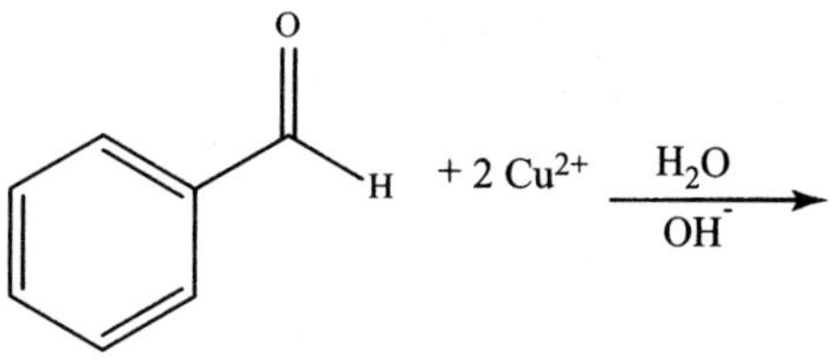

A)

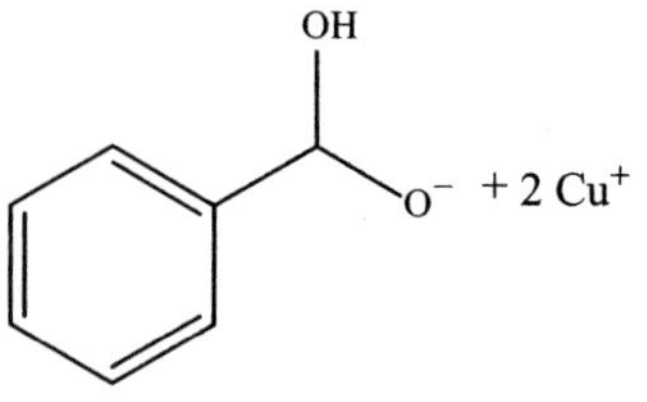

B)

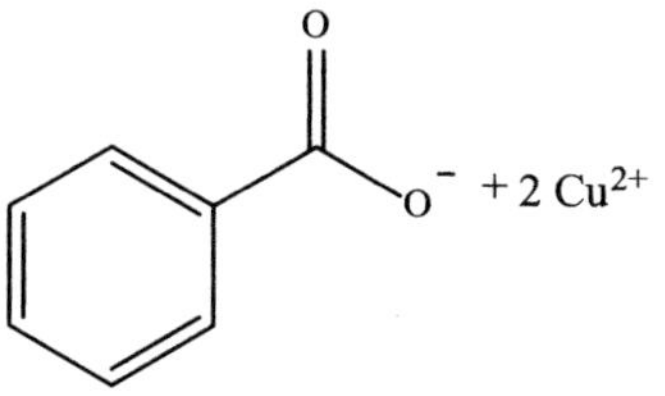

C)

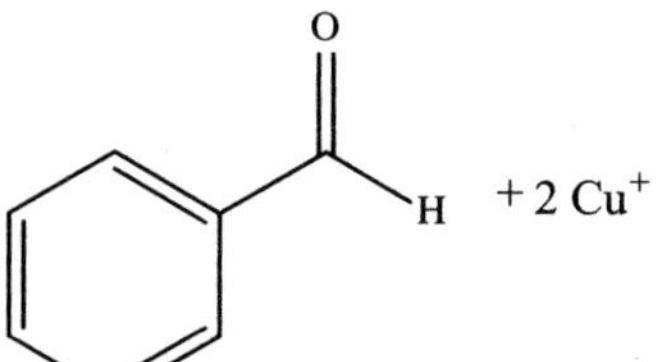

D)

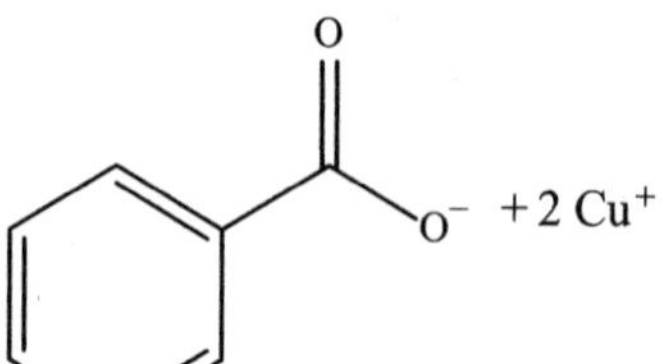

3. A peptide bond is the intramolecular force between two amino acids formed in a catalytic reaction that releases water. What is another name for a peptide bond?

A) Hydrogen bond
B) Amide bond
C) Phosphodiester bond
D) Glycosidic bond

4. Which of the following would result from the treatment of β-D-galactopyranosyl-(1→4)-D-glucose, the disaccharide more commonly known as lactose, with NaBH$_4$?

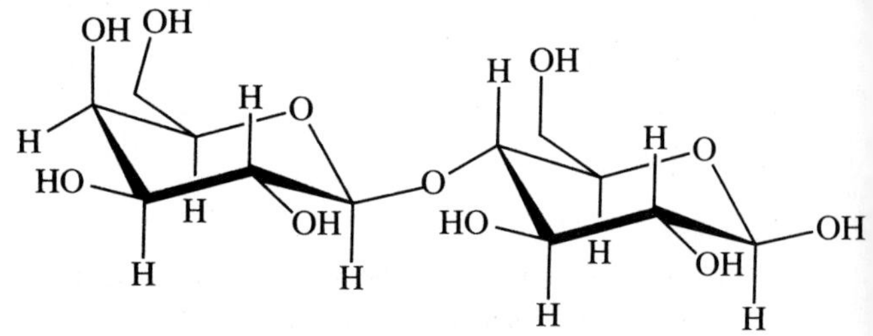

A) Reduction of C-1 of the glucose residue to yield an acyclic primary alcohol
B) Reduction of C-1 of the glucose residue to yield a cyclic ether
C) Cleavage of the glycosidic linkage to yield galactose and glucose
D) No reaction, as all functional groups in lactose are stable to the reaction conditions

5. Given the following reaction, the product(s) will be:

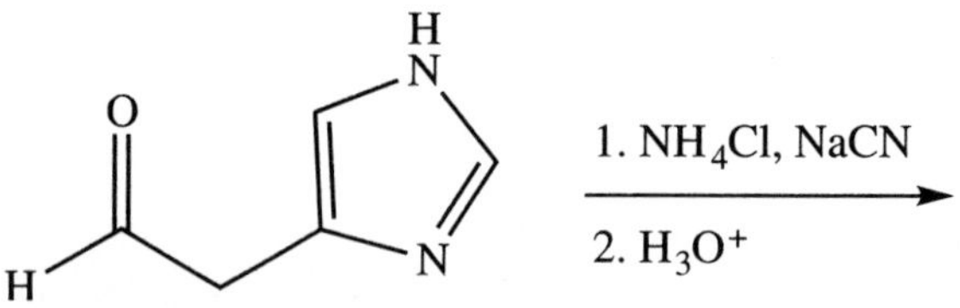

1. NH$_4$Cl, NaCN
2. H$_3$O$^+$

A) enantiomers.
B) optically active.
C) regioisomers.
D) amphipathic.

6. Chitin is a long-chain polymer of *N*-acetyl glucosamine and is the main component of the exoskeletons of arthropods.

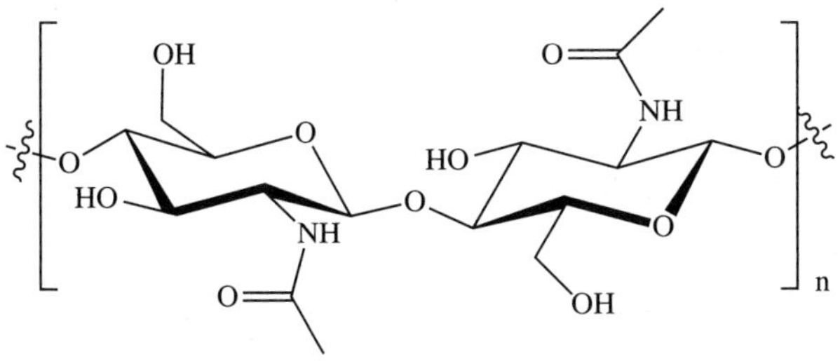

Which of the following best describes the glycosidic linkage in chitin?

A) α-1,2
B) β-1,2
C) α-1,4
D) β-1,4

7. Which of the following best characterizes the differences between fatty acids and phospholipids?

A) Fatty acids have two tails and form micelles; phospholipids have one tail and form membranes.
B) Fatty acids have two tails and form membranes; phospholipids have two tails and form micelles.
C) Fatty acids have one tail and form micelles; phospholipids have two tails and form membranes.
D) Fatty acids have one tail and form membranes; phospholipids have two tails and form micelles.

8. An unknown heptapeptide, Compound I, was subjected to enzymatic cleavage by trypsin and by chymotrypsin. Cleavage of Compound I with trypsin resulted in three peptides with the following amino acid sequences: Ala-Leu, Trp-Arg, and Gly-Tyr-Lys. Cleavage of Compound I with chymotrypsin resulted in three different peptides with sequences Gly-Tyr, Lys-Trp, and Arg-Ala-Leu. What is the amino acid sequence in Compound I?

A) Arg-Ala-Leu-Lys-Trp-Gly-Tyr
B) Gly-Tyr-Lys-Trp-Arg-Ala-Leu
C) Gly-Tyr-Lys-Trp-Leu-Ala-Arg
D) Arg-Ala-Leu-Trp-Lys-Tyr-Gly

BIOLOGICALLY IMPORTANT MOLECULES PRACTICE PASSAGE 1

The Maillard reaction is a nonenzymatic reaction between a reducing sugar and an amino acid, called glycation, characterized in the browning of food. This multi-step reaction is sensitive to heat, pH, water activity, and the presence of other compounds. The reaction results in numerous products, all of which are responsible for the aroma, flavor, and texture of cooked foods.

When asparagine reacts with a reducing sugar in this way, a Schiff base forms. The Schiff base can be irreversibly isomerized and decarboxylated to form acrylamide, which is a known neurotoxin and potential animal carcinogen. The pathway for the formation of acrylamide is shown in Figure 1.

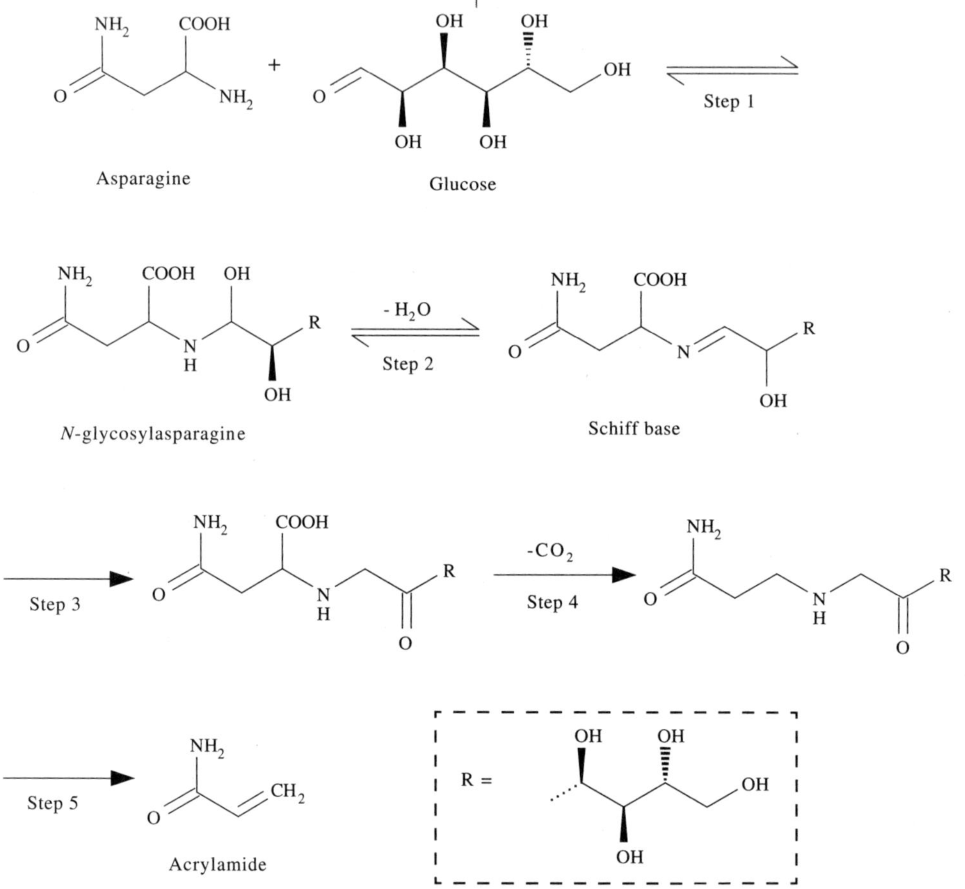

Figure 1 Acrylamide formation

N-linked glycosylation is the name given the endogenous version of the Maillard reaction. *N*-linked glycosylation represents an enzymatic co- or post-translational modification whereby an oligosaccharide chain is linked to the side-chain of an asparagine residue in a protein. The monosaccharides that compose these chains are often D-mannose and N-acetyl-D-glucosamine units assembled into various linear and branched structures. These oligosaccharide chains play important biological roles in intercellular interactions with carbohydrate binding proteins, called lectins.

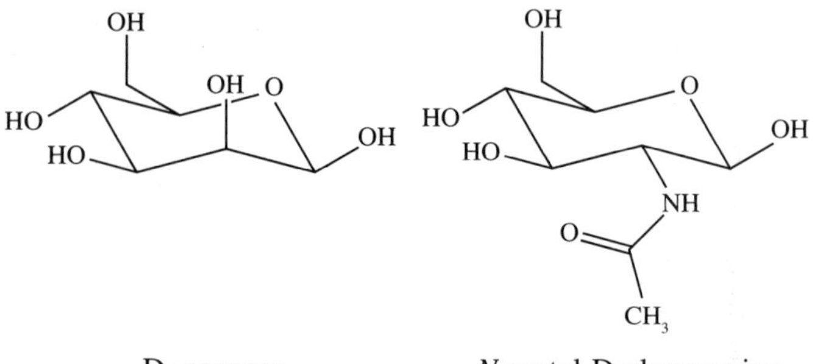

Figure 2 Common monosaccharides found in glycans

1. Which of the following accurately describes D-mannose and *N*-acetyl-D-glucosamine?

A) D-Mannose is shown in the α configuration and *N*-acetyl-D-glucosamine is shown in the β configuration.

B) *N*-acetyl-D-glucosamine can form β-1,4 glycosidic linkages with D-mannose.

C) The *N*-acetyl group in *N*-acetyl-D-glucosamine can form a Schiff base.

D) Mannose is a structural isomer of glucose.

2. How many ^{1}H NMR resonances will be displayed in the spectrum for acrylamide?

A) 2

B) 3

C) 4

D) 5

3. Which of the following reagents would perform the isomerization shown in Step 3 of the reaction?

A) H_2SO_4

B) $NaOCH_2CH_3$

C) CH_3MgBr

D) H_3CCOCH_3

4. Which of the following statements regarding Schiff base formation is true?

A) Under strongly acidic conditions, the rate of the reaction increases.

B) The removal of water from the reaction system decreases the yield of the Schiff base product.

C) The loss of water is the thermodynamic driving force in the reaction.

D) The reaction outcome is under kinetic control, favoring the formation of the Schiff base product.

5. Glycated hemoglobin (hemoglobin-A$_{1c}$) is an adduct that forms when glucose reacts with an amino group in hemoglobin as in the first three steps shown in Figure 1. Which of the following statements about hemoglobin-A$_{1c}$ is FALSE?

A) Glucose and mannose can react to form identical hemoglobin-A$_{1c}$ adducts.

B) A sustained period of hyperglycemia (elevated blood glucose concentration), as in diabetes mellitus, will result in elevated hemoglobin-A$_{1c}$ levels.

C) High-performance liquid chromatography is an effective method of separating hemoglobin-A$_{1c}$ from non-glycated hemoglobin.

D) The isomerization process that ultimately forms hemoglobin-A$_{1c}$ is reversible in an aqueous acidic environment.

6. A biologist researching a particular protein is interested in determining its degree of *N*-linked glycosylation and begins digesting the protein into fragments of various sizes using peptidases. Which chromatographic technique is most appropriate to separate the glycopeptide fragments from the non-glycosylated peptide fragments in the digested mixture?

   I.   Size exclusion chromatography

   II.   Lectin affinity chromatography

   III.   Ion exchange chromatography

A) I only

B) II only

C) I and III only

D) II and III only

BIOLOGICALLY IMPORTANT MOLECULES PRACTICE PASSAGE 2

Glycoconjugates are carbohydrates that have become bonded to other biomolecules, such as proteins, peptides, lipids, and saccharides. Some glycoconjugates function by providing communication between cells and their environment, while others provide recognition sites for extracellular signal molecules like growth factors.

Glycoside hydrolases, or glycosidases, constitute an important class of enzymes that catalyze glycosidic bond hydrolysis, thereby degrading glycoconjugates and oligosaccharides.

Glycosidases are involved in all forms of life; in humans, they reside in the intestinal tract and in saliva where they degrade complex carbohydrates.

Enzyme-catalyzed hydrolysis of glycosidic bonds can proceed with either net inversion or net retention of configuration *via* single- and double-displacement processes as illustrated below (Schemes I and II, respectively).

Scheme I (single displacement)

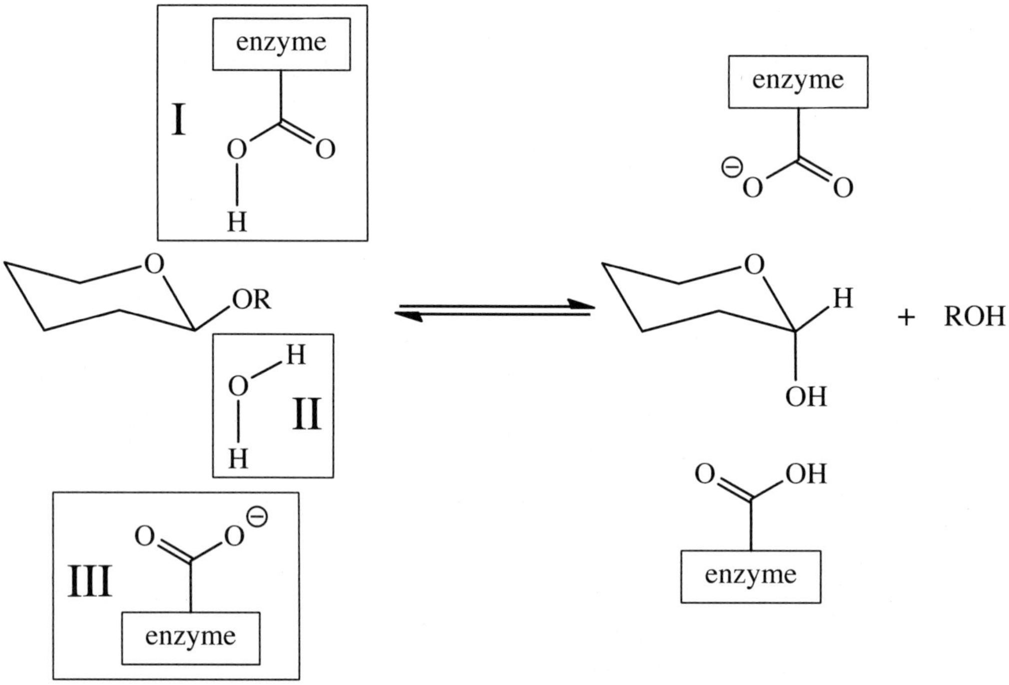

Scheme II (double displacement)

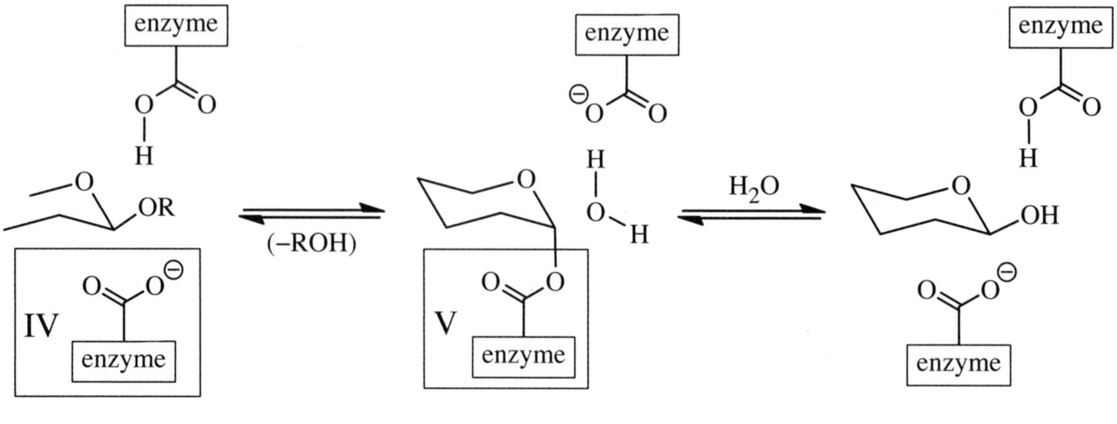

Non-enzymatic acid-catalyzed hydrolysis of cyclic acetals potentially might proceed *via* either endocyclic or exocyclic cleavage of an acetal carbon-oxygen linkage (Mechanisms III and IV, respectively).

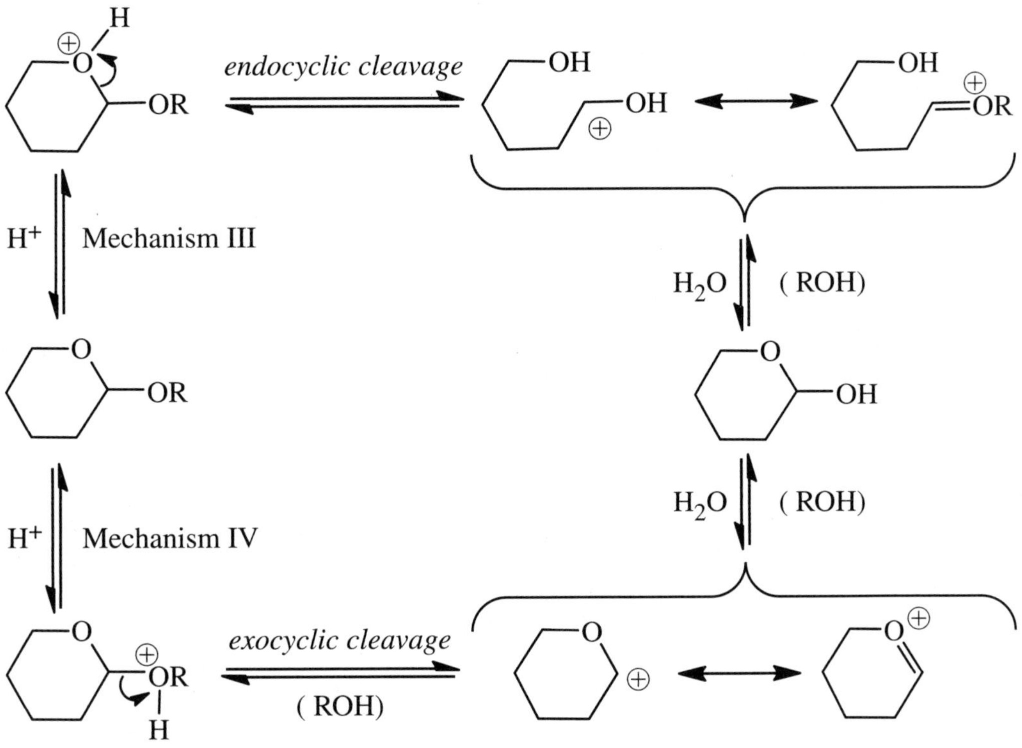

Enzyme-catalyzed hydrolysis of carbohydrate glycosidic bonds that adheres either to Mechanism I or II generally proceeds stereospecifically to afford one of two possible isomeric hemiacetals. However, the corresponding acid-catalyzed process (Mechanisms III or IV) generally produces mixtures of diastereoisomeric hemiacetals.

1. Digoxin, a natural product isolated from a variety of foxglove plant, is used to treat atrial fibrillation and other heart conditions.

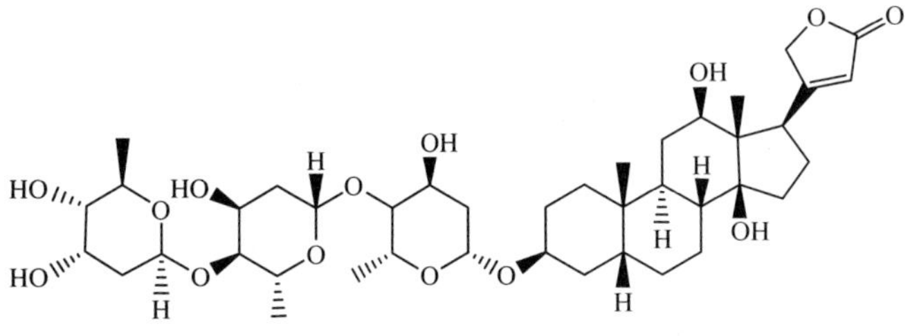

Digoxin

How many fragments are expected to result via acid-catalyzed hydrolysis of digoxin?

A) 3
B) 4
C) 5
D) 6

2. What is the function of species I–V in Schemes 1 and 2 shown in the passage?

	I	II	III	IV	V
A)	Acid	Nucleophile	Base	Nucleophile	Leaving group
B)	Acid	Base	Nucleophile	Base	Leaving group
C)	Leaving group	Nucleophile	Base	Nucleophile	Acid
D)	Leaving group	Base	Nucleophile	Base	Acid

3. Consider the acid-catalyzed equilibrium shown below.

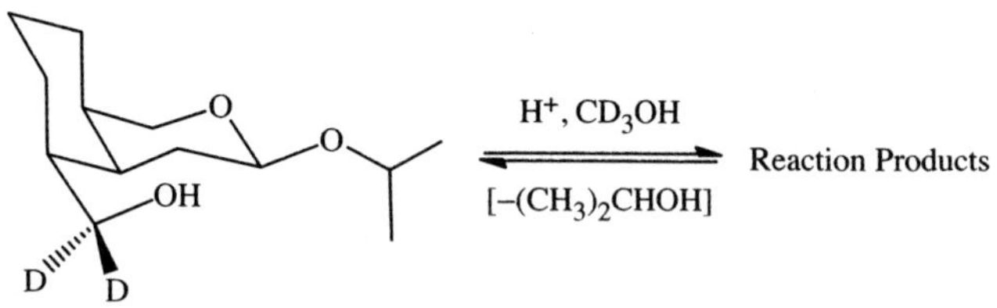

$$H^+, CD_3OH$$

Reaction Products

$$[-(CH_3)_2CHOH]$$

Based on information in the passage, which of the four compounds is/are expected to form as reaction products?

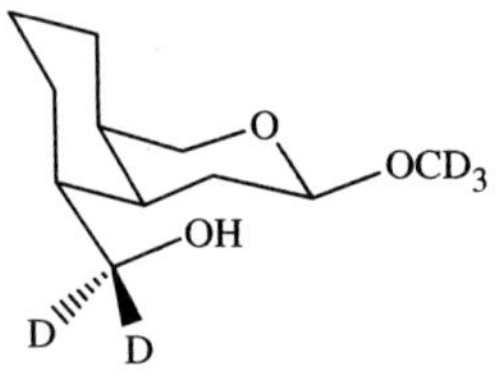

I

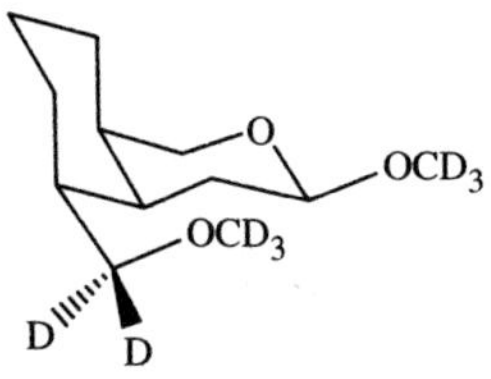

II

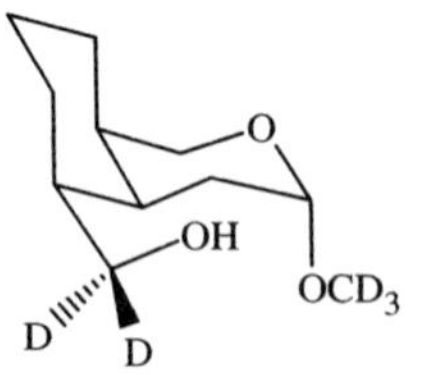

III

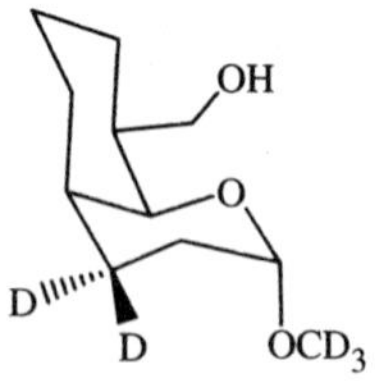

IV

A) I and III only
B) II and IV only
C) I, II, and III only
D) I, III, and IV only

4. Primeverose and vicianose, shown below, are naturally-occurring disaccharides found in several plant species, consisting of D-glucose and either arabinose or xylose.

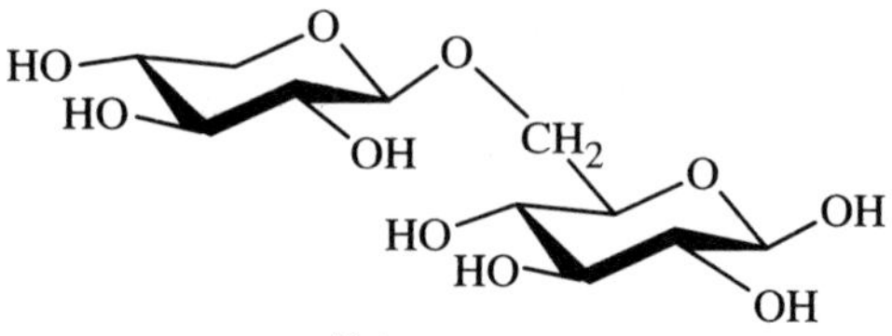

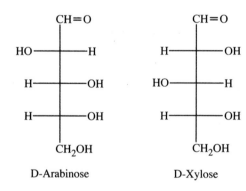

Primeverose

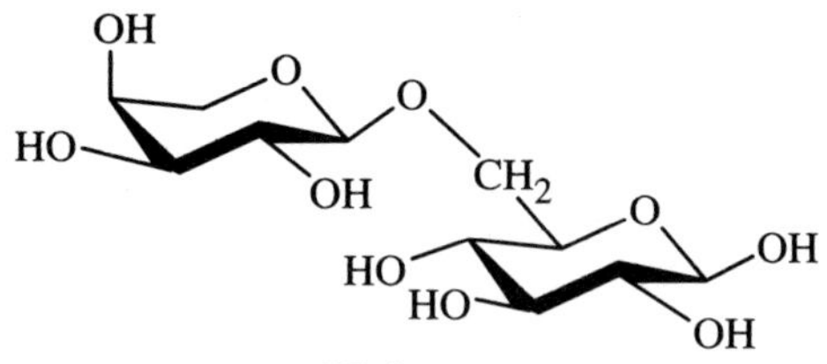

Vicianose

Acid-catalyzed hydrolysis of each disaccharide affords two monosaccharides, one of which is D-glucose and the other either arabinose or xylose, whose Fisher projections are shown below in the D configurations.

CH=O — D-Arabinose

CH=O — D-Xylose

What are the other monosaccharides obtained along with D-glucose upon performing acid-catalyzed hydrolysis of primverose and vicianose, respectively?

A) L-arabinose and D-xylose
B) D-arabinose and D-xylose
C) L-xylose and L-arabinose
D) D-xylose and L-arabinose

5. β-Galactosidase is an essential human enzyme that hydrolyzes the β-glycosidic bond between galactose and glucose units in the disaccharide lactose. This enzyme also promotes transgalactosylation, which converts lactose into allolactose. Hydrolysis of allolactose provides a positive feedback loop for production of β-galactose:

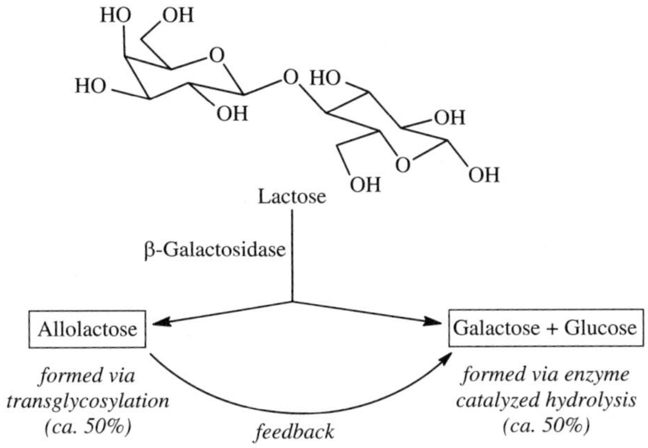

Lactose

β-Galactosidase

Allolactose

formed via transglycosylation (ca. 50%)

feedback

Galactose + Glucose

formed via enzyme catalyzed hydrolysis (ca. 50%)

Based on the information above, which of the following is most likely to represent the structure of allolactose?

A)

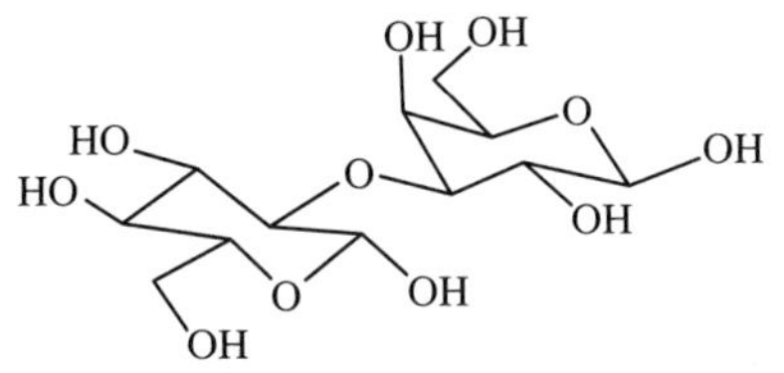

B)

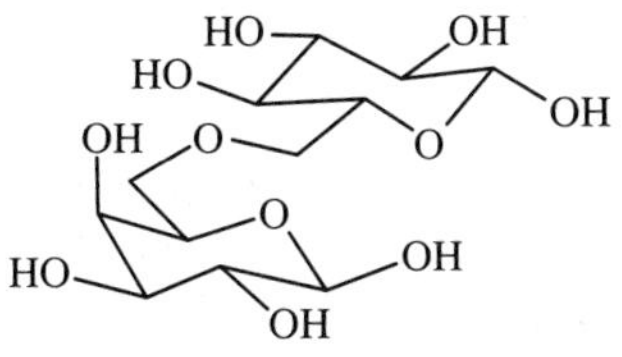

C)

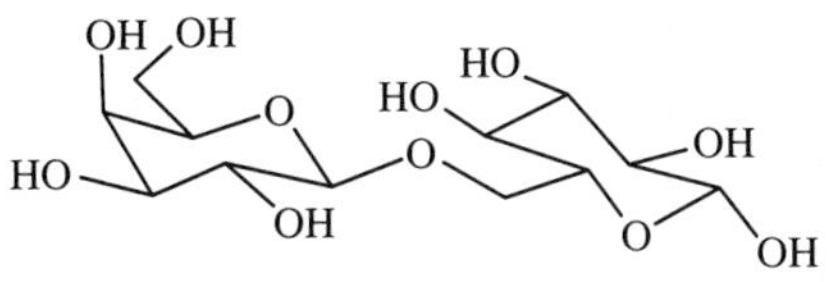

D)

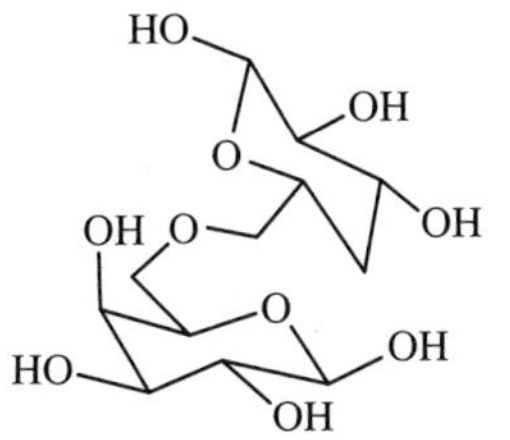

6. Mechanism-based covalently-bound inhibitors have been used to study the mechanism of action of glycosidases. Cleavage of the glycosidic linkage in Compound X (structure shown below) by yeast α-glucosidase affords Aglycone Y, which subsequently reacts with a nucleophilic residue in the enzyme, thereby inhibiting the enzyme irreversibly.

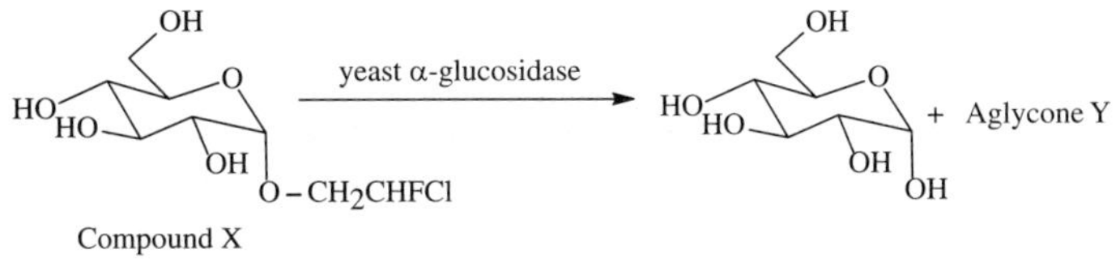

yeast α-glucosidase

+ Aglycone Y

Compound X

Which of the following compounds is most likely to correspond to the aglycone responsible for inactivation of yeast α-glucosidase?

A)

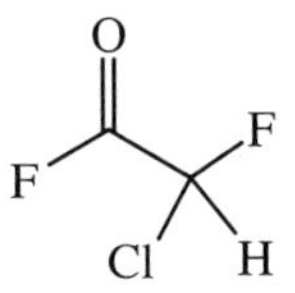

B)

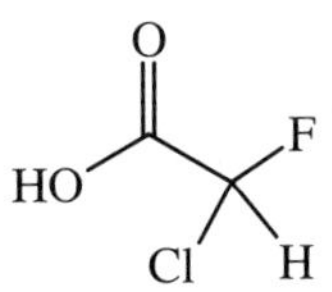

C)

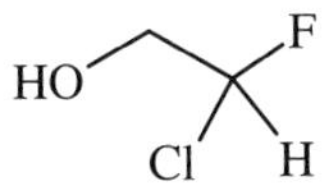

D)

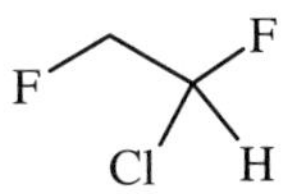

BIOLOGICALLY IMPORTANT MOLECULES PRACTICE PASSAGE 3

Chromatography is used to identify, separate, and purify components of a mixture of compounds. Biologically important molecules, e.g., amino acids, proteins, and nucleic acids, can be separated and purified on the basis of their size, shape, and net electronic charge.

The presence of polar and/or hydrophobic groups on the surface of a protein affects its ability to interact with the stationary phase employed in chromatographic separations. Column chromatographic methods commonly employed for separation and purification of biochemical mixtures that take advantage of molecular characteristics include ion exchange chromatography, size exclusion (gel filtration) chromatography, affinity chromatography, and high performance liquid chromatography (HPLC). In addition to column chromatography, normal- and reverse-phase thin layer chromatography (TLC) and paper chromatography are used commonly to separate and analyze mixtures of compounds.

Gel electrophoresis, which is used to separate and to analyze macromolecules and their degradation products, depends upon the movement of charged species in an applied electric field. The efficiency of separations performed *via* gel electrophoresis is affected by several factors, among which are net charge, molecular size and shape, pH of the medium, viscosity of the porous support (frequently polyacrylamide or agarose), temperature, and voltage across the gel.

1. A sample of a xylanase enzyme, XYN I (molecular mass 19 kDa, pI 5.5) isolated from the fungus *Trichoderma reesei* is contaminated with two other proteins: Protein X (molecular mass 23 kDa, pI 7.5) and Protein Y (molecular mass 120 kDa, pI 5.4). Which one of the following procedures can *best* be used to isolate pure XYN I from this sample?

A) Ion-exchange chromatographic purification of the original sample buffered at pH 6.0 followed by size exclusion chromatographic purification of the eluate

B) Size exclusion chromatographic purification of the original sample followed by sodium dodecyl sulfate-polyacrylamide gel electrophoresis (SDS-PAGE) performed on the eluate

C) Ion-exchange chromatographic purification of the original sample buffered at pH 6.0 followed by gas-liquid chromatographic (GLC) purification of the eluate

D) Size exclusion chromatographic purification of the original sample followed by gas-liquid chromatographic (GLC) purification of the eluate

2. Gel electrophoresis is used to separate a mixture of arginine, tryptophan, and aspartic acid. Relevant pK information is given below:

Amino Acid	pK_1	pK_2	pK_3
Arginine	2.17	9.04	12.48
Tryptophan	2.83	9.39	—
Aspartic acid	1.88	9.60	3.65

Which of the following matrix pH values could *best* be used to separate the mixture of three amino acids into pure components by using gel electrophoresis?

A) pH 2.2
B) pH 3.2
C) pH 6.0
D) pH 10.8

3. A liquid-liquid extraction scheme based on acid-base chemistry employs diethyl ether as the organic phase and 5% dilute aqueous acid or base as the aqueous phase. Which of the following procedures could *best* be employed to separate an ether solution containing a mixture of benzoic acid, phenol, and aniline?

A) Extract the ether solution with 5% HCl, separate the layers, extract the ether layer with 5% NaOH, separate the layers

B) Extract the ether solution with 5% NaOH, separate the layers, extract the ether layer with 5% HCl, separate the layers

C) Extract the ether solution with 5% NaOH, separate the layers, extract the ether layer with 5% NaHCO$_3$, separate the layers

D) Extract the ether solution with 5% NaHCO$_3$, separate the layers, extract the ether layer with 5% HCl, separate the layers

4. A mixture containing five amino acids, Asp, Phe, Met, Trp, and Tyr, was separated *via* reverse-phase HPLC by using isocratic elution with 10% aqueous methanol.

Amino Acid	pI
Asp	2.85
Phe	5.49
Met	5.74
Trp	5.89
Tyr	5.64

What is the expected order of increasing retention time of the components of this mixture?

A) Met < Tyr < Asp < Phe < Trp
B) Trp < Phe < Asp < Met < Tyr
C) Asp < Tyr < Met < Phe < Trp
D) Trp < Phe < Met < Tyr < Asp

5. Diethylaminoethyl cellulose (DEAE-C, structure shown below) is a weak ion-exchange resin used in ion-exchange chromatography for separation and purification of proteins and nucleic acids.

Diethylaminoethyl Cellulose

Which one of the following four statements best describes a property of DEAE-C resin?

A) DEAE-C resin is best used to separate and purify proteins when the pH of mobile phase is buffered above the pK_a of the diethylamino groups.
B) Proteins that bear smaller electric charges are eluted from a column packed with DEAE-C resin more rapidly than those bearing larger electronic charges.
C) Binding of proteins on a column packed with DEAE-C resin is best performed by using a high ionic strength buffer.
D) DEAE-C resin is classed as a weak ion-exchange resin due to its low ability to bind to proteins.

6. A mixture of three compounds (I, II, and III) was spotted on a silica gel TLC plate along with authentic samples of the three compounds that comprise the mixture. The plate was eluted with 10% ethyl acetate in hexane, which resulted in the following chromatogram.

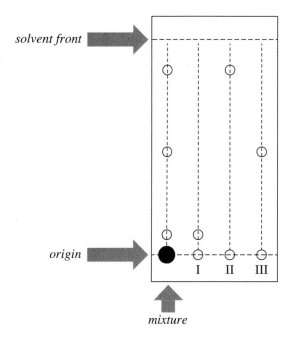

Which of the following statements most accurately reflects a change in the retardation factors (R_f) of spots on the TLC plate (i) if the stationary phase were changed to alumina? (ii) if the mobile phase were changed to 25% ethyl acetate in hexane?

A) (i) The R_f values of all three spots would increase.
   (ii) The R_f values of all three spots would increase.
B) (i) The R_f values of all three spots would decrease.
   (ii) The R_f values of all three spots would increase.
C) (i) The R_f values of all three spots would increase.
   (ii) The R_f values of all three spots would decrease.
D) (i) The R_f values of all three spots would decrease.
   (ii) The R_f values of all three spots would decrease.

SOLUTIONS TO FREESTANDING QUESTIONS: BIOLOGICALLY IMPORTANT MOLECULES

1. **B** Asparagine is a neutral amino acid with two ionizable groups, $-COOH$ and $-NH_3{}^+$:

$$H_3N^+–Asp–COOH \rightleftharpoons H_3N^+–Asp–COO^- \rightleftharpoons H_2N–Asp–COO^-$$

The pH at which asparagine possesses no net charge (also known as the zwitterion form) is the isoelectric point (pI) and can be determined from the given pK_a values. At very low and high pH, asparagine will have a net positive and negative charge, respectively. At a pH between the two pK_a values, asparagine will possess the least net charge, so only choice B is possible. For neutral amino acids, the pI is the average of the pK_a values of the functional groups (pI = 5.4 for asparagine).

2. **D** The reaction conditions shown are those of the Benedict's test for reducing sugars in which Cu^{2+} ions react with aldehydes to form carboxylic acids and Cu^+. It is therefore a redox reaction, and you should expect the aldehyde to gain more oxygen (eliminate choice C) and Cu^{2+} to gain more electrons (eliminate choice B). Choice A can be eliminated because the former carbonyl carbon has been neither oxidized nor reduced.

3. **B** A peptide bond, also known an amide bond, is a covalent bond formed between a carboxyl group and an amino group, with the release of water during the process (choice B is correct). Hydrogen bonds are *inter*-molecular forces, which form the secondary structure (α-helices and β-pleated sheets) in polypeptides, and they are also responsible for base pairing within the DNA double helix (eliminate choice A). Phosphodiester bonds join nucleotides to form the backbone of DNA and RNA (eliminate choice C). Glycosidic bonds join carbohydrate monomers to form di- or polysaccharides (eliminate choice D).

4. **A** $NaBH_4$ is a reducing agent that converts aldehydes and ketones into alcohols. Alcohols, acetals, and hemiacetals do not react with $NaBH_4$, making choice D a tempting answer. However, the hemiacetal group in the glucose residue of lactose is in equilibrium with the open-chain aldehyde form. $NaBH_4$ reduces the aldehyde to the primary alcohol preventing further cyclization (eliminate choice D; choice A is correct). The formation of a cyclic ether would require the removal of the alcohol group of the hemiacetal, which cannot be achieved with $NaBH_4$ (eliminate choice B). Hydrolysis of the glycosidic linkage requires acidic conditions (eliminate choice C).

5. **A** The conditions shown are for the Strecker synthesis of amino acids, and given the reactant, the product will be histidine. This reaction proceeds through an sp^2–hybridized iminium intermediate that when attacked with the cyano group will yield two products with the same connectivity (eliminate choice C).

Regioisomers are constitutional isomers that result from different bond making or bond breaking throughout a reaction. Since there are no chiral centers in the reactant, when the iminium ion is attacked to generate an sp^3-hybridized carbon, both sides of the double bond are susceptible. A racemic mixture of histidine enantiomers is produced because both stereocenters are generated in equal amounts (choice A is correct). Racemic mixtures are optically inactive (eliminate choice B). While histidine is amphoteric, it is not amphipathic. This amino acid is hydrophilic since the imidazole side chain can hydrogen bond with water (eliminate choice D).

6. **D** The glycosidic linkage is between the anomeric carbon of the ring on the left, which is C-1 in the case of an aldose as shown, and C-4 of the ring on the right (eliminate choices A and B). The ring on the right is upside down relative to the ring on the left, so the carbons are numbered counterclockwise starting with the anomeric carbon. The bridging O atom in the glycosidic linkage is up, making this a β linkage (eliminate choice C).

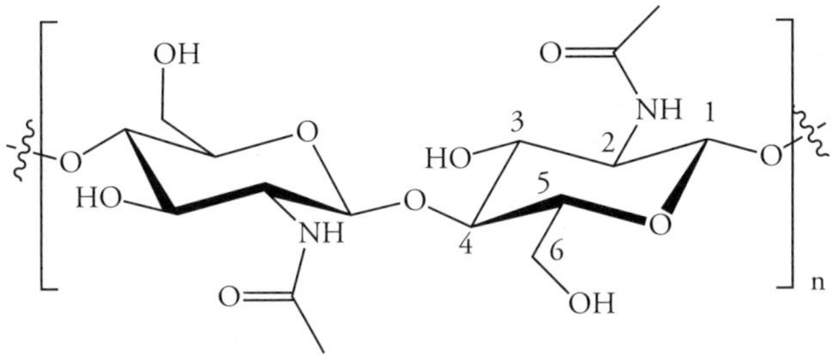

7. **C** This is a 2 × 2 question, which can be attacked based on the number of tails and the type of structure formed by the different lipids. Fatty acids have a single hydrocarbon tail, whereas phospholipids have two hydrocarbon tails (eliminate choices A and B). Because of the structural arrangement of these hydrophobic tails, fatty acids spontaneously form spherical micelles, whereas phospholipids organize into membranes (choice D is wrong; choice C is correct).

8. **B** Trypsin promotes cleavage of peptide chains at the carboxyl side of Lys and Arg (except when either is followed by Pro), and chymotrypsin cleaves peptide bonds at the amide side of aromatic amino acids Tyr, Phe, and Trp. However, it is not necessary to know this in order to arrive at the correct answer. Cleavage with trypsin resulted in a tripeptide Gly-Tyr-Lys, so the full amino acid sequence must contain this fragment (choices A and D can be eliminated). Cleavage with chymotrypsin produced the tripeptide Arg-Ala-Leu, so that must also be found in the full sequence (choice C can be eliminated, and choice B is correct). Note also that the sequence of amino acids can be determined by lining up the various cleavage fragments with the N-terminus at the left as indicated in the following diagram:

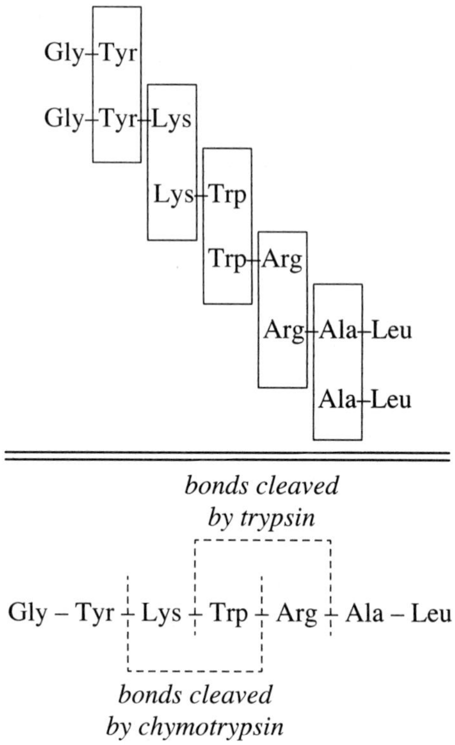

Gly–Tyr
Gly–Tyr–Lys
Lys–Trp
Trp–Arg
Arg–Ala–Leu
Ala–Leu

bonds cleaved
by trypsin

Gly – Tyr ┆ Lys ┆ Trp ┆ Arg ┆ Ala – Leu

bonds cleaved
by chymotrypsin

The correct amino acid sequence appears in choice B.

SOLUTIONS TO BIOLOGICALLY IMPORTANT MOLECULES PRACTICE PASSAGE 1

1. **B** The anomeric carbons of both D-mannose and *N*-acetyl-D-glucosamine are located at C-1 and show a hydroxyl group oriented up; thus both are shown in a β configuration (eliminate choice A). As stated in the passage, D-mannose and *N*-acetyl-D-glucosamine may form linear polymers, which is achieved in a 1,4 glycosidic linkage. Both carbohydrates can potentially form α- and β-1,4 linkages with each other (choice B is correct). The lone pair of electrons on the amide nitrogen in *N*-acetyl-D-glucosamine is involved in resonance with the adjacent carbonyl. Therefore, the nitrogen is less nucleophilic than an amine. Moreover, it is not a primary nitrogen, as required for Schiff base formation (eliminate choice C). Mannose and glucose share a molecular formula and the same atomic connectivity so they are not structural isomers (eliminate choice D). They differ in the spatial orientation of a hydroxyl group about C-2 only, making them epimers.

2. **D**   As the labeled structure shows below, there are a total of five resonances expected from acrylamide. The protons labeled H_d and H_e are non-equivalent because there is no rotation about the C=C π bond. Due to conjugation of the nonbonding pair of electrons of the amide nitrogen with the carbonyl, the amide bond acquires π bond character. This effect removes rotation about the C—N bond, which makes hydrogens H_a and H_b non-equivalent.

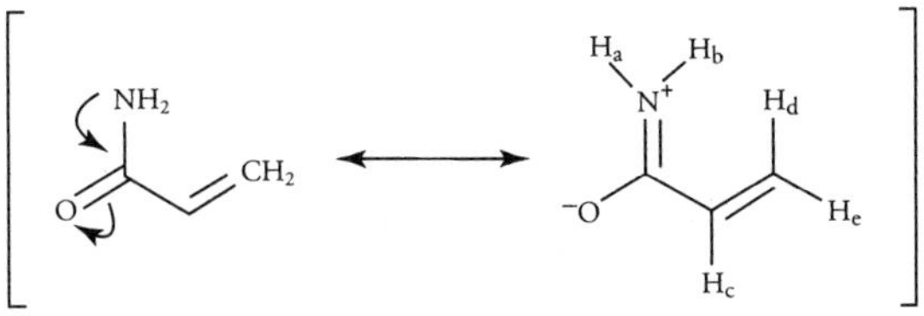

3. **A**   The proton α to the Schiff base is somewhat similar to the α-hydrogen of a carbonyl compound in that it is acidic due to resonance stabilization of its conjugate base. Therefore, under acidic conditions, isomerization of the Schiff base can occur. In the presence of H_2SO_4, the nitrogen will be protonated, increasing the acidity of the α-hydrogen. This allows water to deprotonate the α-hydrogen. This step forms the enol shown below, which tautomerizes under the same acidic conditions to a ketone.

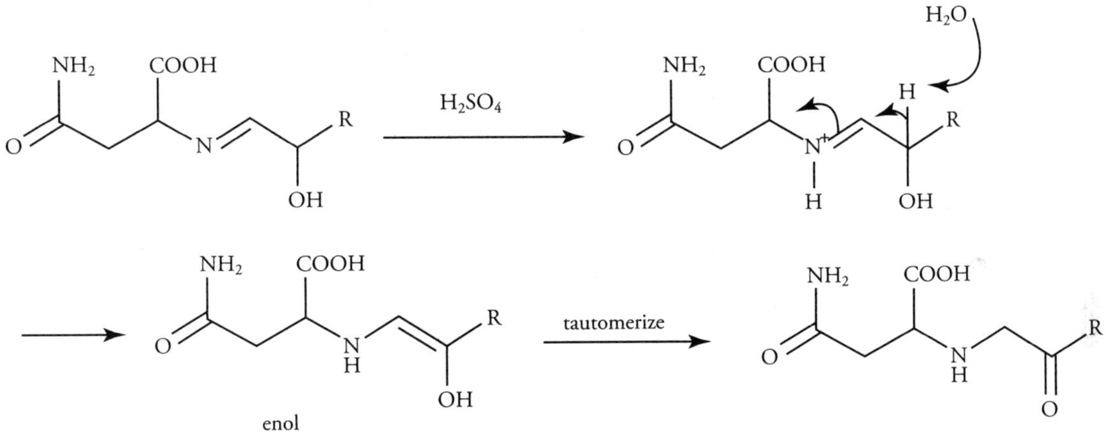

Sodium ethoxide is a base capable of enolizing carbonyls, but imine α-hydrogens are not as acidic as carbon α-hydrogens because the resulting negative charge is on a nitrogen, which is less electronegative than oxygen. Therefore, sodium ethoxide is not capable of the isomerization (eliminate choice B). Methylmagnesium bromide is a Grignard reagent, and thus a strong nucleophile and base; it might react with the imine through nucleophilic addition, but it would definitely be quenched through deprotonation of the acid and alcohol functional groups (eliminate choice C). Acetone is a solvent that does not have acidic or basic properties, so it will not isomerize the Schiff base (eliminate choice D).

4.   **C**   Under strongly acidic conditions the amine will be protonated, converting it to a non-nucleophile, and quickly decreasing the rate of nucleophilic addition to the carbonyl (eliminate choice A). The removal of water would preclude a backward reaction and shift the equilibrium in favor of the Schiff base product (eliminate choice B). Because the reaction is reversible, it is under thermodynamic control; if it were kinetically controlled, it would be unable to reverse (eliminate choice D). In Schiff base formation, water is generated as a by-product. The loss of a stable molecule is an exothermic process, thus favoring the thermodynamics of the reaction and making choice C correct.

5.   **D**   Since the false statement is desired, Process of Elimination is the best approach to this question. As shown in Figure 1 of the passage, the chirality at C-2 in the reducing sugar is destroyed by the time it has completed Step 3. This removes the stereochemical difference between glucose and mannose, therefore, choice A is a true statement and can be eliminated. The isomerization in Step 3 is irreversible, as dictated by the passage text, thus increasing plasma glucose concentration will yield an increase in hemoglobin-A_{1c} levels. This makes choice B a true statement, so it can be eliminated. Because hemoglobin-A_{1c} will have a different hydrophilicity relative to non-glycated hemoglobin due to the addition of a highly polar carbohydrate moiety, choice C is true and can be eliminated. The passage states that the Schiff base is irreversibly isomerized (shown in Step 3 of Figure 1), thus choice D must be false and therefore correct.

6.   **B**   All of the Items appear in exactly two answer choices, so it doesn't matter which you start analyzing. Since digestion of the *N*-linked glycoprotein will yield fragments of various sizes, some of which may contain a carbohydrate chain and some of which may not, an appropriate separation technique must target the carbohydrate-containing components in the digested mixture. Item I will be unreliable in separating glycosylated fragments from non-glycosylated ones as there will be an array of large and small fragments, some containing a carbohydrate chain and some not (choices A and C can be eliminated). Item II must be true since it is in both remaining choices; focus on Item III. Item III is false: Ion-exchange chromatography allows for the separation of components in a mixture with differently charged states. The charged state of each fragment will depend on the composition of the peptide fragment, not on its carbohydrate composition. Carbohydrates show little ionization potential since they lack the necessary amino and carboxylic functional groups (choice D can be eliminated, and choice B is correct). Note that Item II is in fact true: performing lectin affinity chromatography means the stationary phase will adsorb only the glycosylated components in a sample, which is an effective method of separating these fragments from the non-glycosylated fragments.

SOLUTIONS TO BIOLOGICALLY IMPORTANT MOLECULES PRACTICE PASSAGE 2

1. **B**   Digoxin contains three acetal carbons [indicated by dark circles (●) in the drawing shown below], which participate in the formation of glycosidic linkages. [Note that the steroid moiety does not contain an acetal carbon atom.]

    As noted in the passage, acid-catalyzed hydrolysis of sugar acetals generally produces mixtures of diastereoisomeric (anomeric) hemiacetals. This process is summarized below for acid-catalyzed hydrolysis of digoxin.

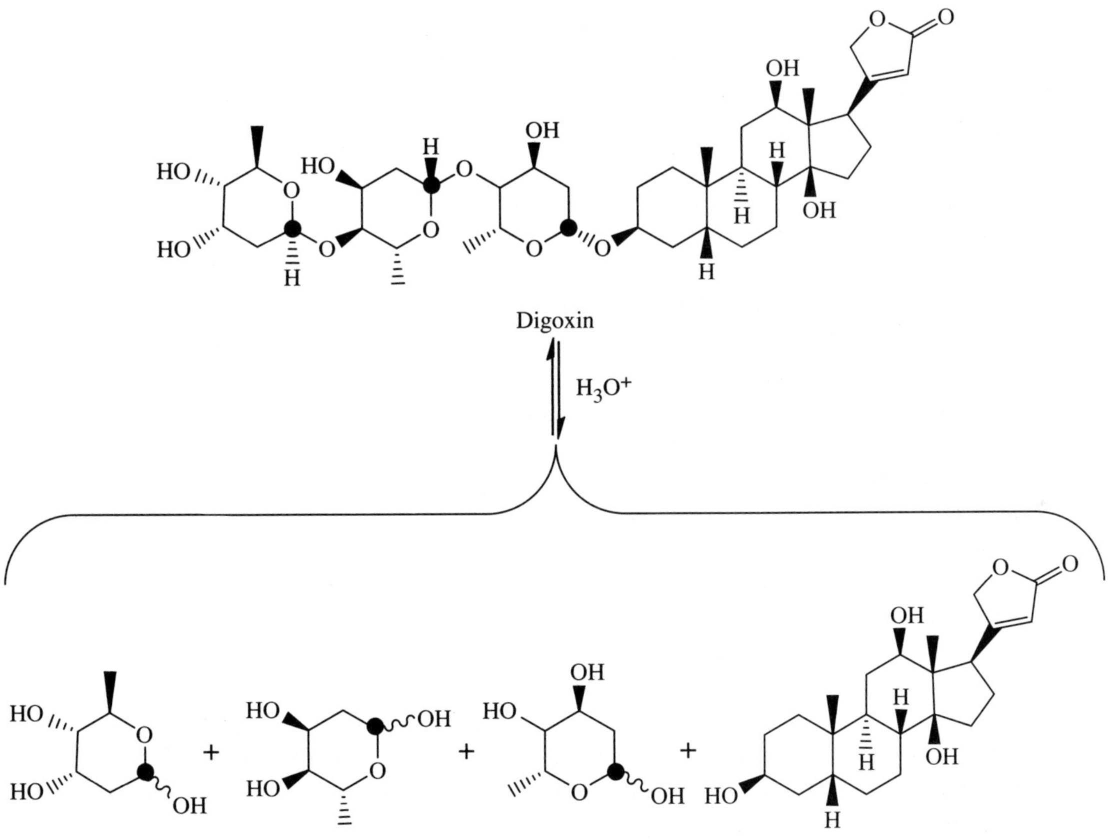

Digoxin

H_3O^+

Four fragments are expected to result via this process (choice B is correct).

2. **A** Inclusion of "electron-pushing" in Schemes 1 and 2 as indicated below helps to clarify the mechanistic function of each of the five species.

Scheme I (single displacement)

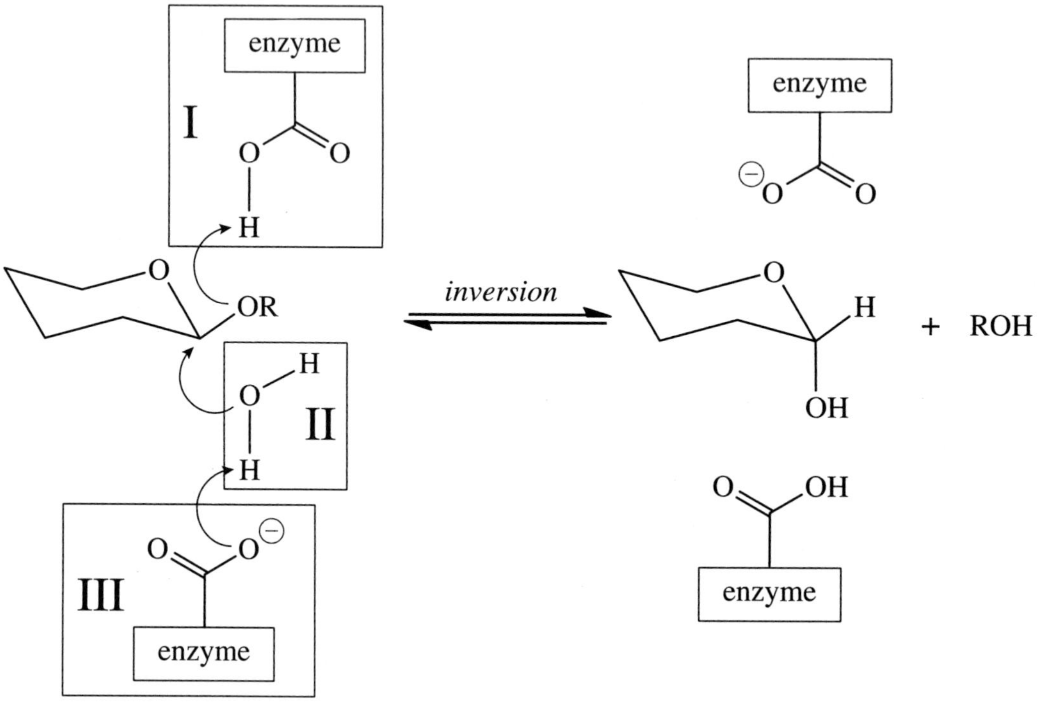

Scheme II (double displacement)

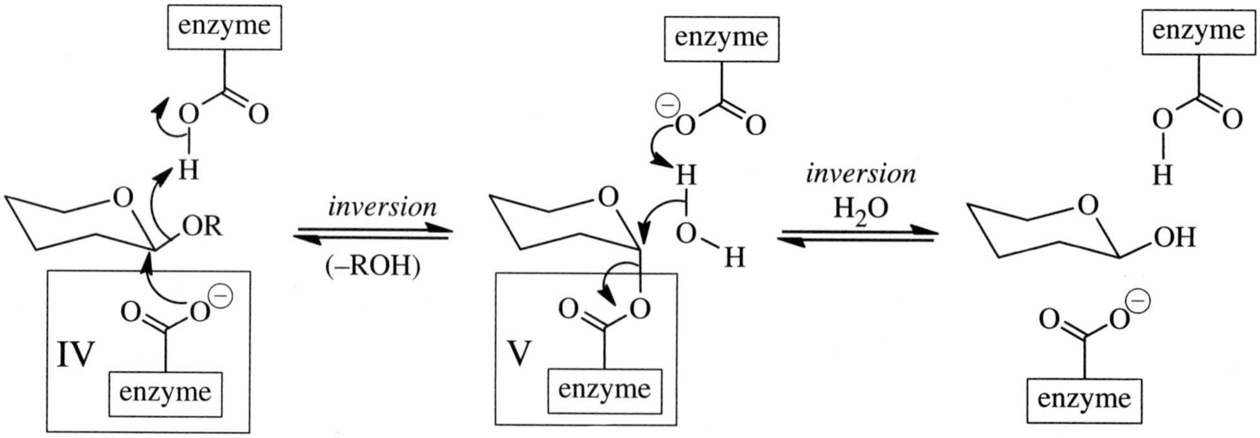

Species I functions as a Brønsted acid by protonating the OR group, which renders ROH a good leaving group.

Water (II) functions both as a nucleophile (by displacing ROH) and as an acid (by protonating III). Choice A is correct; this conclusion is confirmed by assigning the functions of the remaining three species. Species III is protonated by water and thus functions as a Brønsted base. Species IV displaces ROH and thereby functions as a nucleophile. Species V is displaced by OH (from water) and thus serves as a leaving group.

3. **D** The products shown below are expected to result via application of Mechanisms III and IV to the reaction indicated in the stem.

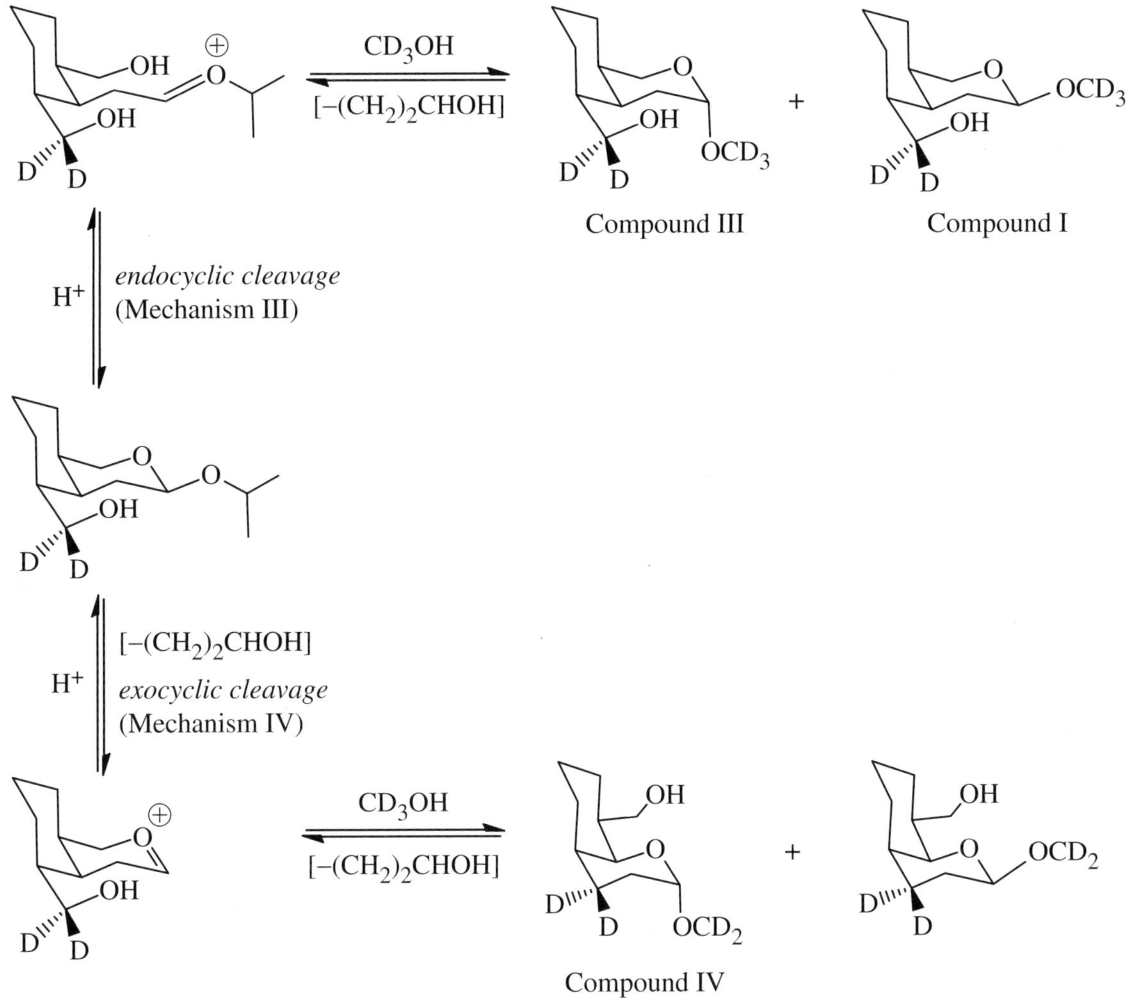

Compound III   Compound I

endocyclic cleavage (Mechanism III)

$[-(CH_2)_2CHOH]$
exocyclic cleavage (Mechanism IV)

Compound IV

Compounds I, III, and IV (choice D is correct, and choice A is wrong) are expected to be formed as reaction products. However, Compound II, in which the primary alcohol group has been replaced by OCD_3, is not expected to be formed via this reaction (choices B and C can be eliminated).

4. **D**   It is helpful to begin by assigning the Cahn-Ingold-Prelog (CIP) *R,S* absolute configuration at C(4) in the aldopentose residues in primeverose and vicianose, respectively.

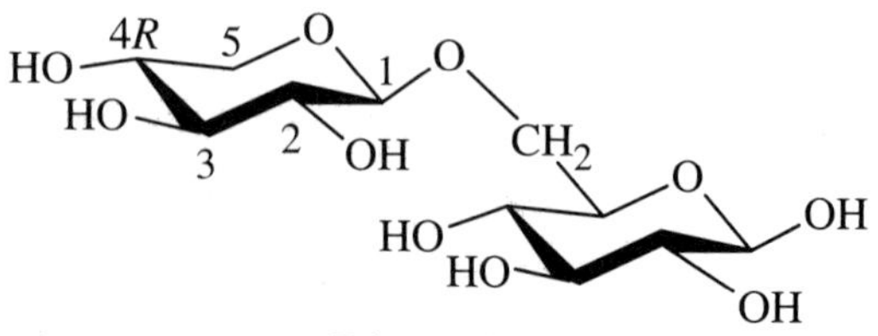

Primeverose

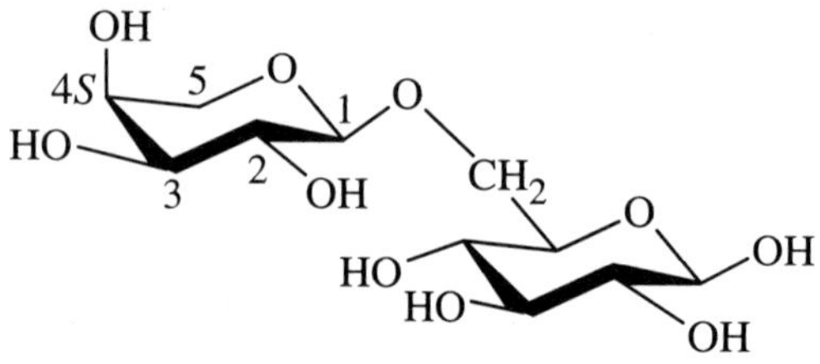

Vicianose

Primeverose contains a D-aldopentose moiety, whereas vicianose contains an L-series aldopentose. Among the four choices offered as responses to this item, only choice D indicates that primeverose contains a D-aldopentose, while vicianose contains an L-aldopentose. Only choice D offers the correct "primeverose/D-aldopentose – vicianose/L-aldopentose" combination.

This can also be seen by assigning the *R,S* absolute configuration to each of the three chiral centers in D-arabinose and in D-xylose.

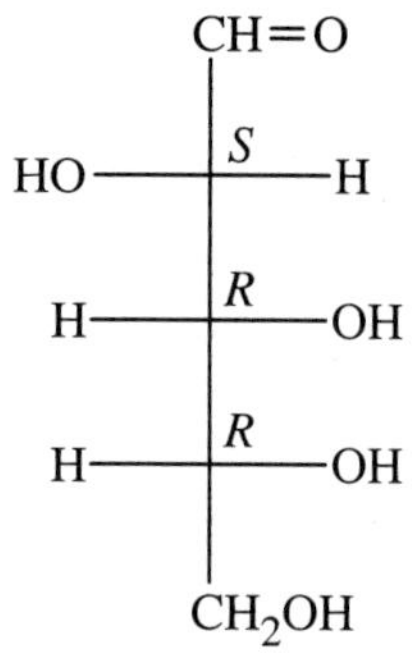

D-Arabinose

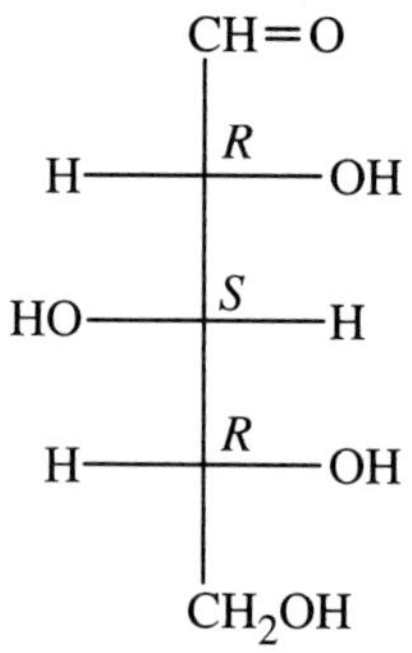

D-Xylose

The corresponding *R,S* configurations at C(2), C(3), and C(4) in the aldopentose moieties in primeverose and vicianose are shown below.

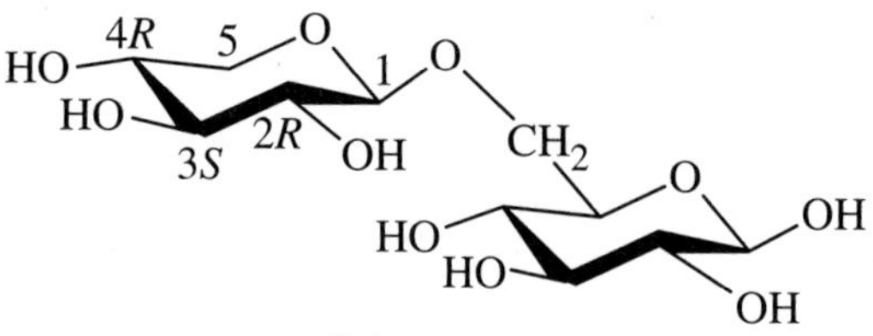

Primeverose

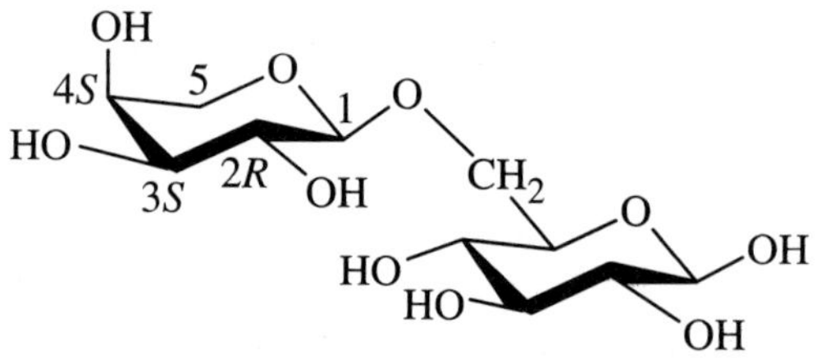

Vicianose

Comparison with the absolute configurations at C(2), C(3), and C(4) in D-arabinose and D-xylose confirms the structures of primeverose [6-O-(β-D-xylopyranosyl)-β-D-glucopyranose] and vicianose [6-O-(α-L-arabinopyranosyl)-β-D-glucopyranose] and also confirms the correct answer, choice D.

5. **C** Only choice C contains a β-glycosidic linkage between glucose and galactose, the two monosaccharide units of which the disaccharide lactose is comprised.

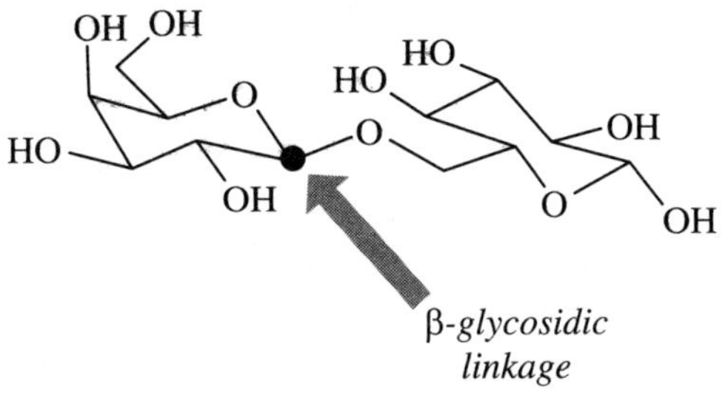

β-glycosidic
linkage

Each of the remaining four choices contains only an ether linkage between monosaccharide units. Choice C is correct.

6. **A** Enzymatic hydrolysis of the glycoside linkage in Compound X results in formation of an unstable geminal halohydrin, which is expected to spontaneously eliminate HF to afford the corresponding acyl fluoride.

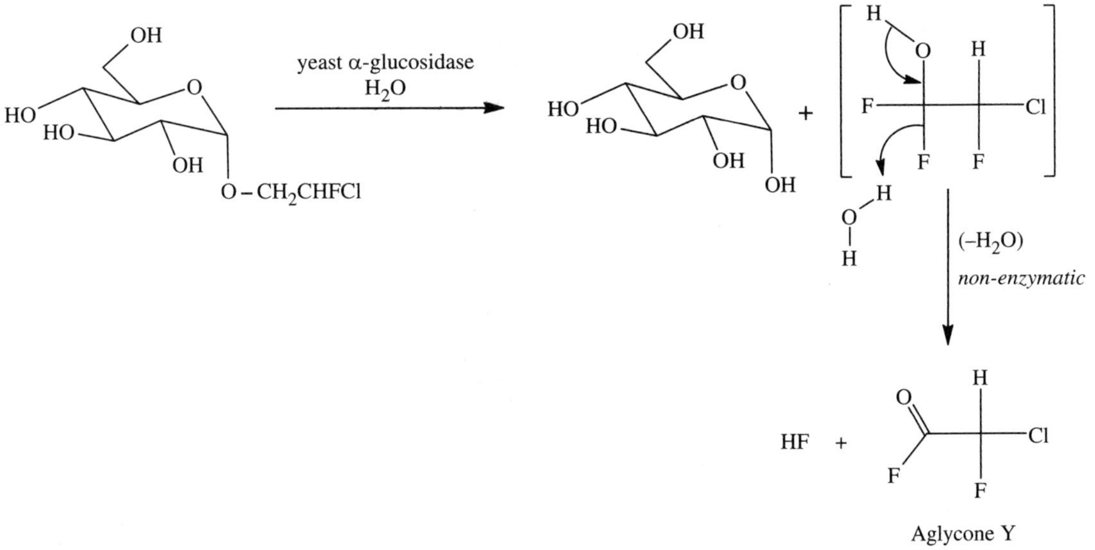

Aglycone Y

Acyl halides are highly reactive and readily undergo an addition-elimination two step reaction sequence with a nucleophilic residue in the enzyme, thereby irreversibly inhibiting the enzyme (choice A is correct).

SOLUTIONS TO BIOLOGICALLY IMPORTANT MOLECULES PRACTICE PASSAGE 3

1. **A** Ion-exchange chromatography offers a separation technique based on charge-charge interactions between the analyte and the cation or anion exchange resin employed as the solid support. The use of ion-exchange chromatography is expected to remove Protein X whose pI differs significantly from that of the xylanase enzyme. Thereafter, size-exclusion chromatography can be used to separate the enzyme (molecular mass 19 kDa) from the much more massive Protein Y (molecular mass 120 kDa). Choice A is the correct answer.

   Choice B utilizes size exclusion chromatography to remove Protein Y. SDS-PAGE separates proteins, which migrate through a gel at different rates under the influence of an applied electrical field. In the presence of the detergent (SDS), all of the proteins have an identical negative charge density. Accordingly, this method, like size exclusion chromatography, relies almost entirely on molecular size as a separation method. After the large Protein Y has been separated by size exclusion chromatography, the remaining xylanase and Protein X, which have similar mass but different pI values, are expected to migrate together as a single band when subjected to polyacrylamide gel electrophoresis containing SDS. Eliminate choice B.

   When the PAGE technique is performed under non-denaturing conditions (i.e., in the absence of SDS), migration toward the cathode or anode is expected to be determined by the analyte's pI. Under these conditions, xylanase enzyme (pI 5.5) and Protein X (pI 7.5) would be expected to migrate at different rates.

   Gas-liquid chromatography (GLC) requires the use of a carrier gas to transport volatile components of a mixture through a heated column. Enzymes and proteins are nonvolatile, heat-sensitive macromolecules for which GLC does not offer a suitable method for separation and purification. Eliminate choices C and D.

2. **C** The nitrogen-containing (basic) functional groups in each amino acid are expected to be protonated when pH < pK, whereas the corresponding carboxylic acid (acidic) groups are expected to be deprotonated when pH > pK. During electrophoresis, amino acids that bear a net positive charge at a given pH value migrate toward the negative electrode, whereas those bearing a net negative charge migrate toward the positive electrode.

   When pH = pI (the "isoelectric point"), the amino acid exists as a (neutral) zwitterion, which does not migrate when an electric field is applied. pI values for the three amino acids of interest can be estimated as indicated below by using pK information contained in the stem.

   pI (arginine) = (9.04 + 12.48) divided by 2 = 10.76

   pI (tryptophan) = (2.83 + 9.39) divided by 2 = 6.11

   pI (aspartic acid) = (1.88 + 3.65) divided by 2 = 2.77

The following species are present in solution at each of the four pH values offered as choices:

	Arginine	Tryptophan	Aspartic acid

pH	Arginine net charge	Tryptophan net charge	Aspartic acid net charge
pH 2.2	+2	+1	0
pH 3.2	+1	0	0
pH 6.0	+1	0	−1
pH 10.8	0	−1	−2

The widest separation among the three amino acids under application of an electric field is made possible when the net charges differ on all three amino acids. Among the four pH values offered as choices, this situation occurs only at pH 6.0. At this matrix, pH arginine and aspartic acid migrate to opposite electrodes while tryptophan remains at the origin. Choice C is the correct answer.

3. **D** The procedure described in choice A is outlined below.

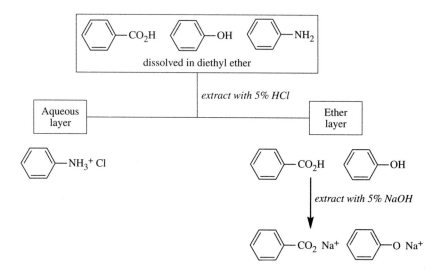

Extraction of an ether solution of the original mixture with 5% HCl permits separation of aniline as anilinium ion, which is transported into the aqueous layer. However, extraction of the remaining ether layer with 5% NaOH is not effective, since both benzoic acid and phenol are soluble in this medium and thus will not be separated. Eliminate choice A.

Extraction of the original ethereal mixture with 5% NaOH is expected to convert benzoic acid and phenol into their corresponding sodium salts, which will be transported into the aqueous layer and cannot be separated further by using the procedure described in either choice B or C, both of which can be eliminated.

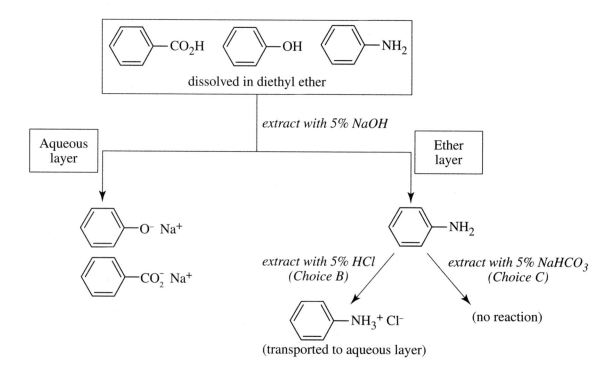

The procedure described in choice D takes advantage of the fact that phenol, a weaker acid than benzoic acid, is soluble in 5% NaOH but insoluble in 5% $NaHCO_3$.

Choice D is the correct answer.

4. **C** Reverse-phase column chromatography utilizes a non-polar stationary phase, which is eluted with a moderately polar aqueous solvent (mobile phase). Amino acids with non-polar, hydrophobic side-chains adhere to the stationary phase most strongly and thus experience the longest retention times (i.e., these species are eluted last).

Relevant properties of the five amino acids of interest are indicated below.

Based upon polarity characteristics and hydrophilicity, Asp and Tyr are expected to display the shortest retention times under reverse-phase HPLC conditions and are thus expected to be eluted first from the column. Methionine is expected to reside on the column for a somewhat longer time. Finally, Phe and Trp, both of which contain non-polar, hydrophobic side chains, are expected to be the last of the five amino acids to be eluted.

Note that Trp contains a non-polar, hydrophobic side chain. This observation is sufficient to permit choices B and D to be eliminated. Choice A indicates incorrectly that Met (less polar) is expected to be eluted more rapidly than either Tyr or Asp (more polar). Eliminate choice A. Choice C is the correct answer.

5.   **B**   DEAE-C resin is employed as the stationary phase in anion-exchange chromatography. When protonated, the diethylamino group bears a positive charge to which negatively-charged proteins will become bound *via* electrostatic interactions.

The pH of the mobile phase must be significantly *below* the pK_a of the dimethylamino group in order for this side-chain to become protonated effectively. Eliminate choice A.

Negatively-charged proteins become adsorbed onto the surface of DEAE-C resin by displacing buffer ions from the mobile phase that balance the charged diethylammonium group in protonated DEAE. There is a continuous, reversible competition between negatively-charged proteins and buffer anions associated with protonated DEAE. Since the primary interaction between proteins and DEAE is electrostatic in nature, it follows that proteins bearing larger electronic charges will be more strongly adsorbed. It follows that proteins bearing smaller electronic charges will be eluted from a column packed with DEAE-C resin more rapidly than those bearing larger electronic charges. Choice B is the correct answer.

The competition between negatively-charged proteins and the buffer ions associated with protonated DEAE is noted above. Thus, increasing the ionic strength of the buffer used in the mobile phase necessarily increases the concentration of buffer anion, which will tend to favor this ion when competing with negatively-charged proteins for binding to protonated DEAE. Eliminate choice C.

As noted in the stem, DEAE-C is a weak ion-exchange resin, which reflects the fact that it is only partially ionized over most pH values. Thus, use of DEAE-C to purify a particular protein requires buffering the mobile phase over a specific and rather narrow pH range. Note that the terms "weak" and "strong" as employed to reference the properties of ion-exchange resins refer to the pH interval over which they are able to maintain their positive or negative charge and *not* to their relative ability to bind to oppositely-charged analytes. Eliminate choice D.

6. **B** The TLC conditions described in the stem are consistent with normal-phase column chromatography, which utilizes a polar stationary phase. The TLC plate is eluted with an organic solvent; more polar analytes are adsorbed more strongly on the surface of the stationary phase and thus have longer retention times than relatively non-polar analytes.

Condition (i) specifies that the stationary phase is changed from silica gel to alumina, a more polar stationary phase. Each compound spotted on the TLC plate is expected to be eluted more slowly (i.e., to present a smaller R_f value) when the stationary phase is rendered increasingly polar. Eliminate choices A and C.

Condition (ii) specifies that the mobile phase is changed from 10% ethyl acetate in hexane to the more polar 25% ethyl acetate in hexane. As the polarity of the mobile phase is increased, analytes become eluted from the polar stationary phase (silica gel) with increasing efficiency. Since all analytes are expected to elute more rapidly with increasing solvent polarity, R_f values will increase. Eliminate choice D; choice B is correct.

Part 7

MCAT Physics

Chapter 33
Kinematics and Dynamics

FREESTANDING QUESTIONS: KINEMATICS AND DYNAMICS

1. A cloud moving at a velocity of w m/s horizontally releases the first batch of raindrops, which hit the ground in t s after leaving the bottom layer of the cloud. If the cloud is y m above the ground, which of the following is the correct expression of the magnitude of the velocity of the raindrops upon touching the ground?

   A) $\sqrt{-2gy+w^2}$

   B) $\sqrt{-2gy+w^2 t^2}$

   C) $\sqrt{2gy+w^2}$

   D) $\sqrt{2gy+w}$

2. Which of the following kinematic descriptions is physically impossible?

   A) An object in motion for a time Δt has zero average velocity but positive nonzero average speed.

   B) An object maintains constant speed for a time Δt but has nonzero acceleration.

   C) An object in motion for a time Δt has zero displacement but nonzero total distance.

   D) An object in motion for a time Δt has an average velocity with a greater magnitude than its average speed.

3. An object is projected from the ground at an angle of 30° above the horizontal and returns to the ground 8 seconds later. What is the object's maximum height?

   A) 40 m
   B) 80 m
   C) 160 m
   D) There is not enough information to solve.

4. Which of the following graphs represents an object making a round trip?

   A)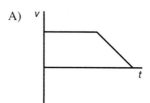

   B)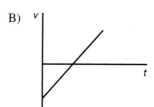

   C)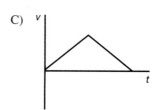

   D)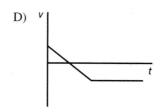

5. Two lead balls of unequal mass are thrown in the vertical direction on the Moon. One ball is thrown directly upwards, and the other is thrown downwards with the same speed. Which of the following statements are true?

   I. The two balls reach the ground with the same speed.
   II. The two balls reach the ground at the same time.
   III. The two balls are attracted to the Moon with a force of equal magnitude.

   A) I only
   B) II only
   C) I and III only
   D) II and III only

6. Which of the following best explains why one can drive a car faster without skidding around a banked curved road than around a level curved road?

A) The greater vertical component of normal force on the banked curve increases the maximum frictional force, which in turn increases the maximum centripetal force.
B) The additional horizontal component of normal force on the banked curve combines with friction from the road to increase the maximum centripetal force.
C) The additional horizontal component of gravity on the banked curve combines with friction from the road to increase the maximum centripetal force.
D) The reduction of the gravitational force on the banked curve means less centripetal force is required to keep the car moving in a curved path than on a level road.

7. In the figure below, the system is in static equilibrium. What is the force of static friction between M and the inclined plane if $M = 16$ kg, $m = 10$ kg, $\theta = 30°$, and $\mu_s = 0.4$?

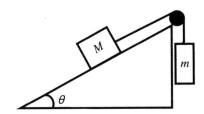

A) 0 N
B) 20 N down the plane
C) 55 N up the plane
D) 55 N down the plane

8. The dwarf planet Pluto has 1/500 the mass and 1/15 the radius of the Earth. What is the acceleration due to gravity near the surface of Pluto?

A) 0.3 m/s²
B) 1.6 m/s²
C) 4.5 m/s²
D) 7.1 m/s²

9. If a satellite undergoes uniform circular motion orbiting the Earth, which of the following statements is/are correct?

I. The larger the satellite's mass, the slower the satellite orbits the Earth.
II. The farther away the satellite is from the center of Earth, the slower the satellite orbits the Earth.
III. If the Earth's mass were to double, so would the speed of the orbiting satellite.

A) I only
B) II only
C) I and II
D) II and III

10. Amanda and Billy want to play on a teeter totter (a plank balanced atop a fulcrum where each child sits on opposite ends of the plank and moves up and down by pushing off the ground in turns). They have a 3 m long, 10 kg plank and a round boulder to serve as a fulcrum. If Amanda weighs 650 N and Billy weighs 300 N, how far from Amanda's seat should they balance the plank in order to make the game as fair as possible?

A) 95 cm
B) 1 m
C) 1.5 m
D) 1.6 m

KINEMATICS AND DYNAMICS PRACTICE PASSAGE

When an object is in contact with a surface, it may experience a frictional force, which resists lateral movement. There are two major kinds of friction: *static* and *kinetic*. The latter applies to an object sliding or skidding along a surface, whereas the former acts when the two surfaces are at rest with respect to each other at their point of contact. Static friction applies not only to two objects that are both totally motionless but also to an object that is rolling without slipping on a surface.

The amount of frictional force experienced by an object depends both on the normal force that the object experiences and on the coefficient of friction, μ, a measure of the molecular-level interactions between the object and the surface and usually corresponding to roughness. The coefficient of friction depends mostly on the materials interacting, though it can also vary with temperature, relative speed, and a variety of other factors. For example, at very high speeds, coefficients of friction are usually reduced.

Coefficients of friction cannot be calculated from fundamental physical equations and must be measured empirically for different surfaces. The following table contains coefficients of friction for certain materials under typical conditions. To test medical tubing commonly used in both home and hospital care (such as catheters) and surgical applications, tests were conducted at constant applied force to a number of different anatomical sites, including palms and posterior forearms, and mean values of coefficients of friction were calculated.

Material	Coefficient of Static Friction	Coefficient of Kinetic Friction
PTFE on PTFE	0.04	0.04
silicone medical tubing on skin (unlubricated)	0.95	0.6
silicone medical tubing on skin (lubricated)	0.7	0.4
zinc on cast iron	0.85	0.21
cast iron on cast iron	1.1	0.15

Table 1   Coefficients of Friction for Certain Materials

Rubber is a polymer (like silicone) that can have an exceedingly high coefficient of friction, as high as 4. One of the properties of rubber is that its coefficient of friction actually decreases with greater normal force. This can be expressed in *Thirion's Law*:

$$\frac{1}{m} = \frac{cF_N}{A} + b$$

Equation 1

in which F_N is the normal force, A is the area of contact between the object and the surface, and c and b are empirically measured constants that depend on the exact types of rubber used.

1. A nurse inserts a catheter into a patient. Assuming that Thirion's Law applies, what should the nurse do to minimize discomfort and shearing damage during the procedure?

A) The nurse should squeeze harder and avoid lubricant to increase the coefficient of friction between the catheter and the patient's tissue.
B) The nurse should squeeze harder and use lubricant to decrease the coefficient of friction between the catheter and the patient's tissue.
C) The nurse should squeeze softer and avoid lubricant to increase the force of friction between the catheter and the patient's tissue.
D) The nurse should squeeze softer and use lubricant to decrease the force of friction between the catheter and the patient's tissue.

2. When a copper pin slides against a copper surface, the force required to keep the pin sliding at constant speed is most likely:

A) zero.
B) greater at high speeds than at low speeds.
C) greater at low speeds than at high speeds.
D) equal at all speeds.

3. Which of the following can be validly concluded from the given data?

A) Lubrication has a more significant effect on the coefficient of static friction than on the coefficient of kinetic friction.
B) If the coefficient of static friction between two materials is greater than that between two other materials, the coefficient of kinetic friction will always follow the same pattern.
C) The coefficient of kinetic friction is always less than or equal to the coefficient of static friction.
D) None of the above can validly be concluded from the given data.

4. Which of the following best approximates the steepest angle at which a flat zinc surface can be tilted before a cast iron pot on it starts to slide?

A) 40°
B) 50°
C) 60°
D) 70°

5. If a rubber object is on a rubber surface, and if the object's mass is increased by adding several weights inside it, which of the following is true of the magnitude of the force required to initiate horizontal movement (F_x) and the weight of the object (w)?

A) The ratio of F_x to w increases.
B) The ratio of F_x to w remains constant.
C) The ratio of F_x to w decreases.
D) The difference between F_x and w remains constant.

6. Which of the following best explains the reason why polytetrafluoroethylene (PTFE), better known by the brand name *Teflon*™, is often used to coat "non-stick" cookware?

A) The toxicity of fumes given off by PTFE-coated pots is less than the toxicity of standard cooking oils.
B) Its extremely low coefficient of friction reduces the occurrence of food sticking to the pans.
C) Its extremely low coefficient of friction reduces the heat lost to friction when food slides on PTFE-coated surfaces.
D) PTFE was also used in the Manhattan Project to coat parts of pipes holding radioactive uranium compounds.

SOLUTIONS TO FREESTANDING QUESTIONS: KINEMATICS AND DYNAMICS

1. **C** To find the magnitude of the final velocity, the horizontal and vertical components of the velocity must be determined first. From the question stem, the horizontal component of the velocity of the raindrops is given, which is the same as the velocity, w, of the cloud. The vertical component of the velocity is determined by the correct freefall equation. The given variables are $v_{0y} = 0$, $y = y$, and $a_y = g$ (taking down to be the positive direction of motion), and you want v_y, so you're missing t. Use Big 5 #5 adjusted for freefall: $v_y^2 = v_{0y}^2 + 2a_y y = 2gy$. The magnitude of the final velocity, v, is then determined by applying the Pythagorean Theorem, $v = \sqrt{v_x^2 + v_y^2} = \sqrt{w^2 + 2gy}$. Therefore, the correct answer is choice C.

2. **D** For a statement to be physically possible, there must be at least one example of its happening. An object moving in a complete circle (or any other closed path) and returning to its starting point would have zero displacement and therefore zero average velocity, but it would have a positive total distance travelled and positive average speed. This eliminates choices A and C. An object undergoing uniform circular motion has constant speed but a centripetal acceleration, eliminating choice B. Choice D is impossible because the maximum value of average velocity is equal to average speed, which happens for travel in a straight line, so that the magnitude of displacement is equal to total distance.

3. **B** The time of the entire flight was given, but since you are looking for the maximum height (that is, the y-displacement traveled during each half of the flight), it is useful to remember the fact that, in the absence of air resistance, time up equals time down. This allows you to focus on either the first half of the trip (the way up) or the second half (the way down). Since you are not given the initial launch velocity, it is easier to look at the second half of the journey, where the initial vertical velocity is zero. Calling the positive y-direction downward, you have $a_y = g$ and $t = 4$ s. You want y and you're missing v_y, so use Big 5 #3: $y = v_{0y} t + (1/2)a_y t^2$; you have $y = 0 + (1/2)(10 \text{ m/s}^2)(4 \text{ s})^2 = 80$ m, or choice B. Alternatively, you would get the same answer by focusing on the way up and using $y = v_y t - (1/2)a_y t^2$. Note that the angle does not factor into the answer.

4. **B** For a round trip, the displacement must equal zero. On a velocity vs. time graph, displacement is represented by the area between the curve and the t-axis when the curve is positive, and is the negative of the area between the curve and the t-axis when the curve is negative. Choice B is the only answer where the area below the axis (negative displacement) is equal to the area above the axis (positive displacement), indicating that the total displacement is zero. Note that choice C would be correct on a position vs. time graph.

5. **A** Since all of the Items appear in exactly two of the answer choices, it doesn't matter which one you start analyzing. Item I is true: the two balls have the same values for the variables v_{0y}, a, and y, so according to Big 5 #5, $v_y^2 = v_{0y}^2 + 2a_y y$, v_y must be the same as well (choices B and D can be eliminated). Since Item II does not appear in either of the remaining choices, it must be false, and you can focus on Item III. Item III is false: since the balls have unequal

mass, the weight mg of the balls would be different (choice C can be eliminated, and choice A is correct). Note that Item II is in fact false. To see why it is false, consider Big 5 #2, $v_y = v_{0y} + a_y t$, which can be rearranged to become $t = (v - v_{0y})/a_y$. Since v_y and a_y are the same with respect to the two balls, only v_{0y} matters. The v_{0y} of the ball thrown downwards would be negative, as opposed to a positive value for the ball thrown upwards. This means that the time for the ball thrown upwards to reach the ground would be longer than that of the ball thrown downwards (this should make intuitive sense to you apart from the math).

6. **B** Process of Elimination is often the best approach to conceptual questions like this: be on the lookout for statements that violate basic physical principles! The vertical component of normal force on a banked curve is $mg \cos \theta$, compared to mg on a level road, so the banking actually reduces the maximum frictional force, $\mu_s F_N$, eliminating choice A. Gravity points down and has no horizontal component, eliminating choice C. Leaning to the side by standing on a bank certainly doesn't reduce an object's weight, so choice D is eliminated. Choice B is correct because the normal force on a banked curve adds a horizontal component that contributes to the horizontal centripetal force while the car turns on the curve.

7. **B** It is not immediately obvious whether static friction is up or down the plane. Therefore, it is useful to determine which direction the system would accelerate if there were no friction. Think of it this way: the weight of mass m [$mg = (10 \text{ kg})(10 \text{ m/s}^2) = 100$ N] is pulling the system one way, while the component of the weight of mass M down the plane [$Mg \sin \theta = (16 \text{ kg})(10 \text{ m/s}^2)(0.5) = 80$ N] is pulling the other way. Since the weight of mass m wins, static friction must be 20 N down the plane in order to maintain static equilibrium. The answer is choice B. Note that μ_s was not needed since the problem stated that the system was in static equilibrium. In the absence of that information, to determine whether the system would move or not, one would calculate the maximum static frictional force, $\mu_s F_N$, to see whether the hanging weight was enough to overcome this friction.

8. **C** This question requires using ratios and proportions, which is the best way to approach all questions involving Newton's Law of Gravitation:

$$\frac{g_{\text{Pluto}}}{g_{\text{Earth}}} = \frac{GM_{\text{Pluto}}/r_{\text{Pluto}}^2}{GM_{\text{Earth}}/r_{\text{Earth}}^2} \rightarrow g_{\text{Pluto}} = g_{\text{Earth}} \frac{M_{\text{Pluto}}/r_{\text{Pluto}}^2}{M_{\text{Earth}}/r_{\text{Earth}}^2} = 10 \frac{\text{m}}{\text{s}^2} \frac{M_{\text{Pluto}}}{M_{\text{Earth}}} \left(\frac{r_{\text{Earth}}}{r_{\text{Pluto}}} \right)^2 = 10 \frac{\text{m}}{\text{s}^2} \frac{1}{500} \left(\frac{15}{1} \right)^2$$

$$g_{\text{Pluto}} = 10 \frac{\text{m}}{\text{s}^2} \left(\frac{225}{500} \right) = 4.5 \frac{\text{m}}{\text{s}^2}$$

9. **B** Since Item I appears in exactly two of the answer choices, start by analyzing it; whether it is true or false, you can immediately eliminate half the answer choices. Item I is false: the centripetal force of the satellite is due to Earth's gravitational pull. Therefore, applying the Universal Law of Gravitation, $GMm/r^2 = mv^2/r$, where M is the mass of Earth and m is the mass of the satellite, the equation becomes: $v = \sqrt{GM/r}$. As expressed in this equation, the velocity of the satellite is independent of its mass (choices A and C can be eliminated). Note that both of the remaining answer choices include Item II; therefore, Item II must be true, and you can focus on Item III. Item III is false: the speed of the satellite is directly proportional to the square root of the mass of Earth, so a quadrupling of Earth's mass would be required to double the satellite's orbital speed (choice D can be eliminated, and choice B is correct). Note that Item II is in fact true: according to the equation above, the distance between Earth and the satellite has an inverse relationship with the speed of the satellite.

10. **B**   The balance point of the teeter totter can be determined either by balancing the torques on either side of the fulcrum, or by finding the location of the center of mass (and placing the fulcrum there). The latter method is a bit more straightforward (use Amanda's location as the reference point):

$$x_{CM} = \frac{m_1 x_1 + m_2 x_2 + m_3 x_3}{m_1 + m_2 + m_3} = \frac{0 + 10 \text{ kg } (1.5 \text{ m}) + 30 \text{ kg } (3 \text{ m})}{65 \text{ kg} + 10 \text{ kg} + 30 \text{ kg}} = \frac{105 \text{ kg-m}}{105 \text{ kg}} = 1 \text{ m}$$

Note that choice A is what you would get if you forgot to include the mass of the plank, and choice C is what you would get if you neglected the weight difference between the two children.

SOLUTIONS TO KINEMATICS AND DYNAMICS PRACTICE PASSAGE

1. **D**   First, consider what actually will cause discomfort and possible tissue damage: it's frictional force, not just the coefficient of friction (after all, you'd rather be rubbed softly by an eraser than very hard by a brick, which has a lower coefficient of friction than a rubber eraser). Thus, choices A and B are eliminated because they don't directly address the issue, and choice C is eliminated because increasing the frictional force is the opposite of the desired effect. The correct answer is choice D. Note that the values in the table show unambiguously that lubrication lowers the coefficient of friction and thus the force of friction for any given applied normal force. Note further that manipulating Thirion's Law yields the following

$$\mu F_N = \frac{A}{c}\left(1 - b\mu\right) = F_{\text{kinetic friction}}$$

Because μ decreases with increasing normal force, squeezing harder increases the frictional force (notice the minus sign before the second term in the parentheses). This isn't a surprising result, obviously, but the fact that Thirion's Law shows that the coefficient of friction decreases with increased normal force does complicate matters (choice B is true but doesn't answer the question asked).

2. **C**   The passage states that coefficients of friction are usually lower at very high speeds. Consequently, the force of kinetic friction is lower at very high speeds. Therefore, the force required to counter kinetic friction is lower at very high speeds. Choice A is a trap, because the net force on an object at constant speed is zero, but there will be a frictional force slowing the object down, so it needs an additional push to keep going. Choice B is backwards. Choice D would be true if the coefficient of friction were constant at all speeds, which is the usual approximation on the MCAT, but the passage indicates that the coefficient of friction should not be considered constant here.

3. **D** You need to be cautious about what you conclude from given data: conclusions from data are more restrictive than facts or tendencies you have memorized. Any big generalization from a small data set is always sketchy. Choice A is wrong because it doesn't even fit the data: the difference in the value of the coefficient of static friction for silicone on skin is greater than for kinetic friction, but the fractional change isn't. Moreover, these are just two data points for silicone and skin (and mean values at that, as the passage indicates), and thus cannot be generalized to all substances. Choice B is contradicted by the last two rows of the table: the coefficient of static friction between cast iron and cast iron is greater than that between zinc and cast iron, but the opposite is true for the coefficients of kinetic friction. Choice C may be tempting, and indeed it does fit the data, but you cannot conclude that it's always true (indeed, several materials used for braking have higher coefficients of kinetic friction than static friction at certain temperatures and normal forces). Choice D is correct.

4. **A** This is an inclined plane problem involving a flat tilted surface. From typical inclined plane analysis, the forces on the pot parallel to the plane are $mg \sin \theta$ down the plane and static friction up the plane. Right before the pot starts to slide, static friction is at its maximum and the two forces are equal, so $mg \sin \theta = \mu mg \cos \theta$, which yields that $\mu = \tan \theta$. From Table 1, the coefficient of static friction between zinc and cast iron is 0.85. Compare this to $\tan(45°)$, which is equal to 1; 0.85 is smaller, so the angle must be less than 45°; Thus, it must be $\tan(40°)$, since 40° is the only choice less than 45° available.

5. **C** First, decipher the wording of the question. The variable F_x refers to the amount of force required to initiate horizontal movement, which means the force required to overcome static friction. The force to overcome static friction is equal to the maximum force of static friction, μF_N, which in turn is equal to μw. The ratio that several of the answer choices talk about is $F_x{:}w$, which is $\mu w/w$, which is the same thing as $\mu/1$. In other words, all that this question is asking is what happens to the coefficient of friction as more weight is added to the rubber object. Now, refer to the passage: Equation 1 describes how the coefficient of friction changes for rubber when the normal force from the surface increases. In particular, the reciprocal of the coefficient of friction increases linearly with the normal force, so the coefficient of friction must decrease with normal force; more weight means less coefficient of friction. Therefore, the ratio goes down.

6. **B** Begin by referring to the passage. PTFE is mentioned in the table, and it has a coefficient of friction of 0.04, which is much lower than anything else in the table. The answer is likely to have to do with this low coefficient of friction. Choice A might be tempting because it suggests that PTFE is not very toxic, but lack of toxicity itself is not a major reason why PTFE is applied to cookware; any other non-toxic substance might equally be applied if that were its only useful property. Choice B addresses the low coefficient of friction and at least is physically possible, because low coefficients of friction enable sliding more easily than high coefficients of friction, and easy sliding means less sticking. Choice C is non-physical: low friction means less heat generated by friction, not less heat lost to friction. Choice D is off-topic; this may or may not have anything to do with cooking.

Chapter 34
Work, Energy, and Momentum

FREESTANDING QUESTIONS: WORK, ENERGY, AND MOMENTUM

1. A basketball player jumps straight up into the air to perform a slam dunk. Neglecting air resistance, which of the following statements correctly describes the motion on the way up?

   I. Total mechanical energy is conserved.
   II. The player's momentum is conserved.
   III. The work being done by gravity is negative.

   A) I only
   B) I and II
   C) I and III
   D) II and III

2. Boxes of the same mass are lifted into the air either on a frictionless ramp with Force $\mathbf{F}_A$ or with a pulley with Force $\mathbf{F}_B$. Both boxes are lifted to a height of 3 meters. Which method requires more work?

   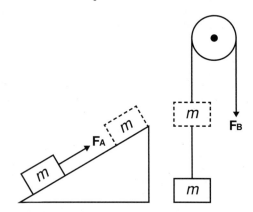

   A) Equal work is required for both methods.
   B) Greater work is required to lift m with the pulley.
   C) No work is required for either method.
   D) Greater work is required to push m up the ramp.

3. Which of the following represents the kinetic energy of an object after it has slid a distance d down a plane inclined at an angle ϕ to the horizontal, assuming a constant frictional force of F, if the object began at rest?

   A) $mgd \sin \phi - Fd$
   B) $mgd \cos \phi + Fd$
   C) $mgd \sin \phi + Fd$
   D) $mgd \cos \phi - Fd$

4. If the acceleration of an object is non-zero, then all of the following could be constant EXCEPT the object's:

   I. speed.
   II. linear momentum.
   III. kinetic energy.

   A) II only
   B) I and III only
   C) II and III only
   D) I, II, and III

5. An object is launched from the top of a 40 m high building with a speed of 10 m/s at an angle of 30° with the horizontal. With what speed does it hit the ground?

   A) 10 m/s
   B) 28 m/s
   C) 29 m/s
   D) 30 m/s

6. An object with mass m is to be pushed up a frictionless inclined plane with angle θ and height H. The figure below shows two possible forces for doing this.

   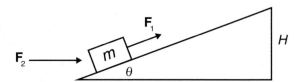

   Which of the following is true about the minimum work required by each force to push the object up the plane and their mechanical advantages?

   A) $W_1 < W_2$ and $MA_1 > MA_2$
   B) $W_1 < W_2$ and $MA_1 = MA_2$
   C) $W_1 = W_2$ and $MA_1 > MA_2$
   D) $W_1 = W_2$ and $MA_1 = MA_2$

7. The Incredible Kazmakarov Twin Brothers perform a circus act where Brother Alexey jumps from a height of 20 m onto a seesaw and launches Brother Boris 10 m into the air. Both brothers weigh 1000 N. Which of the following could contribute to why Boris doesn't get launched to a height of 20 m?

   I. Alexey lands on the seesaw vertically, but Boris launches off at a 45° angle.
   II. Alexey starts with 20 kJ of PE, while Boris starts with 0 kJ of PE.
   III. Not all KE is transferred from Alexey to Boris through the seesaw.

   A) II only
   B) II and III only
   C) I and III only
   D) I, II, and III

8. A car with of mass 250 kg and velocity +10 m/s crashes into a wall over a period of 15 milliseconds before coming to a complete stop. What is the impulse of the collision?

   A) −2500 N·s
   B) 2500 N·s
   C) −375 N·s
   D) 375 N·s

9. A man on a sled is sliding to the right on a frictionless surface with speed 5 m/s. Also on the sled are fifty uniform rocks (1 kg each). The man starts throwing rocks at a speed of 21 m/s to the right (relative to the ground) to slow him down. If the combined mass of the person and sled is 100 kg, how many rocks must the man throw to slow himself and the sled to 1 m/s?

   A) 29
   B) 30
   C) 36
   D) There are not enough rocks to slow the person + sled enough.

10. In which of the following real-world cases is total mechanical energy most nearly conserved?

    A) A sled sliding down an icy bobsled track
    B) A pitched baseball being hit by a bat
    C) A car with the driver slamming on its brakes to avoid a collision
    D) A land mine exploding

WORK, ENERGY, AND MOMENTUM PRACTICE PASSAGE

Jack is running up a hill, at an incline of approximately 30° to the horizontal, along a path that is 450 m long to the top of the hill, as shown in Figure 1. Dr. Jill, his cardiologist, is following close behind, concerned that he is over-exerting himself. Jack weighs 2000 N and Dr. Jill is half his size. Jack makes it halfway up the hill in ten minutes, but takes another twenty minutes to make it all the way to the top.

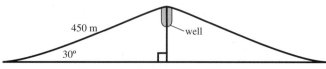

Figure 1   Jack and Dr. Jill's Hill

At the top of the hill is a well; Jack looks severely dehydrated, so Dr. Jill insists they try to fetch a pail of water (she has a pocket kit to test for bacteria). The water level in the well is 15 m below the top, but they cannot see the water. Dr. Jill decides to drop a penny down to check if there is water in the well. They hear a splash, then Dr. Jill lowers the two liter pail using a double pulley system (with two segments of rope attached to the bottom pulley) into the well and draws up a full bucket. After Dr. Jill confirms the drinkability of the water, Jack drinks his fill and then they start jogging back down the hill.

Unfortunately, Jack falls when they are almost at the bottom of the hill and have travelled 440 m from the summit; he slides down the hill for 10 m before coming to a stop at the base of the hill. Dr. Jill, fearing a major heart attack, races down after him. She smartly keeps her footing, and after confirming that Jack is bruised but generally okay, she lifts him onto her shoulders and carries him to his car.

1. Ignoring any frictional effects, how does the mechanical advantage of the hill (considered as an inclined plane) compare to the mechanical advantage of the double pulley system?

A) They are equal.
B) The mechanical advantage of the hill is half that of the double pulley system.
C) The mechanical advantage of the hill is double that of the double pulley system.
D) It is impossible to answer the question without knowing how far up the hill a person walked or how high a mass was lifted by the pulley system.

2. What was Jack's net power output during his entire journey up the hill?

A) 250 W
B) 500 W
C) 2500 W
D) 15 kW

3. How much time passes between when Dr. Jill dropped the penny and when they heard the splash?

A) 0.04 s
B) 0.08 s
C) 1.77 s
D) 3.46 s

4. How much work is done by Dr. Jill in first lowering the empty pail and then lifting the full pail of water out of the well? (Assume the density of water is 1 kg/liter and that the rope has negligible mass.)

A) 30 J
B) 150 J
C) 300 J
D) It is impossible to tell without knowing the mass of the empty pail.

5. Supposing that Jack was moving at 10 m/s when he fell, how much work was done by kinetic friction in stopping him?

A) -10^4 J
B) -2×10^4 J
C) -3×10^4 J
D) -10^5 J

6. Jack gets mad that Dr. Jill is following him around, and out of frustration he throws her portable smartphone ultrasound device (i.e., a non-uniform block of mass m) from the peak of the hill as hard as he can. Neglecting air resistance, which of the following statements are true?

  I. The center of mass of the device will follow a parabolic trajectory until the device strikes the ground.
  II. Assuming the device rotates, it will rotate about its geometric center.
  III. The total displacement of the device from the time Jack throws it to the time it lands depends upon the device's mass.

A) I only
B) I and II only
C) I and III only
D) II and III only

SOLUTIONS TO FREESTANDING QUESTIONS: WORK, ENERGY, AND MOMENTUM

1. **C** Since both Items II and III appear in exactly two of the answer choices, start by analyzing one of them. Whether they are true or false, you can immediately eliminate half the answer choices. Item II is false: gravity is exerting an impulse on the basketball player, causing the player's momentum to decrease over time on the way up (choices B and D can be eliminated). Note that both remaining answer choices include Item I, so it must be true and you can focus on Item III. Item III is true: the displacement points upward and the force of gravity downward, making the work being done by gravity negative (choice A can be eliminated, and choice C is correct). Note that Item I is in fact true: total mechanical energy is conserved because the only force acting on the player is gravity, which is a conservative force.

2. **A** In both the ramp and pulley scenarios, a force is required to lift the mass to a certain height to counteract the force of gravity (choice C is not correct). Because gravity is a conservative force, the change in gravitational potential energy depends only upon the change in a mass's height: $\Delta PE_{grav} = mg\Delta h$. Since there is no mention of a change in kinetic energy, assume that $\Delta KE = 0$, so all the work done on the system goes into increasing the gravitational potential energy. Since the changes in height are the same for both cases, $\Delta h = 3$ m, choice A is correct, and choices B and D are wrong. Note that the force required to push m up the ramp is less than the force required to lift it with the pulley by a factor of $\sin \theta$, but that the distance over which that force is applied is greater by the same factor, so the work equation $W = Fd$ yields the same result.

3. **A** This is a 2×2 question: two answers have sine as the trig function and two have cosine, and different pairs add and subtract the Fd term. The first term, involving mgd, appears to be a potential energy term, and the second term, involving Fd, appears to be the work done by friction. (If it is not clear that this is so, begin with the usual equation for conservation of energy with friction: $KE_i + PE_i + W_{by\,F} = KE_f + PE_f$. Next, the stem of the question states that the object began at rest, so $KE_i = 0$ and let $PE_f = 0$. This means that $KE_f = PE_i + W_{by\,F}$. Thus, the answer needs to be in the form of an "initial potential energy" term and a "work done by friction" term.) Logically, the friction term should be subtracted, because friction is taking energy away from the system and converting it into heat. (Mathematically, the work done by friction is negative, because it is in the opposite direction as the object is moving, so in $W = Fd \cos \theta$, $\cos \theta$ is negative.) Thus, eliminate choices B and C. For the second part of the 2×2, recall that $PE = mgh$, which is nearly what is in the answer choices. However, h, the vertical distance traveled, has been replaced with d, the inclined distance traveled. In this case, $h = d \sin \phi$, because h would be the side opposite ϕ in the right triangle in which d would be the hypotenuse.

4. **A** Item I appears in exactly two of the answer choices, so start by analyzing it. Whether it is true or false, you'll immediately eliminate half the answers. An object undergoing uniform circular motion is accelerating but maintains a constant speed, so Item I is false, eliminating choices B and D. Note that both remaining answer choices include Item II, so it must be true, and you can focus on Item III. Item III is false: reflecting again on Item I, when an object's speed is constant, its kinetic energy, the scalar $(1/2)mv^2$, must be constant as well (choice C can be eliminated, and choice A is correct). Note that Item II is in fact true: if the

acceleration is non-zero, then the velocity is changing. Since linear momentum is the product of mass and velocity, it cannot be constant if the velocity is non-constant.

5. **D** While it is possible to solve this using the kinematics equations, conservation of mechanical energy is easier. With kinematics, you would have to find the final horizontal and vertical velocities separately and then use the Pythagorean Theorem to calculate the magnitude of the total final velocity. Instead, use $KE_i + PE_i = KE_f + PE_f$. Using the ground as the reference and remembering that $KE = (1/2)mv^2$ and $PE = mgh$, you can see that $(1/2)(m)(10\text{ m/s})^2 + (m)(10\text{ m/s}^2)(40\text{ m}) = (1/2)(m)v_f^2 + 0$. Solving for v_f, you get 30 m/s. (Note that the launch angle did not factor into the equation.)

6. **C** As far as work goes, you could use the formula $W = Fd \cos \theta$. While this would be reasonable in finding the work done by $\mathbf{F}_1$, the work done by $\mathbf{F}_2$ would be much more complicated; you would have to split the force into components and figure out which one is equal and opposite to the component of gravity acting down the plane. An alternate way to find work is to remember that the work done by a non-conservative force equals the change in total energy of the system. Since you are looking for the minimum amount of work necessary to push the object up, neither force will be providing any additional kinetic energy, but they would be providing potential energy. Both forces would, in fact, provide mgH of potential energy even though the forces themselves would be different. Therefore, $W_1 = W_2$. This eliminates choices A and B. Mechanical advantage can be written as MA = (resistance force) / (effort force). The resistance force is the force that would be needed without the inclined plane. Since the object is to be lifted, this force is mg in both cases. The effort force would be F_1 or F_2. Since it would be more difficult to push the object up using $\mathbf{F}_2$ than $\mathbf{F}_1$, (because $\mathbf{F}_2$ has a component that is not in the direction of displacement), it must be true that $F_2 > F_1$ and $MA_1 > MA_2$.

7. **C** Since Item I appears in exactly two answer choices, start by analyzing it; whether it is true or false, you'll eliminate half the answers. Item I is true: if you assume that all KE from Alexey is transferred to Boris, you can say $KE_{0a} = KE_{0b}$, thus $\mathbf{v}_a = \mathbf{v}_b$ since their masses are the same. Since Alexey landed vertically, you know that $\mathbf{v}_{ay} = \mathbf{v}_a\sin(90°) = \mathbf{v}_a$. However, if Boris is launching off at a 45° angle, the vertical velocity $\mathbf{v}_{by} = \mathbf{v}_b\sin(45°) = 0.7\mathbf{v}_b$. Since the vertical velocity is reduced, Boris will not travel as high (choices A and B can be eliminated). Since both remaining answers include Item III, it must be true, and you can focus on Item II. Item II states a true fact: comparing their relative heights, you can assign Alexey to start with $PE = mgh = 100\text{ kg} \times 10\text{ m/s}^2 \times 20\text{ m} = 20\text{ kJ}$ and Boris to start with $PE = mgh = mg(0\text{ m}) = 0\text{ kJ}$ of PE. However, that is not an explanation for why energy is lost (evident by Boris's reduced height) because all of Alexey's $PE_{initial}$ is expected to be transferred to Boris. Thus, Item II is wrong (choice D can be eliminated, and choice C is correct). Note that Item III is in fact true: this scenario describes a transfer of energy, in which Alexey's PE transforms into KE, is transferred to Boris as KE, and finally transforms back to PE as he gains height. The simplest explanation for the reduction in PE (again, evident by Boris's reduced height) is that the energy was somehow lost.

8. **A** There are two main equations for impulse, and you must choose the correct one to use given the information in the question. Impulse is $\mathbf{J} = \mathbf{F}\Delta t = \Delta \mathbf{p}$. While the question states that $\Delta t = 15\text{ ms}$, there is no mention of the force, so you cannot use $\mathbf{J} = \mathbf{F}\Delta t$. Instead, use $\mathbf{J} = \Delta \mathbf{p}$, the change in momentum: $\Delta \mathbf{p} = \mathbf{p}_f - \mathbf{p}_i = m\mathbf{v}_f - m\mathbf{v}_i$. Initial velocity of the car is given directly in the question: $\mathbf{v}_i = 10\text{ m/s}$. The question also states that the car comes to a complete

stop: $\mathbf{v}_f = 0$ m/s. Because the final velocity is 0, the final momentum must also be 0, and $\Delta \mathbf{p} = - \mathbf{p}_i = - m\mathbf{v}_i = -(250 \text{ kg})(10 \text{ m/s}) = -2500$ kg·m/s or -2500 N·s. Choice A is correct.

9. **B**   This is a recoil problem, so the total momentum is conserved. Although the man throws the rocks one at a time, you can solve the problem as if he were throwing all the rocks at once. The original mass is 100 kg + (50)(1 kg) = 150 kg. The total mass on the sled after n rocks are thrown is $(150 - n)$ kg. Using $\mathbf{p}_i = \mathbf{p}_f$, you can see that $(150 \text{ kg})(5 \text{ m/s}) = [(150 - n) \text{ kg}]$ $(1 \text{ m/s}) + (n)(21 \text{ m/s})$. Therefore, $750 = (150 - n) + 21n$ or $600 = 20n$. Thus, $n = 30$.

10. **A**   Total mechanical energy is conserved in cases in which kinetic and potential energy transform into each other, without energy lost to nonconservative forces like friction and without other forms of energy entering the picture. The bobsled sliding down the icy track is an example of gravitational potential energy transforming into kinetic energy on a (nearly) frictionless surface. Choice B is wrong because a baseball hitting a bat is an inelastic collision (which deforms the baseball), conserving momentum but not kinetic energy. Choice C is wrong because brakes work by frictional forces, converting kinetic energy to thermal energy. Choice D is wrong because a land mine exploding is an example of non-mechanical chemical potential energy rapidly transforming into kinetic energy.

SOLUTIONS TO WORK, ENERGY, AND MOMENTUM PRACTICE PASSAGE

1. **A**   Mechanical advantage of a simple machine is defined as the ratio of the resistance force (the force required to lift the mass without a machine, in this case the weight) to the effort force put into the machine. In the case of an inclined plane, that is $\text{MA} = \dfrac{mg}{mg \sin \theta}$, which in this case yields MA = 1/0.5 = 2. In the case of the double pulley system, where two tension forces (provided by the person at the top of the well pulling on the rope) oppose the weight, and thus $F_T = mg/2$, that is $\text{MA} = \dfrac{mg}{F_T} = \dfrac{mg}{mg/2}$, which again yields MA = 2. Choice A is correct.

2. **A**   This is a straight calculation question. Recall the formula for power: $P = W / t$. To calculate the work done by Jack, you need to determine how high up the hill he went. Since you know the total time it took for him complete the trip to the top, you can use the full height of the hill, $h = L\sin \theta = (450 \text{ m})(0.5) = 225$ m, where L is the length of the hill (the hypotenuse). Now calculate the work done by Jack: $W_{\text{on system}} = \Delta PE = mg\Delta h = (2000 \text{ N})(225 \text{ m}) = 450{,}000$ J. Next, calculate how much time it took Jack to climb the hill. The passage states that it took Jack 10 minutes to climb halfway and another 20 minutes to climb the rest of the way, for a total of 30 minutes, or 30 min × 60 s/min = 1800 s. Thus, Jack's net power output is $P = W / t = 450{,}000/1800$ J/s = 500/2 W = 250 W, choice A. Choice B is incorrect

because it uses the wrong height of the hill. (It uses the length given in the passage as the height of the hill.) Choice C is incorrect because it mistakes Jack's weight for mass and multiplies by g again. Choice D is incorrect because it uses the time in minutes, not seconds, given in the passage; be careful when reading a passage to check the units.

3. **C** Calculate the total time for the "round trip" for the penny being dropped and then the sound being heard by Dr. Jill. Let t_1 be the time it takes for the penny to hit the water below. Note that this is only part of the trip. The penny is dropped under gravity, so its flight time can be calculated using the freefall equation:

$$y = v_{0y} t_1 + \frac{1}{2} a_y t_1^2$$
$$15 = 0 + \frac{1}{2} g t_1^2$$
$$15 = 5 t_1^2$$
$$t_1^2 = 3$$
$$t_1 = 1.7$$

Given that sound waves travel at 340 m/s as they travel back to Dr. Jill's ear, the total time would be just slightly more than 1.7 s (choice C). (The travel time of the sound would be $t^2 = y/v_{\text{sound}} = (15 \text{ m})/(340 \text{ m/s}) \approx 0.04 \text{ s.}$)

4. **C** First, note that the amount of positive work Dr. Jill does in lifting the mass of the empty pail out of the well is balanced exactly by the amount of negative work she did in lowering it in the first place. Thus, the mass of the empty pail is irrelevant to the question (eliminating choice D). The passage states that the pail has a volume of 2 liters, so given the density in the question stem, the mass of water Jill lifts is 2 kg. Thus, the work she does against gravity is given by $W_{\text{on system}} = \Delta PE = mg\Delta h = (2 \text{ kg})(10 \text{ m/s}^2)(15 \text{ m}) = 300 \text{ J}$ (choice C is correct). Choice A is the answer you get if you forget to multiply mass by g to get weight, and choice B makes the error of factoring in the halved tension force Dr. Jill must exert to lift the mass using the double pulley system while ignoring that she had to pull twice as much rope to do it (mechanical advantage doesn't change the work done, just the force used to accomplish it).

5. **B** The work done by kinetic friction is always negative, as are the answer choices, so that doesn't help. The work cannot be calculated using the product of force and distance without knowing the coefficient of friction, which is not provided. However, you do know the total change in mechanical energy between Jack's initial and final positions and speeds, and that must be equal to the work done by friction: $PE_i + KE_i + W_{\text{fric}} = PE_f + KE_f = 0 \text{ J}$ (presuming $h = 0$ at the bottom of the hill). Thus, the work done by friction is given by $W_{\text{fric}} = -(PE_i + KE_i) = -(mgh + mv^2/2) = -[(200 \text{ kg} \times 10 \text{ m/s}^2 \times 5 \text{ m}) + (200 \text{ kg} \times 100 \text{ m}^2/\text{s}^2/2)]$, noting that we've divided weight by g to get mass and that Jack's height when he fell was half his total distance from the bottom of the hill, because $\sin 30° = 1/2$. This yields $-2 \times 10^4 \text{ J}$, choice B.

6. **A**   Since both Items II and III appear in exactly two of the answer choices, start by analyzing one of them; whether they are true or false, you'll eliminate half the answers. Item II is false: the point is subtle, but the question stem mentions that the device is a *non-uniform* mass, implying that its center of mass is probably not the same as its geometric center. Objects in free rotation rotate about their centers of mass, not their geometric centers (choices B and D can be eliminated). Note that both remaining answer choices include Item I, so it must be true, and you can focus on Item III. Item III is false: the kinematics of ideal projectiles completely lack any mention of mass (choice D can be eliminated, and choice A is correct). Note that Item I is in fact true: ideal projectiles follow parabolic trajectories (or rather, their centers of mass do).

Chapter 35
Thermodynamics

FREESTANDING QUESTIONS: THERMODYNAMICS

1. To cool your coffee before you drink it, you drop an ice cube into your thermos (which prevents heat transfer in or out of the contents), close the lid tightly, and wait for the cube to melt. Which of the following best describes the situation during your waiting period thermodynamically?

A) The total energy of the system (coffee + ice cube) decreased and the entropy remained constant.
B) The total energy of the system (coffee + ice cube) and the entropy both remained constant.
C) The total energy of the system (coffee + ice cube) decreased and the entropy increased.
D) The total energy of the system (coffee + ice cube) remained constant and the entropy increased.

2. A mole of ideal gas undergoes an isochoric process. Which of the following quantities remains constant?

A) Q
B) ΔE
C) T/P
D) PV

3. Oxygen tanks used for breathing in space have a volume of 5000 cm^3 and are filled with pure oxygen at a maximum pressure of 25 kPa. The tanks are well insulated to prevent overpressurization from heating when exposed to sunlight in space. An astronaut is apportioning the oxygen in his tank, which is at maximum pressure, by connecting it to a tank of identical volume that was vented into space and now contains only vacuum. What is the work, W, performed by the oxygen in filling the second tank after the valve between the tanks is opened and what is the change in internal energy, ΔE, of the oxygen after it occupies both tanks?

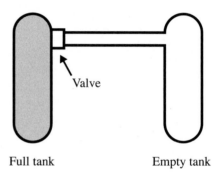

Valve

Full tank   Empty tank

A) $W = 0$ J and $\Delta E = 0$ J
B) $W = 93$ J and $\Delta E = -93$ J
C) $W = 0$ J and $\Delta E = 125$ J
D) $W = 125$ J and $\Delta E = -125$ J

4. Sections of jointed (non-welded) steel railroad track are installed with gaps, called expansion joints, between sections to allow thermal expansion of the track in hot weather. In desert areas during summer, intense sunlight can elevate the temperature of the track well above the local air temperature, causing distortion of the track if the expansion joint is too small. The coefficient of linear expansion, α, for steel is 1.0×10^{-5} /°C. If sections of track were 25 m long when they were laid down in an outdoor temperature of 4 C, and the width of the expansion joint at that time was 10 mm, what must the track temperature be when the expansion joint closes?

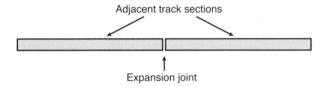

Adjacent track sections

Expansion joint

A) 24°C
B) 40°C
C) 44°C
D) 84°C

5. On a hot, sunny, windless day, you lie on a towel on the sandy beach. After a few minutes, you feel quite a bit warmer. What best explains this phenomenon?

A) Contact with the hot sand transferred heat into you by conduction and the Sun's rays transferred heat into you by radiation.
B) Contact with the hot sand transferred heat into you by conduction and the hot air transferred heat into you by convection.
C) Contact with the hot sand transferred heat into you by convection and the Sun's rays transferred heat into you by radiation.
D) All of your accumulated heat came from conduction by the surrounding air.

6. A perfectly insulated, frictionless piston starts at pressure of 2 kPa with a volume of 0.1 m³, then undergoes a reversible process that follows path 1-2-3-4 on the *P-V* diagram shown below, finally returning to the point where it started:

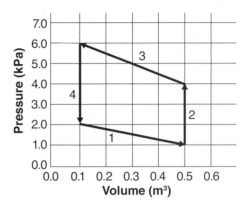

What is the net work done by the gas in the piston?

A) −1400 J
B) 600 J
C) 1400 J
D) 2000 J

THERMODYNAMICS PRACTICE PASSAGE

Thermoregulation is the process by which the body manages heat transfer to maintain a constant core temperature. Metabolic processes required for the body to function release heat as a by-product. The body then releases that heat through radiation, convection, conduction, and evaporation.

For typical values of skin ($T_{skin} \approx 34°C$) and external temperature ($0°C \leq T_{amb} \leq 40°C$), the rate of heat lost by the body via radiation, convection, and conduction can be approximated with very similar expressions:

$$\frac{\Delta Q_{rad}}{\Delta t} = k_{rad} A_{exp} \left(T_{skin} - T_{amb} \right)$$

Equation 1

$$\frac{\Delta Q_{conv}}{\Delta t} = k_{conv} A_{exp} \left(T_{skin} - T_{amb} \right)$$

Equation 2

$$\frac{\Delta Q_{cond}}{\Delta t} = \frac{k_{cond} A_{cov}}{L} \left(T_{skin} - T_{amb} \right)$$

Equation 3

in which A_{exp} is the surface area of the skin that is exposed, A is the surface area of the body that is covered (e.g., with clothing), and L is the thickness of the layer through which heat is conducting (in the case of exposed skin, this thickness is the layer of still air across which there is a temperature gradient between body temperature and ambient temperature, typically 8 mm or less). The total surface area of an adult human is around 2 m². The values and dependencies of k_{rad}, k_{conv}, and k_{cond} differ from each other and depend on a number of parameters external to the body. Note that in Equation 3, different clothing (or hair, or exposed skin) will have different values of k_{cond} and L, so the total rate of heat transfer due to conduction will be a sum of all the different contributions over the total surface area of the body.

The heat loss through radiation is mainly determined by how much clothing is worn, which determines A_{exp}. The value of k_{rad} is approximately constant over typical temperature ranges for skin and ambient temperature, $k_{rad} \approx 5.6 \frac{W}{m^2 K}$. Heat loss through convection depends on both A_{exp} and the speed of the fluid (typically air) flowing across the skin—the greater the speed, the larger the value of k_{conv}. For a slightly breezy day, $k_{rad} \approx 6.1 \frac{W}{m^2 K}$.

Numerous factors contribute to heat loss via conduction. The value of k_{cond} is determined by the material properties of the clothing being worn. For instance, wool has a higher thermal conductivity than cotton, but both are more thermally conductive than still air. Commensurate with experience, wearing thicker clothing will reduce heat loss through conduction. Conduction is also increased if the body is immersed in water instead of air. The body will lose heat via conduction into water about 25 times faster than it will into air at the same temperature.

The rates of radiation, convection, and conduction are mostly determined by factors external to the body, i.e., outside of a person's immediate control (unless there's a swimming pool or lake handy). When the body needs to increase the amount of heat it releases to the environment, it does this primarily through evaporation. When the body gets too warm, it starts to perspire. The sweat on the skin then absorbs heat from the body as it evaporates according to the equation

$$Q_{evap} = mL$$

Equation 4

in which m is the mass of the sweat that is evaporated and $L = 2.43 \times 10^6$ J/kg is the latent heat of vaporization of sweat at normal skin temperature. The body will perspire as long as the core body temperature is above 36.85°C. Even when perspiration isn't perceptible, the body will lose roughly 0.6 kg of moisture from the skin daily.

1. What best explains why people tend to cover most of their bodies with clothing in the winter?

A) To increase the heat created by the body
B) To increase heat loss through conduction
C) To reduce heat loss through conduction
D) To reduce heat loss through radiation and convection

2. If the ambient temperature rises above skin temperature, which of the following best describes what will happen to a person?

A) Since heat can't transfer from lower to higher temperature, the person's body temperature will rise, culminating in heat stroke.

B) The core temperature will initially increase, and in response, the body will increase the amount of heat it radiates to the environment. This will result in cooling of the core temperature to keep it within the acceptable range.

C) Perspiration will increase, as evaporation becomes the only mechanism of heat loss available for the body to maintain its core temperature in the acceptable range.

D) The body will reduce the heat it generates through metabolism to maintain a core temperature within the acceptable range.

3. How much heat will a person release through evaporation on a pleasant and relaxing day when they don't notice any perspiration?

A) 1460 kJ

B) 1460 kW

C) 4050 kJ

D) 4050 kW

4. Which of the following best explains why people who accidently fall into cold water are instructed to remain as still as possible as they wait for assistance?

A) Remaining still reduces the amount of heat generated in the body through metabolism.

B) Remaining still reduces the rate of heat loss via conduction.

C) Remaining still reduces the rate of heat loss via convection.

D) Remaining still reduces the rate of heat loss via radiation.

5. The basal metabolism of a person sitting at room temperature (25°C) with half of their body covered by clothing generates 85 W of heat. Expressed as a percentage of that value, approximately how much heat does that person lose through radiation?

A) 30%

B) 70%

C) 100%

D) 140%

SOLUTIONS TO FREESTANDING QUESTIONS: THERMODYNAMICS

1. **D** First, consider the energy of the system coffee + ice cube: the thermos prevents heat transfer, so $Q = 0$, and the liquid does no work on the environment, so $W = 0$. By the first law, $\Delta E = Q - W = 0$, so the energy of the system did not change. This eliminates choices A and C. The temperature of the coffee does decrease, but that's because some of the energy from the hot coffee went into melting the ice: the overall energy remains constant. Though it is possible to calculate changes in entropy, if you had the initial conditions (temperatures and masses of ice and water, the right constants), the MCAT is unlikely to ask you to do that. It is enough to know (for physics at least) that the entropy change of an irreversible process is always positive (the second law says this). Since the ice cube cannot be reformed once it has melted into the surrounding coffee, the entropy of the system must have increased.

2. **C** Under an isochoric process, volume remains constant, which means that the gas cannot have done any work: $W = P\Delta V = 0$. The first law therefore yields $\Delta E = Q$. Thus, if either of these quantities remained constant, they both would, which eliminates choices A and B. There is nothing keeping heat from entering or leaving the gas, which would mean at constant volume that the pressure would either increase or decrease, respectively. This means that PV need not be constant, eliminating choice D. Choice C is correct, as can be seen using the Ideal Gas Law: $PV = nRT \rightarrow V = nRT/P$, where n and R are constants. If V is constant (as it is for an isochoric process), so must be T/P.

3. **A** The expanding oxygen exerts no force into the volume of the empty tank because there is nothing for it to push against; it only exerts force against the walls of the empty tank. The walls of the tank do not move, therefore, the gas does no work and $W = 0$. The tanks are well insulated so no heat energy, Q, can enter or leave them. Therefore, the internal energy, E, does not change by the First Law of Thermodynamics: $\Delta E = Q - W = 0 - 0 = 0$.

4. **C** The change in length caused by thermal expansion is $\Delta L = \alpha L_0 \Delta T$. To close a 10 mm gap, each adjacent section of track must expand by that amount, since it will expand equally at both ends. The change in temperature for an expansion of 10 mm is $\Delta T = \Delta L/(\alpha L_0) = (0.01 \text{ m})/[(1.0 \times 10^{-5})(25 \text{ m})] = 40°C$. The track was laid down at a temperature of 4°C, so the temperature of the track must be 4°C + 40°C = 44°C for the expansion gap to close.

5. **A** This question tests your recall of the basic definitions of the heat transfer processes: conduction, convection, and radiation. The sand beneath you is essentially a large solid object at a higher temperature than your body, so by the Zeroth Law, heat will flow into you from the sand, via conduction. This eliminates choice C. The rays of the Sun transfer heat via radiation, which is absorbed by the part of your body facing the Sun. Thus, choice A is best. The question mentions that the air is still, so convection is not the primary mechanism of heat transfer, eliminating choice B.

6. **A** Take note of the directions of the processes! When the gas compresses, ΔV is negative, so the gas is having work done on it, according to $W = P\Delta V$. Work done by the gas along path 1 is the area beneath that part of the cycle, which is $W_1 = [(2000 \text{ Pa} + 1000 \text{ Pa})/2][0.5 \text{ m}^3 - 0.1 \text{ m}^3] = 600 \text{ J}$. No work is done by the gas along either section 2 or 4 because the volume

does not change. Work done by the gas along section 3 is the negative area beneath that part of the cycle, which is $W_3 = [(6000 \text{ Pa} + 4000 \text{ Pa})/2][0.1 \text{ m}^3 - 0.5 \text{ m}^3] = -2000 \text{ J}$. The net work by the gas is $W_{net} = W_1 + W_3 = -1400 \text{ J}$.

SOLUTIONS TO THERMODYNAMICS PRACTICE PASSAGE

1. **D** In the winter, people cover their bodies to stay warm, which means that they'd want to reduce heat loss, eliminating choice B. The passage states that heat is generated by the body through internal metabolic processes, which clothing would have little impact on, eliminating choice A. Covering the body would increase A_{cov} and decrease A_{exp}. Increasing A_{cov} would have an ambiguous effect on the heat loss through conduction, because you'd have to know the different thermal conductivities and thicknesses of the garments compared to exposed skin (moreover, the passage mentions that the thermal conductivity of still air is less than that of either wool or cotton, further muddying the waters). This eliminates choice C. On the other hand, heat loss through both radiation and convection unambiguously decrease with a decrease in A_{exp}, making choice D the correct answer.

2. **C** People usually don't succumb to heat stroke until the ambient temperature is well above the typical skin temperature of 34°C, making choice A unlikely. However, it is true that heat will not spontaneously transfer from T_{low} to T_{high} according to the Zeroth Law of Thermodynamics, so choice B is eliminated. Recall, though, that heat does not always result in a temperature change: a phase change such as evaporation also involves heat transfer. Indeed, evaporation is the only mechanism of heat loss mentioned in the passage that is not proportional to $T_{skin} - T_{amb}$ (a negative value in this case, meaning heat would be passing into the body via radiation, convection, or conduction, not out). Thus, choice C is consistent both with the passage and prior knowledge. Although it is possible for the body to reduce the heat it generates through metabolism to reduce the rate at which the core body temperature will rise, there is a base level of metabolic processes necessary to maintaining life, so it will not be able to maintain body temperature solely through this process, eliminating choice D. Choice C is the best answer.

3. **A** The question asks for "how much heat...." Because heat is a form of energy, its units should be in joules, not watts (energy/time), which eliminates choices B and D. Plugging in the values from the passage, 0.6 kg for the mass of fluid loss and $L = 2.43 \times 10^6$ J/kg, into equation 4 yields: $Q = mL = (0.6 \text{ kg})\left(2.43 \times 10^6 \dfrac{\text{J}}{\text{kg}}\right) = 1.46 \times 10^6 \text{ J} = 1460 \text{ kJ}$, choice A.

4. **C** The passage states that the body loses heat via conduction at a rate 25 times faster to water than to air. This means that the body would be in danger of losing too much heat and experiencing hypothermia; if anything, you'd want your body to generate more heat to counteract this effect, eliminating choice A. Although the rate of heat loss via conduction into water is higher than that for air, the passage does not indicate that this rate is dependent on motion, eliminating choice B. Likewise, heat loss via radiation is not dependent on motion, eliminating choice D. Moving increases the speed of the water flowing across the skin, which according to the

passage, would increase k_{conv}, and thus the rate of heat loss via convection. So minimizing motion would reduce the rate of heat loss via convection, making choice C correct.

5. **B** Plugging the numbers from the passage into equation 1 yields:

$$\frac{\Delta Q_{rad}}{\Delta t} = k_{rad}A_{exp}\left(T_{skin} - T_{amb}\right) = \left(5.6\ \frac{W}{m^2K}\right)\left(\frac{1}{2}\left(2\ m^2\right)\right)\left(34°C - 25°C\right) \approx 60\ W,\ \text{which is}$$

closest to choice B. Note that temperature differences on the Celsius and kelvin scales are

equivalent, so it's not necessary to convert the temperature to kelvins. Since the person is

generating 85 W of heat, the percent lost through radiation is 60 W/85 W $\approx$ 70%.

Chapter 36
Fluids and Elasticity
of Solids

FREESTANDING QUESTIONS: FLUIDS AND ELASTICITY OF SOLIDS

1. A person in physical therapy stands on a scale while submerged up to their waist in water. What physical quantity will the scale read?

A) The weight of the person
B) The mass of the person
C) The normal force of the scale on the person
D) The normal force of the scale on the person minus the buoyant force acting on the person

2. A column of liquid with specific gravity = 2.0 fills part of a pipe as shown in the figure below. The pipe is sealed at the top and open at the bottom, then is immersed in a reservoir of the same liquid. The liquid only partially fills the pipe and the vapor pressure is negligible in the volume above the column of liquid. When the atmospheric pressure is 100,000 Pa, what is the height, h, of the liquid in the pipe above the surface of the reservoir?

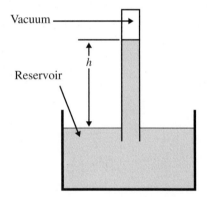

A) 0.5 m
B) 2.0 m
C) 5.0 m
D) 10.0 m

3. An object is placed in a tank of fluid. If the density of the object is three times the density of the fluid, what is the object's acceleration when it is half submerged in the fluid?

A) $3g/2$
B) $5g/2$
C) $3g/4$
D) $5g/6$

4. Your little brother pinches the tube of a hose to spray you with water more effectively. What effect does this have on the water as it moves past the constriction?

A) Its flow speed increases and pressure increases.
B) Its flow speed increases and pressure decreases.
C) Its flow speed decreases and pressure increases.
D) Its flow speed decreases and pressure decreases.

5. At a distance d below the surface of pure water, a balloon experiences buoyant force F_b. If the balloon is submerged to distance $4d$, what is the magnitude of the buoyant force that it experiences? (Assume no atmospheric pressure, that the density of water is constant, and that the volume of the balloon is inversely proportional to the pressure being exerted on it.)

A) $0.25F_b$
B) $0.5F_b$
C) F_b
D) $4F_b$

6. On Earth, an object of mass 67 kg and volume 2000 cm^3 sinks at a rate of approximately 6 m/s^2 in ideal, non-viscous mercury, which has a density of 13500 kg/m^3. On Mars, the acceleration due to gravity is roughly 3.7 m/s^2. At approximately what rate will the object sink through the same mercury on Mars?

A) 0.67 m/s^2
B) 2.3 m/s^2
C) 3.7 m/s^2
D) 6 m/s^2

7. A tank contains a layer of fluid with specific gravity 0.6 sitting on top of a layer of water. An object of uniform density is dropped into the tank and achieves equilibrium when one quarter of it is submerged in the fluid and three quarters is submerged in the water. What is the specific gravity of the object?

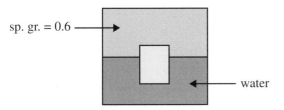

sp. gr. = 0.6

water

A) 0.4
B) 0.8
C) 0.85
D) 0.9

8. A system of pipes circulates water in a two-floor building. If water flows on the second floor through the pipe with a diameter of 3 cm with a speed of 4 m/s and the pressure 300 kPa, what would be the pressure on the first floor 2.5 m below if the pipe expands to the diameter of 6 cm?

A) 75 kPa
B) 300 kPa
C) 333 kPa
D) 485 kPa

9. Suppose a 10 m rope of Young's modulus $E = 10^8$ N/m^2 is run over a massless, frictionless pulley and is attached at either end to resting masses of 100 kg. If the pulley is steadily lifted so that the masses leave the ground, by how much will the rope stretch? Assume the cross-sectional area of the rope to be 5 cm^2.

A) 0.02 mm
B) 0.2 cm
C) 0.2 m
D) 20 m

10. Suppose a steel girder of the Oakland Bay bridge is 20 m long with a cross-sectional area of 0.1 m^2 when manufactured and installed at a temperature of 25°C, flush with adjacent pylons. The coefficient of thermal expansion of steel is $\alpha = 11 \times 10^{-6} \frac{1}{°C}$, and the Young's modulus is $E = 20 \times 10^{10} \frac{N}{m^2}$. If the temperature increases to 30°C, how much force does the girder exert on an adjacent pylon (neglect expansion of the area)?

A) 10^2 N
B) 2×10^4 N
C) 5×10^5 N
D) 10^6 N

FLUIDS AND ELASTICITY OF SOLIDS PRACTICE PASSAGE

When a solid object is subjected to a force tangential to one of its faces while the opposite face is held in a fixed position, it is said to experience a *shear stress*. This stress is equal to F/A, where F is the applied force and A is the cross-sectional area. The resulting deformation is characterized by *shear strain*, which is equal to $\Delta x/L$, where Δx is the distance the sheared face moves and L is the original length of the solid.

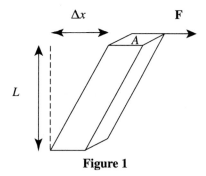

Figure 1

For small forces, the ratio of shear stress to shear strain is a constant, known as the *shear modulus*, which depends on the material. This relationship is known as *Hooke's Law*. Loosely speaking, the more the bend, the more effort required. Hooke's Law breaks down for large forces.

Fluids, by contrast, do not support a shearing stress. However, fluids do offer some resistance to shearing motion due to their *viscosity*. For liquids, viscosity is the result of frictional forces between adjacent layers of fluid as they slide past each other. Figure 2 below shows two plates of glass separated by a layer of homogeneous fluid. The bottom plate is held in place while the top plate moves to the right with speed, v, due to an applied force, **F**. If we divide the fluid into several layers, each layer has a different speed, decreasing from top to bottom.

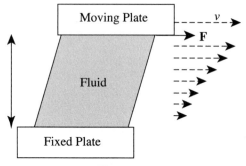

Figure 2

The *coefficient of viscosity*, η, of the liquid is defined as the ratio of the shearing stress to the rate of change of the shear strain. Since strain = $\Delta x/L$, the rate of change of strain = $(\Delta x/L)/\Delta t = v/L$. Therefore,

$$\eta = \frac{F/A}{v/L} = \frac{FL}{Av}$$

Equation 1

The viscosity of liquids decreases exponentially with temperature. In contrast, the viscosity of gases increases with temperature and is independent of density unless the density is very low. *Amorphous solids*, such as glass, will flow at large stresses and therefore have large viscosity coefficients.

An experiment is designed to measure the coefficient of viscosity of a liquid. A metal plate of area 0.20 m² is connected to a 10 g block by a string that passes over a massless and frictionless pulley. A lubricant with a thickness of 0.3 mm is placed between the plate and surface. When the block is released, the system moves with a constant speed of 0.10 m/s.

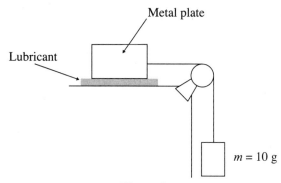

Figure 3

1. For a solid experiencing a small shear force, a graph of strain vs. stress is drawn with strain on the vertical axis. What does the slope of the graph represent?

A) The shear modulus
B) The reciprocal of the shear modulus
C) The product of stress times strain
D) The coefficient of viscosity

2. What is the coefficient of viscosity of the lubricant in Figure 3?

A) 1.5×10^{-4} Pa·s
B) 1.5×10^{-3} Pa·s
C) 1.5 Pa·s
D) Cannot be determined without knowing the mass of the plate

3. One possible explanation of why the viscosity of gases increases with temperature is that, at higher temperatures, the individual molecules:

A) spread out and therefore interact with each other less often.
B) move closer together and therefore interact with each other more often.
C) have greater kinetic energy and therefore have a greater effect on each other's motion.
D) have greater kinetic energy and therefore have a smaller effect on each other's motion.

4. Bernoulli's Equation would not apply to the fluid in Figure 2 because:

   I.   the flow is turbulent.
   II. the liquid is compressible.
   III. some kinetic energy is converted to heat.

A) I only
B) II only
C) III only
D) II and III

5. If the solid in Figure 1 were replaced by one made of the same material but with twice the length and twice the cross-sectional area, what would need to change in order to keep the strain the same?

A) The applied force would need to double.
B) The distance the top face moves would need to stay the same.
C) The shear modulus would need to be cut in half.
D) The stress would need to double.

6. If the fluid in Figure 2 were water and the plates were metal, which of the following changes to the experiment would decrease its viscosity?

A) Increasing the area of the plates
B) Decreasing the thickness of the fluid
C) Increasing the speed of the top plate
D) Placing equal and opposite charges on the plates

SOLUTIONS TO FREESTANDING QUESTIONS: FLUIDS AND ELASTICITY OF SOLIDS

1. **C**   Scales always read the normal force (choices A, B, and D can be eliminated). Choice D is a trap choice: in this particular case, the normal force will be equal to the weight of the individual minus the buoyant force of the submerged portion of the person.

2. **C**   At equilibrium, Pascal's Law states that at the level of the surface of the liquid in the reservoir, the gauge pressure of the column of liquid in the pipe is equal to the atmospheric pressure. Therefore, at the level of the reservoir surface, $P_{gauge} = \rho_f g D = \rho_f g h = P_{atm} = 100,000 \text{ N/m}^2$, where ρ_f is the density of the liquid. A liquid with a specific gravity of 2.0 has a density twice that of water, or 2000 kg/m^3. So $h = P_{atm} / \rho_f g = (100,000 \text{ N/m}^2) / [(2000 \text{ kg/m}^3)(10 \text{ m/s}^2)] = 5$ m.

3. **D**   The object is denser than the fluid and hence will start to sink. You can eliminate choices A and B because the acceleration of the object cannot be greater than g: a buoyant force will be acting in the direction opposite that of gravity. When the object is half submerged in the fluid, its net force equation can be written as $F_{net} = m_o a = m_o g - \rho_f V_{sub} g$, where $V_{sub} = V_o / 2$. Substituting the product of density and volume for the mass of the object gives $F_{net} = \rho_o V_o a = \rho_o V_o g - \rho_f (V_o / 2)g$. Canceling out the volumes and substituting in $\rho_o = 3\rho_f$ yields the following simplified equation: $3\rho_f a = 3\rho_f g - \rho_f g / 2$, so $3a = 3g - g / 2 = 5g / 2$, or $a = 5g / 6$.

4. **B**   The first portion of this 2 × 2 question tackles the velocity of the water. Assuming that the flow rate of water is the same, $f = Av$ tells you that, as the hose is blocked and area decreases, the velocity will increase. That eliminates choices C and D. According to the Bernoulli effect, an increase in flow speed corresponds to a decrease in pressure (so long as height doesn't change), eliminating choice A.

5. **A**   The gauge pressure is directly proportional to the depth of submersion ($P_{gauge} = \rho_{fluid} g d$); therefore, if the depth increases four times, then the pressure increases four times as well. Since pressure and volume are inversely related ($P \propto 1/V$), a fourfold increase in pressure experienced by the balloon means the volume of the balloon decreases four times. Archimedes' principle ($F_b = \rho_{fluid} V_{sub} g$) states that if the volume of the balloon decreases four times, then the buoyant force decreases four times as well. Therefore, the answer is $F_b / 4 = 0.25 F_b$.

6. **B**   Solve first for the acceleration of the sinking object. The forces acting on it are buoyancy and gravity. With the sinking direction defined as positive, $F_{net} = ma$ becomes $w - F_B = ma$. Specifying weight and buoyant force, $mg - \rho_f V_{sub} g = ma$, and dividing by mass, $a = g - \dfrac{\rho_f V_{sub} g}{m}$. At this point, you could plug in the mass of the object, its volume, the density of the mercury, and the acceleration due to gravity on Mars, doing a whole variety of unit conversions and a bunch of math, and the answer would come out. However,

this doesn't take advantage of the fact that the question stem gives what the acceleration rate is on Earth and asks what it is on Mars, where the only difference is the value of g. Factor g out of the right side of the equation to get $a = (1 - \dfrac{\rho_f V_{sub}}{m})g$. Despite the complicated proportionality constant, it appears that a is just directly proportional to g. If the acceleration due to gravity on Mars is 3.7 m/s^2 instead of 9.8 m/s^2, it is a bit more than one-third of its value on Earth, so the acceleration of the object through the fluid should be a bit more than one-third its value on Earth. That's 2.3 m/s^2.

7. **D**   Conceptually, the object's specific gravity should be somewhere between the specific gravities of the fluids. This eliminates choice A. It also follows that, since more of the object is submerged in water, its specific gravity should be closer to 1.0 than 0.6. This eliminates choice B. Since the object is in equilibrium, the upward buoyant force should equal the object's weight. The buoyant force has two contributions:

$F_{buoyant} = \rho_{fluid} V_{sub,fluid}\, g + \rho_{water} V_{sub,water}\, g = (0.6\rho_{water})(0.25 V_{object})g + (\rho_{water})(0.75 V_{object})g = (0.9)(\rho_{water} V_{object}\, g)$. The weight of the object is $mg = \rho_{object} V_{object}\, g$. Setting these expressions equal, you see that $\rho_{object} = 0.9 \rho_{water}$.

8. **C**   This question uses the continuity and Bernoulli equations. Ideal fluids have constant flow rate through the pipe given by $A_1 v_1 = A_2 v_2$, meaning that v is inversely proportional to A. As the diameter of the pipe doubles, the area quadruples, and hence the speed of water on the bottom floor is a quarter of the speed on the second floor: $v_1 = 1$ m/s and $v_2 = 4$ m/s. Bernoulli's Equation provides the pressure:

$$P_1 + \rho g h_1 + 1/2\, \rho v_1^2 = P_2 + 1/2\, \rho v_2^2 + \rho g h_2 \rightarrow P_1 = P_2 + 1/2\, \rho\, (v_2^2 - v_1^2) + \rho g(h_2 - h_1)$$

Substituting in values yields $P_1 = 3 \times 10^5$ Pa + 1/2 (1000 kg/m^3)[(4 m/s)^2 − (1 m/s)^2] + (1000 kg/m^3)(10 m/s^2)(2.5 m) = (300,000 + 7500 + 25000) Pa = 332,500 Pa ≈ 333 kPa.

9. **C**   First, note that supporting a 100 kg mass requires a tension of $F_T = mg = (100\text{ kg})(10\text{ m/s}^2) = 1000$ N. Don't be fooled by the presence of two masses: a force diagram for the place where the rope is attached to either mass will show a balance between the rope's tension force and the weight of one mass. With the force determined, the Young's modulus formula of stress / strain yields:

$$E = 10^8\, \tfrac{N}{m^2} = \frac{F_T / A}{\Delta L / L} = \frac{10^3\, N / 5 \cdot 10^{-4} m^2}{\Delta L / 10\ m} = \frac{2 \cdot 10^7\, \tfrac{N}{m}}{\Delta L} \rightarrow \Delta L = \frac{2 \cdot 10^7\, \tfrac{N}{m}}{10^8\, \tfrac{N}{m^2}} = 0.2\ m.$$

Miscalculations are likely the result of forgetting to convert units correctly, such as 5 cm^2 to 5×10^{-4} m^2.

10. **D** Recall the linear thermal expansion equation (or figure it out using unit analysis):

$$\Delta L = \alpha L \Delta T = \left(11 \times 10^{-6}\, \tfrac{1}{°C}\right)\left(20\text{ m}\right)\left(5\ °C\right) = 1.1 \times 10^{-3}\text{ m},\text{ or about 1 mm. This amount of}$$

thermal expansion will result in a force exerted on the adjacent pylon given by the Young's

modulus equation: $E = \dfrac{F/A}{\Delta L/L} \rightarrow 20 \times 10^{10} = \dfrac{F/10^{-1}}{10^{-3}/20} = 2 \times 10^{5} F \rightarrow F = 10^{6}\text{ N}.$

SOLUTIONS TO FLUIDS AND ELASTICITY OF SOLIDS PRACTICE PASSAGE

1. **B** The slope of any line is given by "rise-over-run"; in other words, the quantity represented by the vertical axis divided by the quantity represented by the horizontal axis. Since strain is on the vertical axis, the slope = strain/stress. In the passage, the shear modulus is defined as the ratio of stress to strain. Therefore, the slope represents the reciprocal of the shear modulus.

2. **B** Equation 1 states that the viscosity coefficient = FL/Av. Since the system moves with constant speed (i.e., acceleration is zero), the tension in the string must be equal to the weight of the hanging mass: $(0.010\text{ kg})(10\text{ m/s}^2) = 0.1$ N. This force therefore pulls the plate to the right. Using Equation 1, you have that $\eta = [(0.1\text{ N})(3 \times 10^{-4}\text{ m})] / [(0.2\text{ m}^2)(0.1\text{ m/s})] = 1.5 \times 10^{-3}\,\text{Pa} \cdot \text{s}$. (Note that the mass of the metal plate does not directly matter in this calculation.)

3. **C** You can answer this question by eliminating the wrong choices. Choice B is false because the density of a gas decreases with an increase in temperature. However, the passage states that the viscosity of gases is, in most cases, independent of density, so choice A can also be eliminated. The passage also states that viscosity arises from the forces between molecules, so choice D can be eliminated. Greater kinetic energy would increase interaction and therefore increase viscosity.

4. **C** Since Items II and III appear in exactly half the answer choices, start by analyzing one of them; whether they are true or false, you'll be able to eliminate half the answers. Item II is false: under normal circumstances, liquids are approximately incompressible; that is, the density is constant (choices B and D can be eliminated). Note that you only have to evaluate one of the remaining Items to get to the correct answer. Item I is false: the fluid is non-turbulent (choice A can be eliminated, and choice C is correct). For completeness, Item III is in fact true: Bernoulli's Equation is conservation of energy (density) for fluids. It applies to *ideal* fluids: incompressible, non-turbulent, non-viscous fluids with steady flow. The fluid in the passage has viscosity, which is related to friction. Since friction dissipates energy as heat, Item III is correct.

5. **A**   The question states that the strain must stay the same. Since strain = $\Delta x/L$, and L doubles, Δx must also double. This eliminates choice B. The question states that the new solid is made of the same material. Since the shear modulus depends only on the material, it must remain the same, eliminating choice C. In addition, since strain/stress must remain constant, a constant strain will require a constant stress. This eliminates choice D. The correct answer is choice A. Since stress = F/A, doubling A requires F to double if the stress is to remain the same.

6. **D**   You can eliminate choices A, B, and C without fully understanding why choice D is the correct answer. While Equation 1 seems to imply that choices A, B, and C are correct, remember that this equation is only used to measure the value of the viscosity coefficient. The coefficient itself is determined by the fluid. The only fluid property mentioned in the passage that affects viscosity is temperature. As to why choice D is correct: placing opposite charges on the plates creates a voltage across them. Since water is a good conductor, current will flow through it from one plate to the other. All conductors have resistance. Therefore, power will be dissipated as heat. This heat will increase the temperature of the water, which in turn will decrease its viscosity.

Chapter 37
Electrostatics, Electricity, and Magnetism

FREESTANDING QUESTIONS: ELECTROSTATICS, ELECTRICITY, AND MAGNETISM

1. Two negative charges are separated by a fixed distance of 4 cm, and the electric force between them is 1.6×10^{-9} N. If the distance between the two particles is halved, then which of the following represents the resulting electrical potential energy of the system?

A) 1.3×10^{-10} J
B) 8.0×10^{-10} J
C) 1.3×10^{-8} J
D) 8.0×10^{-8} J

2. Two isolated charges, one 2 nC and the other −3 nC, are separated by a distance of 2 m. Which of the following could be the magnitude of the electric field at a point an equal distance from the charges? (Note: $k = 8.99 \times 10^9$ Nm²/C².)

   I.   30 N/C
   II. 45 N/C
   III. 60 N/C

A) II only
B) III only
C) I and II only
D) II and III only

3. A muon is particle with the same charge as an electron but with greater mass. If the kinetic energy of an electron orbiting a stationary proton with radius r is K_1 and the kinetic energy of a muon orbiting a stationary proton with the same radius is K_2, which of the following is true?

A) $K_1 < K_2$
B) $K_1 = K_2$
C) $K_1 > K_2$
D) The relationship between K_1 and K_2 cannot be determined without knowing the mass of the muon.

4. If the resistance of the 3 Ω resistor in the circuit below is quadrupled, how will the total current in the circuit be affected?

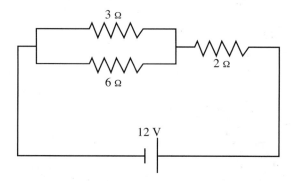

A) The total current through the circuit will decrease by a factor of $\frac{2}{3}$.
B) The total current through the circuit will decrease by a factor of $\frac{1}{4}$.
C) The total current through the circuit will increase by a factor of $\frac{2}{3}$.
D) The total current through the circuit will remain unchanged.

5. An electron travels between two uniformly charged capacitor plates separated by a distance of 3 cm, aligned so that the top plate is positively charged. If the voltage difference between the two plates is equal to 12 V, then the electric force that the electron experiences will be equal to which of the following?

A) 6.4×10^{-17} N upward
B) 4.0×10^{-2} N downward
C) 6.4×10^{-17} N downward
D) 4.0×10^{-2} N upward

6. Capacitor C_1 has a capacitance of 5 F and holds an initial charge $Q_{1,o} = 40$ C. Capacitor C_2 has a capacitance of 15 F and holds an initial charge $Q_{2,o} = 60$ C. The two capacitors are in a circuit with an open switch S between them, as shown in the figure below. When the switch closes, the charges on the capacitors will redistribute. What is the quantity of charge, $Q_{1,f}$ and $Q_{2,f}$, on each capacitor a long time after the switch closes?

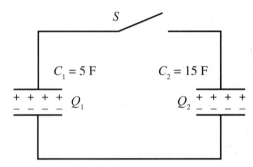

A) $Q_{1,f} = 25$ C, $Q_{2,f} = 75$ C
B) $Q_{1,f} = 75$ C, $Q_{2,f} = 25$ C
C) $Q_{1,f} = 50$ C, $Q_{2,f} = 50$ C
D) $Q_{1,f} = 40$ C, $Q_{2,f} = 60$ C

7. Four resistors with equal resistance are arranged in parallel and connected to a battery that provides a constant voltage. How do the total power dissipated over the resistors and the total current change if the resistance of each resistor is halved?

A) Power is doubled and current is halved.
B) Power is doubled and current is doubled.
C) Power is halved and current is halved.
D) Power is halved and current is doubled.

8. For the circuit shown, each resistor has the same resistance, R. Switch S_1 has been closed and switch S_2 has been open for a long time, and the circuit is in a condition of steady state with the battery supplying a constant power output, P_1. In steady state, no current flows into the capacitor. At a later time, S_2 is also closed (while keeping S_1 closed), and the battery's power output changes. Compared to P_1, what is P_2, the battery's power output when the circuit has reached a new steady state?

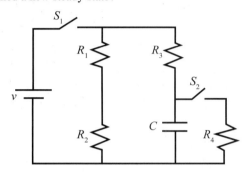

A) $P_2 = P_1$
B) $P_2 = 2P_1$
C) $P_2 = P_1/2$
D) $P_2 = 4P_1/3$

9. Consider the following circuit:

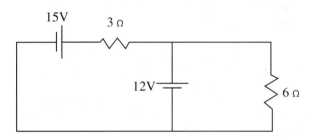

If the 15 V source were replaced with an 18 V source, which of the following is NOT true?

A) The current across the now 18 V source would increase.
B) The current across the 3 Ω resistor would increase.
C) The current across the 12 V source would decrease.
D) The current across the 6 Ω resistor would increase.

10. A 10-volt battery charges a capacitor, storing 20 μJ on it. What voltage battery would be required to double the energy stored on the same capacitor?

A) 14 V
B) 16 V
C) 20 V
D) 40 V

ELECTROSTATICS, ELECTRICITY, AND MAGNETISM PRACTICE PASSAGE

A cloud chamber is a device for studying subatomic particles. It is called a cloud chamber because it is filled with a pressurized vapor. When a charged particle enters the vapor, it ionizes the atoms that it passes by. These ions cause the vapor to condense into droplets, leaving a track behind the charged particle. Photographs of these tracks are taken and used to study the particles. Heavier particles, like alpha particles and protons, interact more strongly with the vapor, causing more droplets to form. This results in alpha particles and protons leaving thicker tracks than electrons. However, the stronger interaction causes the heavier particles to lose energy and come to a stop more quickly. Also, the greater the charge of a particle the more strongly it will interact with the vapor, causing more atoms to ionize.

Placing the cloud chamber in a constant magnetic field causes the charged particles to curve in a circular path of radius

$$r = \frac{mv}{qB}$$

where m is the mass of the particle, v is its speed, q is its charge, and B is the strength of the magnetic field. Positive and negative charges will curve in opposite directions. To make it possible to determine the direction of the particles' motion from the photograph, a thin lead plate is placed in the chamber. When the particles pass through the plate they slow down, causing their radii of curvature to decrease on the opposite side of the lead plate.

A cloud chamber with a magnetic field and lead plate was used to discover the positron, the electron's antiparticle. Antiparticles have the same mass as their counterparts but opposite charge. Figure 1 is a diagram of what a photograph from such an experiment might look like. In this picture, the magnetic field points into the page.

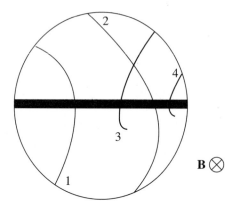

Figure 1   Photograph from a cloud chamber experiment

1. Which of the tracks in Figure 1 was most likely left by a positron?

   A) 1
   B) 2
   C) 3
   D) 4

2. If an electron and a proton have the same kinetic energy, then the proton will:

   A) curve in a smaller circle and have a longer track length.
   B) curve in a larger circle and have a shorter track length.
   C) curve in a smaller circle and have a shorter track length.
   D) curve in a larger circle and have a longer track length.

3. Suppose the magnetic field was turned off and was replaced with an electric field pointing from left to right. Which track would curve in the opposite direction from that in which it curved with the magnetic field?

   A) None of them
   B) 1 only
   C) 2, 3, and 4 only
   D) All of them

4. Suppose an electric field, of strength E, pointing from left to right was added to the experiment in addition to the magnetic field pointing into the page. If a negatively charged particle were observed to move in a straight line it would:

   A) be moving upward with speed E/B.
   B) be moving upward with speed B/E.
   C) be moving downward with speed E/B.
   D) be moving downward with speed B/E.

5. If q is the charge of the particle, d is the distance traveled, and m is the mass of the particle, which formula would most accurately describe the kinetic energy loss of a charged particle as it passes through the vapor?

A) $\Delta KE \propto q^2 d$

B) $\Delta KE \propto \dfrac{q^2}{d}$

C) $\Delta KE \propto \dfrac{q^2 d}{m}$

D) $\Delta KE \propto \dfrac{md}{q^2}$

6. Compared to a proton with the same momentum, an alpha particle will leave:

   I.   a track with a larger radius of curvature.
   II. a wider track.
   III. a shorter track.

A) I only
B) III only
C) II and III
D) I, II, and III

SOLUTIONS TO FREESTANDING QUESTIONS: ELECTROSTATICS, ELECTRICITY, AND MAGNETISM

1. **A** This question gives you the magnitude of the electric force, so write down the formula for electric force: $F = \dfrac{kQq}{r^2} = 1.6 \times 10^{-9}$ N. In this case, you need information about the electric potential energy of the system, so write down the relevant formula: $PE_{electric} = \dfrac{kQq}{r}$. Note that if you know the force between the two particles, you only need to multiply the force by r in order to find the potential energy of the system. Here, $r = 4$ cm, or 4×10^{-2} m. Therefore, the potential energy of the system is $\left(1.6 \times 10^{-9} \text{ N}\right)\left(4 \times 10^{-2} \text{ m}\right) = 6.4 \times 10^{-11}$ J. The magnitude of the potential energy of the system is proportional to $\dfrac{1}{r}$, so if the distance between the two particles is halved, the potential energy of the system will double. Thus, the new potential energy of the system will be $2\left(6.4 \times 10^{-11}\right) \approx 1.3 \times 10^{-10}$ J.

2. **C** First, consider the situation. The greatest possible electric field strength an equal distance from the two charges occurs at the position at which the field vectors point in exactly the same direction (and therefore the magnitudes just add, whereas elsewhere some components will add and some will subtract from each other). This means that the maximum field strength at a point equidistant from the two charges is exactly halfway between the two charges, on a straight line from charge to charge. At this point, the field vector from the positive charge and the one toward the negative charge both point in exactly the same direction. Next, calculate what that maximum field strength is $E = k\dfrac{q}{r^2}$ for each charge, so the total electric field is given by $E_{tot} = (9 \times 10^9)\dfrac{2 \times 10^{-9}}{1} + (9 \times 10^9)\dfrac{3 \times 10^{-9}}{1} = 45$ N/C. Eliminate choices B and D, because 60 N/C is impossible: it is greater than the maximum. Finally, consider the wording of the question: it just says "an equal distance from the charges," not "halfway between the charges." Anything less than 45 N/C is also possible if the point under consideration is farther away (eliminate choice A also).

3. **B** For a particle orbiting a proton in a circular path, the centripetal force is provided by the electrostatic force of attraction. Since the magnitude of the charges of the proton, electron and the muon is e, you can say that $ke^2/r^2 = mv^2/r$, where m is the mass of the orbiting particle. Canceling a factor of r and multiplying each side of the equation by $1/2$, you can see that $(1/2)ke^2/r = (1/2)mv^2$. Since the right side of this equation is kinetic energy, and the left side of the equation is the same for both the electron and the muon in orbit, the answer must be choice B.

4. **A** This question asks about the total current in the circuit, so use Ohm's Law: $I = \dfrac{V}{R}$. Since there is an inverse relationship between current and resistance, increasing the resistance will decrease the current. This eliminates choices C and D. The total resistance determines the current.

To calculate total resistance, note that the $2\ \Omega$ resistor is in series with the parallel configuration of the $3\ \Omega$ and $6\ \Omega$ resistors. Therefore, $R_{eq} = 2\,\Omega + \dfrac{(6\,\Omega)(3\,\Omega)}{6\,\Omega + 3\,\Omega} = (2\,\Omega + 2\,\Omega) = 4\,\Omega$.

Thus, the total current is equal to $\dfrac{12\ \text{V}}{4\ \Omega} = 3$ A. However, if the $3\ \Omega$ resistor is exchanged for a $12\ \Omega$ resistor, then $R'_{eq} = 2\,\Omega + \dfrac{(6\,\Omega)(12\,\Omega)}{6\,\Omega + 12\,\Omega} = (2\,\Omega + 4\,\Omega) = 6\,\Omega$. The new current is

$I' = \dfrac{V}{R} = \dfrac{12\ \text{V}}{6\ \Omega} = 2$ A. Thus, if the $3\ \Omega$ resistor is exchanged for a $12\ \Omega$ resistor, the current will drop from 3 A to 2 A, a decrease by a factor of $\dfrac{2}{3}$, so the correct answer is choice A.

5. **A** This is a 2×2 question: determining whether the force will be upward or downward eliminates two answers, as does determining the magnitude of the force to be 6.4×10^{-17} N or 4.0×10^{-2} N. Begin by figuring out the direction of the force. Since the particle is an electron, it is negatively charged, so it will be attracted to the positively charged plate. Thus, the force must be upward, eliminating choices B and C. Now calculate the magnitude of the force using the equation $F = qE$, where for an electron q is the elementary charge, $e = 1.6 \times 10^{-19}$ C (the sign is irrelevant because the direction of the force has already been determined). To find the electric field, use Ed's formula, $V = Ed$. Thus, you have $E = \dfrac{V}{d} = \dfrac{12\ \text{V}}{3\ \text{cm}} = \dfrac{12\ \text{V}}{3 \times 10^{-2}\ \text{m}} = 4 \times 10^2$ N/C, and

$F = \left(4 \times 10^2\ \text{N/C}\right)\left(1.6 \times 10^{-19}\ \text{C}\right) = 6.4 \times 10^{-17}\ \text{N}$.

6. **A**   The sum of the charges, Q_{tot}, on the two capacitors is 100 C. After Switch S is closed, capacitors C_1 and C_2 are connected together and must have the same terminal voltage, V. Q_{tot} remains 100 C. After a long time, the charge has become redistributed between the two capacitors. If the final charge on C_1 is $Q_{1,f}$, then the final charge on C_2 is $Q_{2,f} = Q_{tot} - Q_{1,f}$. Therefore, $V = Q_{1,f} / C_1 = Q_{2,f} / C_2 = (Q_{tot} - Q_{1,f}) / C_2$. Solving for $Q_{1,f}$ gives $Q_{1,f} = Q_{tot} / 4 = 25$ C and $Q_{2,f} = 75$ C.

7. **B**   This is a 2 × 2 question, so establishing the change in one quantity eliminates two of the four answer choices. Initially the equivalent resistances are calculated by $1/R_{eq} = 1/R + 1/R + 1/R + 1/R = 4/R \rightarrow R_{eq} = R/4$. After the resistances are halved, the equivalent resistance will be given by $1/R_{eq} = 2/R + 2/R + 2/R + 2/R = 8/R$, or $R_{eq} = R/8$. The total power dissipated is $P = IV = V^2 / R_{eq}$, so P is inversely proportional to the equivalent resistance. The equivalent resistance is halved and hence the power is doubled, eliminating choices C and D. The current is inversely proportional to the equivalent resistance, according to Ohm's Law ($V = IR$). Therefore, as the equivalent resistance is halved the current is doubled, which eliminates choice A.

8. **B**   The battery supplies power to the circuit according to the equation $P = V^2 / R_{eq}$, where R_{eq} is the equivalent resistance of the circuit. When S_2 is open and the circuit is in steady state, no current flows through R_3 or R_4, since no current can flow through either the charged capacitor or the open switch. Thus, the equivalent resistance of the circuit results from R_1 and R_2 connected in series, $R_{eq} = R + R = 2R$, so $P_1 = V^2 / 2R$. When S_2 is closed and the circuit reaches steady state, current now flows through all four resistors (but still not through the charged capacitor), since there is now a path for the current to flow through the branch including R_3 and R_4. R_3 and R_4 are connected in series, so the equivalent resistance of that branch of the circuit is also $2R$. The two branches of the circuit are connected in parallel, so $R_{eq} = (2R)(2R) / (2R + 2R) = R$. Thus, $P_2 = V^2 / R = 2P_1$.

9. **D**   In either case, the voltage across the 6 Ω resistor is 12 V, because it is in parallel with the 12 V battery. Ohm's Law, $V = IR$, yields 12 V = 6 Ω × I, and the current will be 2 A in both cases. Thus, choice D is correct (in that the statement is false). To see why the other choices make true statements, consider the following. The right side of the 3 Ω resistor is at 12 V, while its left side is at 15 or 18 V. The current in the left loop must be big enough that the 3 Ω resistor drops the voltage from the output of the 15 or 18 V to 12 V. For the 15 V source, $\Delta V = 3$ V so 3 V = 3 Ω × I and I is 1 A. For the 18 V source, $\Delta V = 6$ V and $I = 2$ A, making choices A and B true (here the notation ΔV is used simply to clarify the explanation: V is still taken to mean the potential difference across a circuit element). Note that the battery and the 3 Ω resistor are in series, and thus carry the same current. If choice A were untrue, choice B would also be untrue, and vice versa; since they can't both be the answer, they could be eliminated on that basis alone. Contrary to intuition, the current across the 12 V source is reduced, making choice C true. The two sources must provide a total of 2 A to the junction above the 12 V source, because in either case the 6 Ω resistor takes 2 A. The more current provided by the 15 or 18 V source, the less provided by the 12 V source.

10. **A**   This is set up like a proportion problem. There are several formulas for the energy stored on a capacitor: $1/2\ QV$, $Q^2/(2C)$, and $1/2\ CV^2$. Between the two trials, PE, V, and Q change, but C remains the same. To determine the proportional relationship requires an equation containing only PE (the given change), V (the asked-for change) and constants. Therefore, the equation $PE = 1/2\ CV^2$ is the appropriate one to relate E to V, and E is proportional to V^2. To double E, V must increase by square root of 2, that is, a factor of 1.4. 1.4 × 10 V = 14 V.

SOLUTIONS TO ELECTROSTATICS, ELECTRICITY, AND MAGNETISM PRACTICE PASSAGE

1. **A** The positrons are lightweight particles like electrons, so they will leave long thin tracks. This eliminates choices C and D. Due to the decrease in the radius of curvature after crossing the plate, you can tell that the direction of Track 1 is up and Track 2 is down. Using the right hand rule, and that the magnetic field points into the page, you can see that a positive charge moving down would curve to the right. This eliminates choice B, leaving choice A as the correct answer.

2. **B** This is a 2 × 2 question, meaning that there are two different quantities in the answer and two choices for each quantity. The best way to solve these questions is to solve the easy quantity first, eliminating two of the choices. In this case, the easy quantity is the track length. The passage states that heavier particles will interact more strongly and thus come to a stop more quickly. Thus, the proton will leave a shorter track, eliminating choices A and D. Setting the kinetic energies equal, you have $\frac{1}{2}m_p v_p^{\,2} = \frac{1}{2}m_e v_e^{\,2}$, giving $v_p = \sqrt{\frac{m_e}{m_p}}v_e$. Thus, $m_p v_p = \sqrt{m_p \cdot m_e} \cdot v_e > m_e v_e$ and the proton moves in a larger radius because its momentum is larger.

3. **B** If the electric field is pointing left to right, then positive charges will move to the right while negative charges will move to the left. Track 1 is moving upwards (the radius of curvature is smaller above the plate); using the right hand rule, you can see that it is positive. Since it is positive, it would move to the right under the electric field, thus switching directions (this eliminates choices A and C; they don't include Track 1 switching directions). Using the same analysis, you see that Track 2 is negative, and that both Tracks 3 and 4 are positive. Thus, Track 2 will still curve to the left and Tracks 3 and 4 will still curve to the right. Thus, the correct answer is choice B.

4. **A** This is another 2 × 2 question. The electric field points from left to right, so a negatively charged particle will be pulled to the left by the electric field. For the particle to move in a straight line, the net force on it must be zero so the magnetic force must point to the right. Using the right hand rule and flipping directions (or using the left hand rule), the negatively charged particle must be moving upwards. This eliminates choices C and D. Setting the electric force equal to the magnetic force, you have $qE = qvB$. This gives $v = E/B$.

5. **A** There is no way to derive this formula from the information given, so eliminate answers that contradict the information in the passage. Choice B can be eliminated because it has the distance in the denominator. The farther the particle travels through the vapor the more energy it will lose. The passage states that heavier particles and particles with more charge

interact more strongly and lose their energy sooner, so choice C can be eliminated because it has the mass in the denominator, and choice D can be eliminated because it has the charge in the denominator. Therefore, the correct answer must be choice A.

6. **C** Since Items I and II both appear in exactly two answer choices, start by analyzing one of them; whether they are true or false, you'll eliminate half the answers. Item I is false: the proton and the alpha particle have the same momentum, so the only thing influencing the radius of curvature is the charge. The alpha particle has more charge; thus, its radius of curvature is smaller (choices A and D can be eliminated). Note that both remaining answer choices include Item III, thus it must be true, and you can focus on Item II. Item II is true: the alpha particle consists of two protons and two neutrons. Since the alpha particle is heavier and has more charge than the proton, it will leave a thicker and shorter track (choice B can be eliminated, and choice C is correct).

Chapter 38
Oscillations, Waves, and Sound

FREESTANDING QUESTIONS: OSCILLATIONS, WAVES, AND SOUND

1. A string fixed at each end is vibrating in its third harmonic mode. A second string, with the same tension and linear mass density but 4 cm longer, is vibrating in its fourth harmonic mode. If the frequencies of the two strings are identical, what is the length of the shorter string?

A) 16/3 cm
B) 8 cm
C) 12 cm
D) 16 cm

2. A hot wheels racetrack uses a compressed spring ($k = 1000$ kg/s^2) to launch a toy car along the racetrack. The track is arranged so that after launch the 10 g toy car first climbs a gradual 3 m long incline to a height of 1 m, then travels down the incline on the other side. Assume friction can be ignored. The launching mechanism loses 0.7 J of energy with each launch. What is the minimum compression of the spring required for the car to reach the top of the incline?

A) 0.2 cm
B) 1 cm
C) 4 cm
D) 6 cm

3. A cube with side length 10 cm and mass 2 kg is hung from a vertical spring, causing the spring to stretch 12 cm beyond its rest length. The block is pulled downward and released, oscillating vertically. The entire system is then immersed in water and the experiment is repeated. Assuming drag is negligible, which of the following is true about the immersed system's equilibrium position and frequency?

A) The equilibrium position is 6 cm beyond the spring's rest length, but the frequency is the same.
B) The equilibrium position is 6 cm beyond the spring's rest length, and the frequency has increased.
C) The equilibrium position is 6 cm less than the spring's rest length, but the frequency is the same.
D) The equilibrium position is 6 cm less than the spring's rest length, and the frequency has increased.

4. A block of mass m is attached to a horizontal spring with spring constant k, and it oscillates on a frictionless surface between points $-A$ and A. If the speed of the block at point A is equal to v, which of the following represents the mass of the block?

A) $\dfrac{A}{v}\sqrt{k}$

B) $\dfrac{kA^2}{v^2}$

C) $\dfrac{v^2}{kA^2}$

D) $\dfrac{v}{A}\sqrt{k}$

5. An insect with mass m lands lightly (with no impulse) on the bob of mass $3m$ of a simple pendulum that is initially oscillating with the frequency f. How does the pendulum's new frequency compare to the original?

A) f increases by a factor of 2.
B) f decreases by a factor of 2.
C) f decreases by a factor of 3.
D) f stays the same.

6. A mass hangs vertically from a heavy rope of uniform linear mass density. A wave is generated at the top of the rope. As the wave travels downward toward the mass, which of the following is true? (Note: $v = \sqrt{F_T/\mu}$ where v is the speed of a wave in a rope or string, F_T is tension, and μ is linear mass density).

A) The frequency and speed are constant.
B) The frequency is constant, but the speed decreases.
C) The frequency is constant, but the speed increases.
D) Both the frequency and the speed decrease.

7. A sound traveling from one medium to another loses 40% of its intensity. By approximately how much does the sound level decrease?

A) 2 dB
B) 12 dB
C) 22 dB
D) 32 dB

8. If M represents mass, T represents time, and L represents length, which of the following represents the dimensions of sound intensity?

A) Unitless
B) ML/T^3
C) M/LT^3
D) M/T^3

9. A motorcyclist is traveling at 10 m/s when he hears an ambulance siren approaching from behind at a rate of 40 m/s. If the siren frequency detected by the ambulance driver is 700 Hz, which of the following is closest to the frequency detected by the motorcyclist? (The speed of sound in air is approximately 340 m/s.)

A) 600 Hz
B) 636 Hz
C) 770 Hz
D) 817 Hz

10. How does a hollow cylindrical pipe that is open on both ends compare to the exact same pipe with one end closed off?

A) Increasing the length of both of the pipes will increase the fundamental harmonic frequency of both pipes.
B) Sound propagates more quickly through the pipe that has both ends open than in the pipe with one end closed off.
C) The pipe that has both ends open will never have any of the same resonant frequencies as the closed pipe.
D) Over a large, but finite, range of frequencies, the open pipe has more resonant frequencies than the closed pipe.

OSCILLATIONS, WAVES, AND SOUND PRACTICE PASSAGE

Therapeutic ultrasound has a range of treatment applications. These include the breakdown of kidney and gallstones, delivery of drugs both transdermally and through targeted pulses that increase penetration of drugs into certain tissues, musculoskeletal and soft pain relief and scar tissue breakdown, and non-invasive destruction of tumors. Ultrasound technology has been used in medical applications for over six decades, and its uses continue to expand and be refined. However, perhaps its most common application, for pain relief and soft-tissue injury recovery (generally applied by physical therapists or chiropractors), is not well justified by randomized controlled trial studies over placebo effects.

Therapeutic ultrasound involves the use of sound wave frequencies between 0.8 and 3.5 MHz, well beyond the human hearing range (which has a maximum at ~20 kHz). In typical ultrasound therapies, a *transducer,* which converts electrical energy into sound energy, is placed against the skin to which an aqueous gel has been applied (to maximize transmission of the sound energy into the body). The sound energy is absorbed by soft tissues, preferentially connective tissues, generally between depths of two to five centimeters of efficacy; the intensity of the ultrasound attenuates with depth according to a negative exponential function,

$$I = I_0 e^{-2\alpha z}$$

Equation 1

where I_0 is the intensity at the surface, α is the attenuation constant, and z is the depth of tissue into which the waves have traveled. The following table provides the attenuation constants for various tissues in decibels/cm at a frequency of 1 MHz (attenuation constants increase linearly and proportionally with frequency):

Tissue	Attenuation constant (dB/cm at 1MHz)
Blood	0.18
Fat	0.63
Liver	0.5–0.94
Kidney	1.0
Muscle	1.3–3.3
Bone	5.0

Table 1

When ultrasound energy is absorbed, it has two primary non-mechanical effects on tissue. The first and most common of these is thermal: the absorbed sonic energy is transformed into thermal energy, increasing the temperature of the absorbing tissues. The second is *cavitation*, the formation and often subsequent rapid collapse of bubbles of gas in a fluidic medium by large, rapid changes in pressure. These collapses generate *shock waves* that mechanically disrupt adjacent tissue.

High-intensity Focused Ultrasound (HIFU) is a relatively new form of ultrasound treatment used to destroy tumors, cysts, and fibroids. The ultrasound waves are focused using an acoustic lens, so that an array of multiple ultrasound waves converge and constructively interfere at a small region of tissue. Using 250 kHz to 2 MHz waves, HIFU gives rise to rapid temperature increases in the targeted tissue up to a range of between 65°C and 85°C, inducing tissue death.

1. The wavelength of HIFU treatment places a physical limit on the precision to which it can be applied. Taking the speed of sound in tissue to be 1500 m/s, what is the minimum tissue size that can be targeted by the indicated HIFU frequencies? (Assume that the limit on one dimension applies in all three dimension, i.e., a cube of side x.)

A) 0.43 mm
B) 0.75 mm
C) 1.9 mm
D) 6 mm

2. Which of the following would NOT be a plausible reason why physical therapy patients receiving ultrasonic therapy for muscle sprain experience short-term relief?

A) The heating of tissue increases blood flow to the area, speeding healing.
B) The vibration of deep muscle tissue has an effect similar to a physical massage.
C) The placebo effect associated with having one's symptoms taken seriously and treated increases the patients' expectations that they will begin feeling better.
D) Polarized ultrasound waves realign scar tissue to its pre-injury condition.

3. Through approximately how many centimeters of bone would an ultrasound signal of 1 MHz have to pass for its intensity to have decreased by a factor of 100?

A) 2 cm
B) 4 cm
C) 50 cm
D) 500 cm

4. Which of the following explains a condition under which shock waves due to cavitation would be most likely to occur?

A) A high intensity, high frequency ultrasound wave creates microbubbles within the rarefaction region of the sound wave and then collapses those bubbles within its compression region.
B) A low intensity, high frequency ultrasound wave creates microbubbles within the rarefaction region of the sound wave and then collapses those bubbles within its compression region.
C) A high intensity, low frequency ultrasound wave creates microbubbles within the compression region of the sound wave and then collapses those bubbles within its rarefaction region.
D) A reflected ultrasound wave creates a standing wave pattern where pressure nodes lead to the creation of microbubbles, which build up over time.

5. What minimum attenuation through muscle tissue would one expect for a 3 MHz ultrasound signal?

A) 0.43 dB/cm
B) 1.3 dB/cm
C) 3.9 dB/cm
D) 9.9 dB/cm

SOLUTIONS TO FREESTANDING QUESTIONS: OSCILLATIONS, WAVES, AND SOUND

1. **C** The frequency for a string attached at each end vibrating in its nth harmonic mode is given by $f_n = vn/2L$, where v is the speed of the wave and L is the length of the string. The frequency of the original string can therefore be written as $3v/2L$. Since the second string has the same tension and linear mass density as the first string, the wave speed is the same ($v = \sqrt{F_T/\mu}$, where F_T is the tension and μ is the linear mass density). For the second string, the frequency can be written as $4v/2(L + 4\text{ cm})$ if you leave lengths in centimeters. Setting the two expressions for frequency equal, you get $3v/2L = 4v/2(L + 4\text{ cm})$ or $3/L = 4/(L + 4\text{ cm})$. Cross-multiplying, you get $3L + 12\text{ cm} = 4L$ or $L = 12\text{ cm}$.

2. **C** The elastic potential energy of the spring is converted into the gravitational potential energy of the toy car, with some energy being lost in the launching mechanism. This can be expressed as *elastic potential energy = gravitational potential energy + energy lost*. The elastic potential energy is $(1/2)kx^2$, where k is the spring constant and x is the displacement of the spring. The gravitational potential energy is mgh, where m is the mass of the car and h is the height of the car. Notice that the length of the incline is extraneous. So the gravitational potential energy = $(0.01\text{ kg})(10\text{ m/s}^2)(1\text{ m}) = 0.1\text{ J}$. The main energy equation so far is $(1/2)(1000\text{ kg/s}^2)x^2 = 0.1\text{ J} + 0.7\text{ J} = 0.8\text{ J}$. Solving for x^2 the equation becomes $x^2 = (0.8\text{ J})(2)/(1000\text{ kg/s}^2) = 1.6/1000 = 0.0016\text{ m}^2$ and $x = 0.04\text{ m} = 4\text{ cm}$. The correct answer is choice C.

3. **A** The frequency of a mass on a spring is always $1/2\pi \sqrt{k/m}$ regardless of whether the spring is vertical or horizontal. All gravity does for a mass on a vertical spring is shift the equilibrium position. With the system immersed in water, the buoyant force acts on the mass as well. This reduces the effect of gravity. This changes the equilibrium position, but not the frequency. This eliminates choices B and D. Comparing the remaining choices, you can see that the difference between them is the effect of the buoyant force. In choice A, gravity would have to be stronger than the buoyant force, causing the string to stretch (although not as much as before the system was immersed). In choice C, the buoyant force would have to be stronger than gravity, causing the spring to compress upward. So you need to compare these two forces. Gravity is given by $mg = (2\text{ kg})(10\text{ m/s}^2) = 20\text{ N}$. The buoyant force is given by $\rho_{water}V_{sub}g$. Since the entire object is submerged, $V_{sub} = V_{object} = (0.10\text{ m})^3 = 10^{-3}\text{ m}^3$. So the buoyant force is $(1000\text{ kg/m}^3)(10^{-3}\text{ m}^3)(10\text{ m/s}^2) = 10\text{ N}$. Since gravity is stronger, choice A is the correct answer.

4. **B** Use conservation of energy: $KE_i + PE_i = KE_f + PE_f$, or $\frac{1}{2}mv_i^2 + \frac{1}{2}kx_i^2 = \frac{1}{2}mv_f^2 + \frac{1}{2}kx_f^2$.

   Assume that the block's initial position is at the equilibrium point, and that its final position is at $x = A$. At the equilibrium point, $x = 0$, so $\frac{1}{2}kx_i^2 = 0$. At the point $x = A$, the block is turning around, and therefore $v = 0$, so $\frac{1}{2}mv_f^2 = 0$. Now $\frac{1}{2}mv_i^2 = \frac{1}{2}kx_f^2$. Divide both sides by $\frac{1}{2}$ to get $mv_i^2 = kx_f^2$. Finally, divide both sides by v_i^2 to find that $m = \dfrac{kx_f^2}{v_i^2}$. Here, you are looking at the block when $x = A$, so the correct answer is choice B. You could also solve this by analyzing the units involved: mass units are kilograms, so you need an answer in which all of the units except kilograms cancel out. Here, A is in meters, v is in m/s, and the spring constant k is in N/m, or kg/s^2. Hence, the correct answer must have a linear term k in the numerator of the fraction, since k is the only variable with kilograms in its units. Only choice B fits this description.

5. **D** The frequency of a simple pendulum is given by $f = \dfrac{1}{2\pi}\sqrt{\dfrac{g}{L}}$, where L is the length of the pendulum string. Since the frequency is not dependent on the mass of the pendulum, the change in mass does not affect the frequency of the pendulum. Choices A and B are likely to be trap answers; mass appears as a factor in the expression for the frequency of an oscillating spring, not in the expression for the frequency of a pendulum.

6. **B** The second Big Rule for wave speed states that the frequency of a wave remains constant, even if it passes into a new medium. Consider that at any point on the string, the number of pulses coming toward it per second must equal the number of pulses moving away from it per second. This eliminates choice D. Since the rope is heavy, the tension must decrease as the wave moves down the string. Since every point on the string is "responsible" for supporting the total weight beneath it, the top of the rope must support rope + mass, while as you move down, there is less rope to support. Since speed increases with tension, it must decrease as it travels down the rope. The correct answer is choice B.

7. **A** If 40% of the intensity is lost, then 60% is transmitted, so the intensity is now 0.60I. This value is between $I/10 < 0.60\ I < I$. By the sound level equation, $\beta = 10 \log(I/I_o)$, any decrease in intensity by a factor of ten subtracts 10 dB from the sound level. Hence, β decreases by 10 dB if the intensity is divided by a factor of 10. Since intensity decreases by a factor less than ten in this case, β reduces by an amount between 0 dB and 10 dB, eliminating all answers but choice A.

8. **D** Intensity is given by $I = P/A$. Power is work/time, which is equivalent to force × length/time, which in turn equals mass × length/time^2 × length/time, or dimensions of ML^2/T^3. Area (in the denominator) has dimensions of L^2. Therefore, intensity has dimensions of M/T^3, which is represented by choice D. Choice A is a trap: sound intensity is not the same as intensity or sound <u>level</u>, which is measured in dimensionless dB.

9. **C** This question asks about the difference between the frequency that an observer detects and the frequency that a source detects, so use the formula for the Doppler effect: $f_D = f_S \left(\dfrac{v \pm v_D}{v \mp v_S} \right)$. In order to decide whether to add or subtract in the numerator and the denominator, consider the motion of each object separately. The motorcyclist (the detector) is moving away from the ambulance, so use the bottom sign in the numerator (this makes sense, because motion that increases the distance between source and detector should decrease the detected frequency, which means subtraction in the numerator). The ambulance driver (the source) is moving <u>to</u>ward the motorcyclist, so use the <u>top</u> sign in the denominator, (this makes sense, because motion that decreases the distance between source and detector should increase the detected frequency, which means subtraction in the numerator). This yields

$$f_D = f_S \left(\frac{v - v_D}{v - v_S} \right) = \left(700\,\text{Hz} \right) \left(\frac{340\ \text{m/s} - 10\ \text{m/s}}{340\ \text{m/s} - 40\ \text{m/s}} \right) = \left(700\ \text{Hz} \right) \left(\frac{330\,\text{m/s}}{300\,\text{m/s}} \right) = \left(700\,\text{Hz} \right) \left(\frac{11}{10} \right) = 770\ \text{Hz}.$$

Overall, the ambulance is getting closer to the motorcyclist, which means the frequency that the motorcyclist hears should be higher than the frequency that the ambulance driver hears. Therefore, you can immediately eliminate choices A and B. The correct answer is choice C.

10. **C** For standing waves, the resonant frequencies are inversely proportional to the length of the rod ($f_n = nv/2L$ for an open pipe, while $f_n = nv/4L$ for pipes with one end closed). Therefore, increasing the lengths of the pipe will cause the fundamental harmonic frequency (f_1) to decrease in both the pipes, eliminating choice A. The propagation of sound (or its velocity) through the pipes will depend only on the medium that is filling the pipe, and not whether the pipe is open or closed, eliminating choice B as well. Choice C is correct since the open pipe has resonant frequencies that are multiples of half wavelengths, while the closed rod has resonant frequencies that are odd-integer multiples of quarter wavelengths. These two sets of resonance frequencies do not overlap. Choice D is false since the occurrence of standing waves depends on the counting integer n in the equations $f_n = nv/2L$ and $f_n = nv/4L$. The first equation is defined by $n/2$ (with $n = 1, 2, 3, \ldots$), while the second equation has $n/4$ ($n = 1, 3, 5, \ldots$). At first it may seem that the $n/4$ will have twice as many standing waves as $n/2$, due to the larger denominator, but this does not occur because for $n/4$, $n = 1, 3, 5, \ldots$ (and not $n = 1, 2, 3, \ldots$). Ultimately, both rods end up having the same number of resonant frequencies over a finite frequency range.

SOLUTIONS TO OSCILLATIONS, WAVES, AND SOUND PRACTICE PASSAGE

1. **B**   This is a calculation question requiring the wave speed equation and the maximum HIFU frequency (for the minimum wavelength) given in the last paragraph of the passage.

$$v = \lambda f \rightarrow \lambda = \frac{v}{f} = \frac{1500 \, \frac{m}{s}}{2 \, \text{MHz}} = \frac{15}{2} \times \frac{10^2}{10^6} \, \text{m} = 7.5 \times 10^{-4} \, \text{m},$$ which corresponds to choice B

(the power of ten doesn't really matter once you see the coefficient must be 7.5).

2. **D**   Sound waves are longitudinal waves and cannot polarize, making choice D a false statement about ultrasound and thus the correct answer. All of the other answer choices are implied by the passage: ultrasound can have both mechanical and thermal effects on tissue, and of course the placebo effect is nearly always a medical possibility in patient treatment (and is alluded to in the first paragraph).

3. **B**   Recall the relation between sound level in dB and intensity in W/m²: for each decrease in intensity by a factor of ten, you subtract 10 dB from the sound level. Thus, in this case, a decrease in intensity by a factor of 100 (10 × 10) corresponds to a decrease of 10 dB + 10 dB = 20 dB (note the word "decrease" here: we're subtracting 20 dB, not adding). According to Table 1, each centimeter of bone decreases the ultrasound level by 5 dB, so a decrease of 20 dB requires 4 cm of bone (choice B is correct).

4. **A**   The passage states that shock waves are associated with the collapse of cavitation bubbles, not their accumulation, so choice D is eliminated (moreover, one would expect pressure antinodes to be associated with cavitation, where the pressure can drop to a very low level suddenly, not remain constant over time). Cavitation itself is associated with "large, rapid changes in pressure," implying a large amplitude ultrasound wave with a high frequency (eliminating choice C; note also that one would expect bubbles in a fluid to form when the pressure dropped, not when it rose, also eliminating choice C). Since intensity is proportional to the square of amplitude, large amplitude implies high intensity, eliminating choice B.

5. **C**   Just above Table 1, the passage states that attenuation constants increase as a linear proportion with frequency. Since the table provides values for 1 MHz, an increase to 3 MHz implies an increase in the value of α by a factor of 3. The minimum value provided for the attenuation constant α for muscle is 1.3 dB/cm, which multiplied by 3 is 3.9 dB/cm (choice C is correct).

Chapter 39
Light, Optics, and Quantum Physics

FREESTANDING QUESTIONS: LIGHT, OPTICS, AND QUANTUM PHYSICS

1. A spectroscope is a device for determining the composition of incandescent objects. In one design, light enters a spectroscope and passes through a diffraction grating, producing a pattern of spectral lines at frequencies characteristic of the elements in the source. If a distant galaxy is moving toward an astronomer who is studying it with a spectroscope, which of the following statements is true?

A) Observed spectral lines in the light emitted from the galaxy are shifted toward the blue end of the visible spectrum.
B) Observed spectral lines in the light emitted from the galaxy are shifted toward the red end of the visible spectrum.
C) The observed spectral lines are the same as what they would be if the galaxy were stationary with respect to the Earth.
D) The observed spectral lines of visible light are brighter than they would be if the galaxy were stationary with respect to the Earth.

2. Every color of light has a slightly different index of refraction, which gives rise to rainbows. A beam of white light is incident on a pool of water at 42 degrees. The red light is refracted such that it is closest to the surface of the water, with yellow light in the middle, and blue light deepest into the water. Which color of light travels fastest in water?

A) Red
B) Yellow
C) Blue
D) They travel at the same speed.

3. You are swimming in a pool of water and you shine a light with an angle of 30 degrees to the surface of the water. What angle out of the water (with respect to the surface of the water) will the light ray appear if the index of refraction of water is 4/3 and the index of refraction of air is 1?

A) arcsin (1/3)
B) arcsin (1/√3)
C) arcsin (2/3)
D) None of the above

4. A hyperopic individual is considered to be farsighted, a condition in which images of some objects would come into focus behind the retina rather than at the retina. Which of the following accurately describes the appropriate corrective lens for such an individual?

A) A converging lens is appropriate, due to its positive power.
B) A converging lens is appropriate, due to its negative power.
C) A diverging lens is appropriate, due to its positive power.
D) A diverging lens is appropriate, due to its negative power.

5. Two lenses, the first converging with a focal point of 20 cm, the second diverging with a focal point of −40 cm, are placed side by side. What is the effective focal point of the lens combination?

A) Diverging, focal point = −20 cm
B) Diverging, focal point = −10 cm
C) Converging, focal point = 20 cm
D) Converging, focal point = 40 cm

6. Which photon would be most likely to knock an inner-shell electron out of a tungsten atom?

A) A gamma ray, because it has the most energy
B) A gamma ray, because it can also rearrange the nucleus
C) An X-ray, because it has the most energy
D) A visible ray, because it is tuned to the resonant frequency

7. What is the magnification of the image formed of an object 20 cm from a mirrored sphere with a diameter of 20 cm?

A) 5
B) 0.2
C) − 0.2
D) − 5

8. The minimum size of an object visible through an optical microscope is approximately equal to the shortest wavelength of the light used for illumination. Compared to optical microscopes, electron microscopes have a much higher resolution but are also limited because electrons used for imaging have a wavelength as a result of wave-particle duality. Like photons, the wavelength of an electron is $\lambda = h/p$. Here, p is the momentum of a photon or the relativistic momentum of an electron, and h is Planck's constant. Which of the following statements is true?

A) The wavelength of an imaging electron is much greater than the wavelength of red light.
B) The momentum of an imaging electron is much less than the momentum of blue light.
C) The momentum of an imaging electron is much greater than the momentum of blue light.
D) The wavelength of an imaging electron is between the wavelengths of red and blue light.

9. Light emitting diodes are electronic devices that emit light when electrons in a high energy state, called the conduction band, enter a low energy state called a valence band. Planck's constant is 4.14×10^{-15} eV-seconds. When an electron falls from the conduction to the valence band of aluminum gallium arsenide, which has a band gap of 1.6 eV, what is the wavelength of emitted light?

A) 0.77×10^{-7} m
B) 0.77×10^{-6} m
C) 0.77×10^{-5} m
D) 0.77×10^{-4} m

10. If a second electron binds to a hydrogen atom (making H⁻) in the ground state, will both electrons have the same energy?

A) No, because the Pauli Exclusion Principle forbids two electrons having the same energy.
B) Yes, because the Pauli Exclusion Principle allows a maximum of two electrons with the same energy.
C) Yes, but the two electrons must have opposite spin to satisfy the Pauli Exclusion Principle.
D) No, the Pauli Exclusion Principle makes both energies uncertain, so they cannot be equal.

LIGHT, OPTICS, AND QUANTUM PHYSICS PRACTICE PASSAGE

In radiation therapy, tumor cells are destroyed by X-ray or gamma radiation (photon therapy), or by particle therapy (e.g., proton therapy). The aim of radiotherapy is to destroy the tumor completely, while having minimal effect on the surrounding healthy tissues. Protons have different dosimetric characteristics than photons used in radiation therapy. Once a proton beam enters tissue, it shows an increasing energy deposition with depth, leading to a maximum called the *Bragg peak*. Beyond this point, the dose falls to zero within millimeters (Figure 1). Photons, however, deliver their maximum dose shortly after they have entered the body. After this region, the dosage exponentially decreases and will not reach zero before it exits the patient's body.

Proton depth dose curves

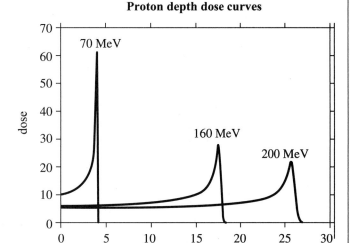

Figure 1   Proton depth dose curves for beams of various energies

The physical absorbed dose (or just "dose") at a point in a radiation field is quantified as the energy absorbed per unit target mass. It is measured in J/kg, which is also named the gray, or Gy. A typical therapy dose used to destroy a tumor is roughly 60 Gy and is delivered in fractional doses throughout several days of treatment. A whole-body dose of 1–2 Gy causes radiation sickness within a few hours, usually with recovery in a few weeks. A whole body dose of 2–6 Gy is usually fatal within 2 months.

In proton therapy, proton beams of up to 230 MeV are generated in particle accelerators, usually cyclotrons or synchrotrons. Both are circular accelerator rings that use magnetic fields to deflect charged particles that are given greater kinetic energy by electric fields. Cyclotrons use constant magnetic and electric fields to accelerate charged particles in increasing-radius spirals until they eject with fixed energies. Synchrotrons use time-

varying electromagnetic fields to accelerate particles within a fixed-radius ring to higher and higher energies, until they are ejected by steering magnets. Because of this synchronization of field strength and particle energy, these accelerators are called synchrotrons. This technique allows the production of proton beams with a variety of energies (unlike the cyclotron, which has a fixed extraction energy).

Type	Synchrotron (rapid cycle)	Synchrotron (slow cycle)	Cyclotron
Energy level selection	Continuous	Continuous	Fixed
Size (diameter) [m]	10	6	4
Average Power (beam on) [kW]	200	370	300
Repetition Frequency [Hz]	60	0.5	Continuous

Table 1   Accelerator technology comparisons for some parameters

Adapted from Paganetti & Bortfeld, Proton Beam Radiotherapy, MGH Boston 2005; J. Wilkens, *Therapy with Protons and Ion Beams*, Biomedical Physics Lecture, Technische Universität München 2013.

1. Using radiation therapy, what is the approximate amount of energy required to destroy 99% of the mass of a tumor weighing 10 grams?

A) 0.6 J
B) 6 J
C) 60 J
D) 6 kJ

2. Which type of radiation would most likely be best for treating tumors 17 cm within a patient's body?

A) X-ray beam
B) 70 MeV proton beam
C) 160 MeV proton beam
D) 200 MeV proton beam

3. Which of the following is true regarding X-ray and proton beams used in radiation therapy?

A) Both X-ray beams and proton beams can be deflected within an external magnetic field.
B) The speed of an X-ray beam in tissue can be controlled by the radiation source.
C) An X-ray beam will refract in tissue if its angle of incidence is greater than 0°.
D) An X-ray beam will have a lower exit dose compared to a beam of protons.

4. Which of the following could be a good reason a radiologist might decide to treat a tumor with beta radiation instead of a proton beam?

A) There is less risk of side scatter (deflection in a different direction than the original collimated beam) for beta particles than a proton beam.
B) Negatively charged particles are more ionizing than positively charged particles, therefore requiring a smaller dose.
C) A beam of beta particles will ionize tumor tissue via the photoelectric effect, which is more finely tuned than the bulk ionization of proton therapies.
D) The tumor in question is close to the surface of the patient's skin, meaning that less penetrative beta particles will be less likely to do damage to deep tissues along the beam's path.

5. What is the approximate speed of a 0.7 MeV beam of protons in air? (Note: use mass of proton $m_p = 1.67 \times 10^{-27}$ kg, and 1 MeV $= 1.60 \times 10^{-13}$ J)

A) 1.7×10^9 m/s
B) 3.0×10^8 m/s
C) 1.2×10^7 m/s
D) 2.5×10^6 m/s

6. Which of the following graphs best represents how the dosage of an X-ray beam changes according to depth in a patient's body?

A)
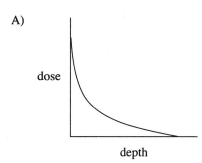

B)
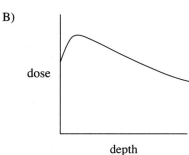

C)
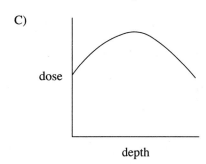

D)
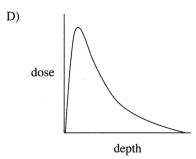

SOLUTIONS TO FREESTANDING QUESTIONS: LIGHT, OPTICS, AND QUANTUM PHYSICS

1. **A** For a source that approaches the observer, the Doppler effect increases the frequency of detected light compared to what was emitted. Blue light is at the high frequency end of the visible spectrum and red light is at the low frequency end, so spectral lines from the approaching galaxy are "blue shifted." Choice B is incorrect because it describes a "red shift," which occurs when a galaxy recedes from Earth. Choice C is incorrect because the Doppler effect produces a frequency shift whenever there is relative motion between the source and detector. Choice D is incorrect because intensity is a function of distance from the source, irrespective of relative motion.

2. **A** Snell's Law states that $n_1 \sin\theta_1 = n_2 \sin\theta_2$. Since n_1 is 1 in air, the angle of refraction decreases as the index of refraction increases. Therefore, red light must have a smaller index of refraction. The index of refraction is equal to $n = c/v$. Thus, red light must have the largest velocity in water.

3. **D** Using Snell's Law, and remembering that the angles are with respect to the vertical, you can find that

$$n_1 \sin\theta_1 = n_2 \sin\theta_2$$
$$\tfrac{4}{3} \sin 60° = 1\sin\theta_2$$
$$\tfrac{4}{3} \left(\tfrac{\sqrt{3}}{2}\right) = \sin\theta_2$$

However, this is not an acceptable equation, as it states that $\sin\theta_2$ is greater than one. If you check the critical angle in this instance, it is less than 60°, meaning that you cannot see out of the water because the light rays will be totally internally reflected.

4. **A** This is a 2 × 2 question, as knowledge of which lens type is associated with positive/negative power allows two answer choices to be eliminated, and knowledge of the effect of converging/diverging lenses allows for the remaining two answer choices to be distinguished. Converging lenses are always associated with positive powers, whereas diverging lenses are associated with negative powers (choices B and C can be eliminated). The goal of the appropriate corrective lens should be to focus the light closer to the retina, forward in the eye, and therefore a converging lens is appropriate.

5. **D** Lenses can be combined by adding their powers. The first lens is $f = 0.2$ m, so the power is $1/0.2 = 10/2 = 5$ D. The second lens is $f = -0.4$ m, so the power is $1/-0.4 = -10/4 = -2.5$ D. Combining these powers, the effective power of the lens combination is 5 D $+ -2.5$ D $= 2.5$ D. So the effective focal point of the lens combination is $1/2.5 = 4/10 = 0.4$ m. Since the focal point is positive, the lens is converging. The correct answer is choice D.

6. **A** The topic of this question is unfamiliar, so it can be difficult to select the right answer by direct reasoning. In such cases, Process of Elimination is often a fruitful strategy. Gamma ray photons have more energy than either X-ray photons or visible light photons, so choice C can be eliminated. A collision between a photon and an electron need not involve the nucleus, so choice B can be eliminated. Nothing in the question or prior knowledge supports choice D.

7. **B** The object distance is given, so to get the image distance, you need the focal length. First, note that a mirrored sphere must be convex (unless you're inside it), so the focal length will be negative. The rule for spherical mirrors is that the absolute value of the focal length is half the radius of curvature. The diameter is given, so compute:

$$d = 2r \rightarrow r = 10 \text{ cm} \rightarrow |f| = \frac{r}{2} \rightarrow f = -5 \text{ cm}.$$

Now the mirror/lens equation can be applied to find i:

$$\frac{1}{o} + \frac{1}{i} = \frac{1}{f} \rightarrow \frac{1}{20} + \frac{1}{i} = \frac{1}{-5} \rightarrow \frac{1}{i} = -\frac{1}{5} - \frac{1}{20} = -\frac{4+1}{20} \rightarrow \frac{1}{i} = -\frac{1}{4} \rightarrow i = -4 \text{ cm}.$$ Finally, apply the magnification equation: $m = -\frac{i}{o} = -\frac{-4}{20} = \frac{1}{5}$ (choice B is correct, and choice A is wrong). Note that convex mirrors do not form real images or real objects, and since real images are inverted, convex mirrors will never produce negative magnifications. This eliminates choices C and D.

8. **C** The momentum of an electron is $p = h/\lambda$. An electron microscope has much higher resolution than an optical microscope; therefore, the wavelength of the electron that illuminates the object being viewed is much smaller than the wavelength of light, which requires a much greater momentum for the electron. Choice A is incorrect because an electron microscope has much higher resolution than an optical microscope; therefore, the wavelength of an electron must be much shorter than the wavelength of red light, which is in the visual spectrum used for optical microscopes. Choice B is incorrect because wavelength is inversely proportional to momentum. To have a wavelength shorter than light in the visual spectrum, which includes blue, an electron must have a momentum greater than photons in the visual spectrum. Choice D is incorrect because red and blue are both in the visual spectrum, and the wavelength of an electron must be shorter than either of them.

9. **B** Despite the unfamiliarity of the material (or because of it!), this is actually a straightforward calculation problem. The emitted light has energy equal to the band gap energy that the electron loses when entering the valence band. $E = hf = hc/\lambda$; therefore $\lambda = hc/E$. The energy lost by the electron is 1.6 eV, and the wavelength $\lambda = [(4.14 \times 10^{-15} \text{ eV-seconds}) (3.0 \times 10^8 \text{ m/s})]/(1.6 \text{ eV}) = 0.77 \times 10^{-6}$ m. Notice that you're really only trying to get the order of magnitude of the answer, so pay attention to the powers of ten and not the coefficients.

10. **C** The Pauli Exclusion Principle allows states with two electrons in which at least one quantum number is different. Even the ground state, with only one value of quantum numbers l and m, can contain two electrons if their spins are different. Choice A is incorrect because different states, allowed by Pauli, can have the same energy if their quantum states are different. Choice B is incorrect because for all shell numbers n greater than 1 there are more than two states at the same energy (recall from chemistry that for the second shell and higher level shells, larger numbers of electrons than two can be contained). Choice D is incorrect because the Pauli Exclusion Principle does not deal with uncertainty.

SOLUTIONS TO LIGHT, OPTICS, AND QUANTUM PHYSICS PRACTICE PASSAGE

1. **A** According to the information in paragraph 2, the dose required to destroy a tumor is around 60 Gy or 60 J/kg. You can round the 99% to 100% because it will not really affect the calculation for this question. The tumor is 10 grams (0.01 kg), so the energy required is (0.01 kg) (60 J/kg) = 0.6 J.

2. **C** Choice A can be eliminated, since according to paragraph 1, Bragg peaks are a property of proton beams, not X-rays. Look for the radiation type that has its Bragg peak close to 17 cm. According to Figure 1, the Bragg peak for the 200 MeV proton beam forms at 25 cm depth (eliminating choice D) and that for the 70 MeV proton beam forms at 4 cm (eliminating choice B). The Bragg peak for the 160 MeV is somewhere between 15 cm and 20 cm deep, making choice C correct.

3. **C** Choice A is incorrect because only charged particles in motion can experience a magnetic force (remember $F_{\text{magnetic}} = qvB$). Electromagnetic waves (or photons) such as an X-ray beam are not charged, so they will not experience an external magnetic force and will not be deflected in a magnetic field. Protons are charged particles; therefore, a beam of protons will experience a magnetic force and will be deflected. Choice B is wrong; according to the first Big Rule for Waves, the speed of a wave only depends on the type of wave (sound, electromagnetic, …) and the medium. So the speed of X-rays in tissue is always going to be the same. Choice D is incorrect; according to paragraph 1, the dosage of protons drops to zero immediately after the Bragg peak, but X-rays may exit the body. This leaves choice C, which is correct because in general, electromagnetic waves refract upon transmission into another medium (in this case, from air into tissue).

4. **D** Answering this question correctly relies heavily on outside knowledge of types of radioactive decay. Beta particles are electrons or positrons, much less massive than protons but with the same magnitude of charge. Because they are so much smaller than protons, they are much more likely to be deflected from their original paths upon interaction with matter, eliminating choice A. Choice B is false: there's no reason to think that negative particles are more ionizing than positive. Choice C might be tempting if you remember that the photoelectric effect involves electrons, but this choice defines the effect incorrectly. The photoelectric effect refers to the ejection of electrons upon absorption of high energy photons, not other electrons (the photoelectric effect is a concern with X-ray or gamma ray treatment). Choice C is therefore eliminated. That leaves choice D. Choice D is correct: beta particles are not as penetrative as protons because they have less kinetic energy and momentum due to their smaller mass (because of the restrictions of special relativity, it is technically difficult to impart energies in the high MeV range to electrons).

5. **C** Choice A is incorrect since nothing can travel faster than the speed of light in vacuum (3×10^8 m/s). Choice B is also wrong because protons are not electromagnetic waves and will always travel slower than the speed of light in vacuum. To answer this question, you can assume that 0.7 MeV is the kinetic energy of the proton and $KE = (1/2)mv^2$. In this equation, KE is in joules, mass is in *kg*, and v is in m/s. So: (0.7 MeV) $\times$ (1.6×10^{-13} J/MeV) = $(1/2)(1.67 \times 10^{-27}$ kg$)v^2$. You can simplify the math by canceling the 1.6 on the left side of the equation with the 1.67 on the right side of the equation. Handling the powers of 10, you get $1.4 \times 10^{14} = v^2$. Taking the square root of both sides, you get $v = 1.2 \times 10^7$ m/s.

6. **B** According to paragraph 1, X-rays (photons) will reach their maximum dose "shortly after" they have entered the body. This eliminates graphs A and C. Then, the dosage decreases but will not reach zero, therefore, choice D is incorrect. Choice B is correct: X-rays interact with the skin (again eliminating choice D), interact more over a short distance, then drop off as a decaying exponential before leaving the body.

Part 8

MCAT
Critical Analysis and Reasoning Skills

Chapter 40
CARS Practice Passages

CARS PRACTICE PASSAGE 1

We freeze some moments in time. Every culture has events so important they transcend the normal flow of news.

In 1945, people gathered around radios for the news [of President Roosevelt's death], and stayed with the radio to hear more about their fallen leader. Newspapers [and magazines] filled their columns with detail for weeks afterward. Something similar happened in 1963, but with a newer medium. The immediate news of John F. Kennedy's assassination came for most via television. As in the earlier time, newspapers and magazines added detail and context. September 11, 2001, followed a similarly grim pattern. We watched—again and again—the airplanes exploding into the skyscrapers, thanks to the television networks.

But something else, something profound, was happening this time around: news was being produced by regular people who had something to say, and not solely by "official" news organizations. This time, the first draft of history was being written in part by the former audience, in blogs and other forms of social media. It was possible—it was inevitable—because of new publishing tools available on the Internet. We were witnessing—and in many cases were part of—the future of news.

In the 20th century, making the news was almost entirely the province of journalists, newsmakers, and marketing people. The economics of publishing and broadcasting created large, arrogant institutions—call it Big Media. Big Media treated the news as a lecture. We told you what the news was. You bought it, or you didn't. Tomorrow's news reporting and production will be more of a conversation. The lines will blur between producers and consumers. The communication network itself will be a medium for everyone's voice, not just the few who can afford to buy multimillion-dollar printing presses or win the government's permission to squat on the public's airwaves.

When anyone can be a journalist, many talented people will try—and they'll find things the professionals miss. Politicians and business people, the newsmakers, are learning this every day. The people at the edges of the communications and social networks can be a newsmaker's harshest, most effective critics. But they can also be the most fervent and valuable allies, offering ideas to each other and to the newsmaker as well.

Big Media enjoys high profit margins. For Wall Street, however, no margin is sufficiently rich, and next year's profits must be higher still. Wall Street's demands on Big Media are dumbing down the product itself. This has led to a hollowing-out syndrome: newspaper publishers and broadcasting station managers have realized they can cut the amount and quality of journalism in order to raise

profits. In case after case, the demands of Wall Street and the greed of investors have subsumed the "public trust" part of journalism…. Consolidation makes it even more worrisome. Media companies are merging to create ever larger information and entertainment conglomerates. In too many cases, serious journalism—and the public trust—continue to be victims. All of this leaves a journalistic opening, and new journalists— especially citizen journalists—are filling the gap.

Who will do big investigative projects, backed by deep pockets and the ability to pay expensive lawyers when powerful interests try to punish those who exposed them, if the business model collapses? At a more prosaic level, who will serve, for better or worse, as a principal voice of a community or region? Flawed as Big Media may be in the business of journalism, anarchy in news is not my idea of a solution. Credibility matters. People need, and want, trusted sources—and those sources have been, for the most part, serious journalists. Instead of journalism organizations with the critical mass to fight the good fights, we may be left with the equivalent of countless pamphleteers and people shouting from soapboxes. We need something better.

It won't be immediately workable for the people who already get so little attention from Big Media. Today, citizen journalism is mostly the province of what former newspaper editor Tom Stites calls "a rather narrow and very privileged slice of the polity—those who are educated enough to take part in the wired conversation, who have the technical skills, and who are affluent enough to have the time and equipment." However, with the proliferation of social media a larger and larger percentage of the population is finding the means to make their views known; to our discredit, we in Big Media have not listened to them as well as we should. The rise of the citizen journalist will help us listen. The ability of anyone to make the news will give new voice to people who've felt voiceless— and whose words we need to hear. They are showing all of us—citizen, journalist, newsmaker—new ways of talking, of learning. In the end, they may help spark a renaissance of the notion, now threatened, of a truly informed citizenry.

Adapted from D. Gillmor, *We the Media: Grassroots Journalism, By the People, For the People.* © 2004 by O'Reilly Media, Inc.

1. According to the passage, the frozen moment after which the production of "the first draft of history" changed drastically was:

A) the emergence of the Internet.
B) Franklin Roosevelt's death.
C) JFK's assassination.
D) the September 11th terrorist attacks.

2. The author would most likely agree that which of the following voices has too much strength in today's current model of Big Media news production?

A) An intelligent blogger
B) A serious journalist
C) A wealthy media mogul
D) A loud pamphleteer

3. In May 2008, accurate news of a devastating earthquake in China was reported by a blogger an hour before any major news outlets began confirming and then reporting it. According to the author of the passage, this is likely an example of the influence of:

A) "a narrow and very privileged slice of the polity."
B) "people shouting from soapboxes."
C) "the few who can afford to buy multimillion-dollar printing presses."
D) "a principal voice of a community."

4. The main idea of the passage is that:

A) advertisers should also provide revenue for citizen journalists.
B) shifts in how consumers get information are affecting the status quo of news production.
C) in order to be heard, journalists need wide exposure rather than an investigative angle.
D) the emergence of widespread blogging and other "democratic" media is the main contributor to the decline in serious journalism.

5. The author suggests that "hollowing-out syndrome" results in:

A) newspapers laying off staff reporters to save money.
B) a loss of credibility in broadcast and printed news stories.
C) cutting the length of printed stories in newspapers to make room for more ads.
D) consumers becoming overwhelmed by the amount of information constantly available.

6. Based on the passage, the author would most likely agree with which of the following statements?

A) Big Media has caused irreparable damage to the news industry and should be replaced entirely.
B) The suppositions and misinformation provided by blogs and social media make it hard to find credible information.
C) It is always preferable to get news from bloggers rather than from news anchors.
D) Bloggers and other citizen journalists can be useful to politicians and business leaders.

7. Which of the following developments would most strengthen the author's argument about the effect on journalism of Big Media's current business plan?

A) In their attempts to beat other networks to the big scoops, thereby gaining more viewers and more advertising dollars, news networks will broadcast stories without waiting to verify the information they get, which can result in the dissemination of inaccurate or wrong information.
B) Despite the efforts of Middle Eastern governments to block news of government protests from leaving their countries, citizens of the countries in turmoil will still able to get news of the events to the rest of the world through social media.
C) Independent viral news sites created and maintained by citizen journalists begin to grow rapidly, a few becoming the fastest-growing media companies in the world.
D) Major newsmagazines and newspapers, after steadily losing subscribers and advertisers, begin to cease publication of their print editions and go to all-digital formats.

CARS PRACTICE PASSAGE 2

The word *myth* belongs with the terms that Humpty Dumpty says deserve extra pay for doing so much work. To its detractors, such as David Bidney, the word suggests that which is unreal and untrue. Bidney admits that as a cultural force myth must be taken seriously, but "only in order that it may be gradually superseded in the interests of the advancement of truth and the growth of human intelligence." To Bidney, myth is an outdated and inauthentic form of religious expression. Yet I would argue that it is unnecessary to discredit myth by linking it to lies and deception. It is not important to measure the stories in Genesis against scientific discoveries. The empires of the past that used myth to enslave the religious sensibilities of countless millions no longer have any claim on the population. In our modern maturity we should not reject the old stories but rather recollect and learn from them in tranquility.

To its defenders, such as Mircea Eliade, myth is the source of reality and truth inasmuch as it provides human beings with models and patterns of behavior thought to be divinely established. Myth, then, is not simply another form of religious expression—it is religion—complete, authentic, and ineradicable.

Eliade's conclusion is that myths are sacred, exemplary, and significant. Instead of leading humanity away from reality, myths provide safe passage into reality; instead of promoting social delusions, myths, by encouraging imitation of preexisting models, promote social cohesion; instead of alienating people, myths put them in touch not only with themselves but with the entire cosmos. Myths serve an aetiological function. This cannot be denied. They tell, surely, how the leopard got its spots, why man must work by the sweat of his brow, why women must bring forth children in pain, and so forth; but in light of the foregoing discussion, this explanatory function must be understood ontologically, as an attempt to understand the question of how all things came, fundamentally, to be the way they are. "To be or not to be," Hamlet said, reducing the world's most profound question to six exact monosyllables.

The comparative mythologist Joseph Campbell in his four-volume study of world mythology, *The Masks of God,* argues that myth serves four primary functions—the mystical, the cosmological, the sociological, and the psychological. First, by opening back into the mystery of things, into the "eternal myth," it helps reconcile our own consciousness with the preconditions of its own existence; second, it provides an image of the cosmos acceptable to the science of time; third, it tells us who we are in the social scheme; and fourth, it helps us through various crises in life, from birth to death. This fourth function, Campbell says, is the most important since it supports the other three.

Campbell showed that the adventures of all the great heroes of myth are remarkably similar. Behind all the bewildering disguises, the thousand faces of the hero, is the single, unchanging face, the true hero of myth and legend. Understood psychologically, the hero story is the depiction, in symbolic terms, of the quest of the human soul for complete realization. The true hero is the self, that is, me. I am the hero.

To speak about Western history as a story of demythologization is to create another myth, the myth of demythologization.

Adapted from M. W. Sexson, "Myth: The Way We Were or the Way We Are?" from *Introduction to the Study of Religion.* © 1978 by Harper & Row.

1. Which of the following definitions of *aetiological* would best fit its usage in the passage (paragraph 3)?

A) Explaining the origin of pain in childbirth
B) Explaining the cause of a contemporary situation by means of an ancient story
C) Delineating the empirical causes of a disease
D) Promoting social cohesion

2. Bidney would most likely agree with which one of the following statements about myth?

A) It is a comprehensive symbolic form that orients people to all dimensions of reality.
B) It is an important factor in our relationship to reality.
C) It is a primitive form of religious thought destined to be outgrown.
D) It reveals the deep structures of the mind.

3. Which of the following would Campbell agree is the most significant function of myth?

A) Psychological, because it upholds both our understanding of how we fit socially and the reconciliation of our consciousness with the circumstances of our existence.
B) The psychological, because it shows that the self is the true hero.
C) The sociological, because it offers us some understanding of the difficulties that we inevitably must encounter in our social lives.
D) The sociological, because it supports who we are in the social scheme.

4. With which of the following statements would Eliade most likely agree?

A) Myth enables humans to achieve complete self-understanding.
B) Myth makes it easier to cope with truth, but myths are not themselves actually true.
C) Myth can serve a useful psychological purpose for people today.
D) Myth can help us understand the world in which we live.

5. The author most likely quotes Hamlet (paragraph 3) in order to:

A) question whether myth represents truth.
B) suggest that we use myth to try to understand the way things are.
C) suggest that stories help us to recognize the value of life.
D) introduce the concept of the myth of demythologization.

6. Plato acknowledged the functional value of myth, claiming that while centaurs and "countless other remarkable monsters of legends" could never be considered literal realities, for certain "crude minds" myths will always be necessary. What relationship, if any, does this information have to the author's argument?

A) It would be inconsistent with the author's support for Eliade's idea that myth is a kind of reality.
B) It would weaken it, since the author finds myth to be relevant to even educated people.
C) It would be consistent with the author's discussion of the myth of demythologization.
D) It would strengthen it, since the author would agree that myths are not literally true.

CARS PRACTICE PASSAGE 3

The "creative process" should cover the entire sequence from the subconscious origins of a literary work to those last revisions which, with some writers, are the most genuinely creative part of the whole.

There is a distinction to be made between the mental structure of a poet and the composition of a poem, between impression and expression. Croce has not won the assent of writers and critics to his reduction of both to aesthetic intuition; indeed, something like the contrary reduction has plausibly been argued by C. S. Lewis. But any attempt to definitively separate "experience" and "poetry," after the fashion of Kilthey, also fails to satisfy. The painter sees as a painter; the painting is the clarification and completion of his seeing. The poet is a maker of poems; but the matter of his poems is the whole of his percipient life. With the artist, in any medium, every impression is shaped by his art; he accumulates no inchoate experience.

Of the creative process itself, not much has been said at the degree of generalization profitable to literary theory. We have the individual case histories of particular authors; but these of course will be authors from comparatively recent times only, and authors given to thinking and writing analytically about their art (authors like Goethe and Schiller, Flaubert, James, Eliot, and Valéry); and then we have the long-distance generalizations made by psychologists concerning such topics as originality, invention, imagination, finding the common denominator between scientific, philosophical, and aesthetic creation.

Any modern treatment of the creative process should chiefly concern the relative parts played by the unconscious and the conscious mind. It would be easy to contrast literary periods: to distinguish romantic and expressionistic periods which exalt the unconscious from classical and realistic periods which stress intelligence, revision, communication. But such a contrast may readily be exaggerated: the critical theories of classicism and romanticism differ more violently than the creative practices of their best writers.

Can psychology, in its turn, be used to interpret and evaluate the literary works themselves? Psychology obviously can illuminate the creative process. As we have seen, attention has been given to the varying methods of composition, to the habits of authors in revising and rewriting. There has been study of the genesis of works: the early stages, the first drafts, the rejected readings. Yet the critical relevance of much of this information, especially the many anecdotes about writers' habits, is surely overrated. A study of the author's revisions and corrections of the actual work has more which is literarily profitable, since, well used, it may help us perceive critically relevant fissures, inconsistencies, turnings, distortions in a work of art. Analyzing how Proust composed his cyclic novel, Feuillerat illuminates

the later volumes, enabling us to distinguish several layers in their text. A study of variants seems to permit glimpses into an author's workshop.

Yet if we examine even these later revisions and corrections more soberly, we conclude them not, finally, necessary to an understanding of the finished work or to a judgment upon it. Their interest is that of any alternative, i.e., they may set into relief the qualities of the final text. But the same end may very well be achieved by devising for ourselves alternatives, whether or not they have actually passed through the author's mind.

For some conscious artists, psychology may have tightened their sense of reality, sharpened their powers of observation or allowed them to fall into hitherto undiscovered patterns. But, in itself, psychology is only preparatory to the act of creation; and in the work itself, psychological truth is an artistic value only if it enhances coherence and complexity—if, in short, *it is art.*

Adapted from R. Wellek and A. Warren, *Theory of Literature.*© 1942 by Houghton Mifflin Harcourt Publishing Company.

1. What is the main idea of the passage?

A) Psychology can be an art in itself.
B) Studying early, unpublished drafts of a literary work is not necessary to understanding or judging the finished product.
C) A psychological analysis of the creative process has some benefits but is not always or intrinsically useful in the study of a work of art itself.
D) Poets differ psychologically from painters.

2. The authors mention Feuillerat in order to support which of the following points?

A) An examination of an author's drafts is an exercise in futility.
B) A psychological assessment of Proust's creative process is difficult to make.
C) The critical relevance of anecdotes of writer's habits is overrated.
D) Sometimes psychology provides insight into the creative process.

3. The author implies all of the following EXCEPT:

A) literary periods can be easily contrasted.
B) no impression made on an artist escapes being shaped by that artist's art.
C) psychology in itself has limited artistic value.
D) creative practices of the best writers differ more substantially from one another than do the theories of different literary periods.

4. According to the passage, James is:

A) an author who reflected upon his creative process and wrote about the act of writing.
B) a psychologist who made generalizations about creativity.
C) an author whose writing has enabled psychologists to come to general conclusions about imaginative writing.
D) an author of whom the authors of the passage approve.

5. Suppose an early manuscript of James Joyce's novel *Ulysses* is uncovered. In the draft, the final sentence of the novel is "Never a doubt" instead of the simple "Yes" in the published version. The alternate ending leads many Joyce scholars to fundamentally reinterpret the novel and reject many previous understandings of the work. How would the authors of the passage respond to these scholars' actions?

A) They would approve because the study of Joyce's early draft would enable psychologists and literary theorists to gain a new and unique insight into the author's creative process.
B) They would argue that the rejection of previous interpretations is misguided because the study of drafts and revisions is not the only way to gain a valid understanding of a work.
C) They would be scornful because revisions to earlier drafts are irrelevant to an understanding of the finished work.
D) They would suggest that psychologists, not literary scholars, should be the ones reinterpreting the novel.

6. What is the most significant concern in a modern treatment of the creative process, according to the passage?

A) The literary period in which an author is situated
B) The psychological health of the artist
C) The roles played by the unconscious and the conscious mind
D) The drafts and revisions of a text made by an author prior to publication

CARS PRACTICE PASSAGE 4

It is good anthropology to think of ballet as a form of ethnic dance. Currently, that idea is unacceptable to most Western dance scholars. This lack of agreement shows clearly that something is amiss in the communication of ideas between the scholars of dance and those of anthropology.

It has been a long time since anthropologists concerned themselves with unknowable origins, and I will not add another origin theory for dance, because I don't know anyone who was there. About the dance of primeval man we really know nothing. About primitive dance, on the other hand, we know a great deal. The first thing that we know is that there is no such thing as *a* primitive dance. There *are* dances performed by primitives, and they are too varied to fit any stereotype.

Despite all anthropological evidence to the contrary, however, Western dance scholars set themselves up as authorities on the characteristics of primitive dance. Sorell combines most of these so-called characteristics of the primitive stereotype. However, his paternalistic feelings on the one hand, and his sense of ethnocentricity on the other, prompt him to set aside any thought that people with whom he identifies could share contemporarily those same dance characteristics.

Another significant obstacle to the identification of Western dancers with non-Western dance forms, be they primitive or "ethnologic" is the double myth that the dance grew out of some spontaneous mob action and that once formed, became frozen. Apparently it satisfies our own ethnocentric needs to believe in the uniqueness of our dance forms, and it is much more convenient to believe that primitive dances, like Topsy, just "growed," and that "ethnological" dances are part of an unchanging tradition.

Let it be noted, once and for all, that within the various "ethnologic" dance worlds there are also patrons, dancing masters, choreographers, and performers with names woven into a very real historical fabric. The bias which those dancers have toward their own dance and artists is just as strong as ours. The difference is that they usually don't pretend to be scholars of other dance forms, nor even very much interested in them.

I have made listings of the themes and other characteristics of ballet and ballet performances, and these lists show over and over again just how "ethnic" ballet is. Consider, for example, how Western is the tradition of the proscenium stage, the usual three part performance which lasts for about two hours, our use of curtain calls and applause, and our usage of French terminology. Think how our worldview is revealed in the oft recurring themes of unrequited love, sorcery, self-sacrifice through long-suffering, mistaken identity, and misunderstandings which have tragic consequences.

Our aesthetic values are shown in the long line of lifted, extended bodies, in the total revealing of legs, of small heads and tiny feet for women, in slender bodies for both sexes, and in the coveted airy quality which is best shown in the lifts and carryings of the female. To us this is tremendously pleasing aesthetically, but there are societies whose members would be shocked at the public display of the male touching the female's thighs! So distinctive is the "look" of ballet, that it is probably safe to say that ballet dances graphically rendered by silhouettes would never be mistaken for anything else. An interesting proof of this is the ballet *Koshare* which was based on a Hopi Indian story. In silhouettes of even still photos, the dance looked like ballet and not like a Hopi dance.

The question is not whether ballet reflects its own heritage. The question is why we seem to need to believe that ballet has somehow become acultural. Why are we afraid to call it an ethnic form?

Adapted from J. Kealiinohomoku, "An Anthropologist Looks at Ballet as a Form of Ethnic Dance." © 1970, *Impulse* 20: 24–33.

1. From statements in the passage, it can be inferred that the author would claim that ballet:

A) should be more inclusive of cultural diversity.
B) has a distinctive look that places it above other dance forms.
C) should not be understood as transcending the boundaries of a particular culture.
D) differs from other dance forms by including themes of love and suffering.

2. The author's attitude toward the dance scholars mentioned in the first paragraph can be best described as:

A) sympathy toward their lack of knowledge concerning primeval dance.
B) condemnation of their interpretation of ballet principally as an ethnic dance.
C) approval of their attempts to integrate anthropological findings within their scholarship.
D) criticism of their practice of making claims that exceed their scholarly competence.

3. The author discusses the Koshare ballet in order to:

A) demonstrate that ballet does incorporate different cultural perspectives.
B) underscore the distinctive aesthetic of ballet as a dance form.
C) describe a difference between ballet and traditional Hopi dance forms.
D) counter an earlier suggestion ballet is an "ethnological" dance form.

4. An ethnologist who agrees with Sorell about ethnological dance would be most likely to make which of the following claims?

A) The characteristics of primitive dance are significantly different from those of contemporary ballet.
B) The term "primitive" dance is inaccurate and should be avoided.
C) Contemporary dancers would do well to incorporate certain characteristics of primitive dance.
D) Primitive dances incorporate a considerable variety of form and technique.

5. Which of the following claims is made in the passage?

A) Ballet is more distinctive in its forms and themes than are non-Western dances.
B) Western dance scholars are more inclined to make overarching claims about dance than are experts in other dance traditions.
C) The traditions of "ethnological" dances are less likely to undergo change over time than are Western dance traditions.
D) The traditions of "ethnological" dances are more likely to undergo change over time than are Western dance traditions.

6. Suppose that a contemporary anthropologist sought to prove the thesis that dance originated in primeval communities as a ritual expression of suffering and self-sacrifice. How would the author respond to this argument?

A) The author would approve of drawing links between primeval dance and contemporary ballet.
B) The author would encourage Western dance scholars to incorporate this anthropological foundation into their writings on ballet.
C) The author would question whether appropriate evidence is available to draw such conclusions.
D) The author would challenge the ethnocentric bias of identifying any dance form as primitive.

CARS PRACTICE PASSAGE 5

Why do many intelligent, well-meaning, modern, middle-class parents, so concerned about the happy development of their children, discount the value of fairy tales and deprive their children of what these stories have to offer? Even our Victorian ancestors, despite their emphasis on moral discipline and their stodgy way of life, not only permitted but encouraged their children to enjoy the fantasy and excitement of fairy tales.

From an adult point of view and in terms of modern science, the answers which fairy stories offer are fantastic rather than true. As a matter of fact, these solutions seem so incorrect to many adults that they object to exposing children to such "false" information. However, realistic explanations are usually incomprehensible to children, because they lack the abstract understanding required to make sense of them. While giving a scientifically correct answer makes adults think they have clarified things for the child, such explanations leave the young child confused, overpowered, and intellectually defeated. A child can derive security only from the conviction that he understands now what baffled him before—never from being given facts which create new uncertainties. Even as the child accepts such an answer, he comes to doubt that he has asked the right question. Since the explanation fails to make sense to him, it must apply to some unknown problem—not the one he asked about.

We do encourage our children's fantasies; we tell them to paint what they want, or to invent stories. But unfed by our common fantasy heritage, the folk fairy tale, the child cannot invent stories on his own which help him cope with life's problems. All the stories he can invent are just expressions of his own wishes and anxieties. Relying on his own resources, all the child can imagine are elaborations of where he presently is, since he cannot know where he needs to go, nor how to go about getting there. This is where the fairy tale provides what the child needs most: it begins exactly where the child is emotionally, shows him where he has to go, and how to do it. But the fairy tale does this by implication, in the form of fantasy material which the child can draw on as seems best to him, and by means of images which make it easy for him to comprehend what is essential for him to understand.

Because some people withdraw from the world and spend most of their days in the realm of their imaginings, it has been mistakenly suggested that an over-rich fantasy life interferes with our coping successfully with reality. But the opposite is true: those who live completely in their fantasies are beset by compulsive ruminations which rotate eternally around some narrow, stereotypical topics. Far from having a rich fantasy life, such people are locked in, and they cannot break out of one anxious or wish-fulfilling daydream. But free-floating fantasy, which contains in imaginary form a wide variety of issues also encountered in reality, provides the ego with an abundance of material to work with. This rich and variegated fantasy life is provided to the child by fairy stories, which can help prevent his imagination from getting stuck within the narrow confines of a few anxious or wish-fulfilling daydreams circling around a few narrow preoccupations.

If a child is told only stories "true to reality" (which means false to important parts of his inner reality), then he may conclude that much of his inner reality is unacceptable to his parents. Many a child thus estranges himself from his inner life, and this depletes him. As a consequence he may later, as an adolescent no longer under the emotional sway of his parents, come to hate the rational world and escape entirely into a fantasy world, as if to make up for what was lost in childhood. At an older age, on occasion this could imply a severe break with reality, with all the dangerous consequences for the individual and society. Or, less seriously, the person may continue this encapsulation of his inner self all through his life and never feel fully satisfied in the world because, alienated from the unconscious processes, he cannot use them to enrich his life in reality. Life is then neither "a pleasure" nor "a kind of eccentric privilege." With such separation, whatever happens in reality fails to offer appropriate satisfaction of unconscious needs. The result is that the person always feels life to be incomplete.

Adapted from B. Bettelheim, *The Uses of Enchantment: The Meaning and Importance of Fairy Tales.* © 1989 by Vintage Books.

1. The passage indicates that fairy tales are most important in providing:

A) an escape into a fantasy world.
B) fantasy and excitement.
C) emotional and creative inspiration.
D) emotional independence from parental control.

2. Based on the passage, what can be inferred about the Victorians?

A) They preferred fairy tales to other children's stories.
B) They were not concerned with the proper development of their children.
C) They allowed their children to read fairy tales.
D) They believed that fairy tales contributed to moral discipline.

3. What is the main idea of the passage?

A) Many modern parents don't agree with exposing their children to fairy tales.
B) Fairy tales are important for proper psychological development.
C) Fairy tales help children create stories to cope with their emotions.
D) Fairy tales provide a rich and exciting fantasy world for all ages.

4. According to the passage, which of the following will happen when a child is told a realistic story?

    I.   The child will alienate himself from his inner personality.
    II.   The child will invent stories of his own.
    III. The child won't be able to understand it.

A) III only
B) I and II only
C) I and III only
D) II and III only

5. The author uses the example of the Victorians in order to:

A) suggest that our modern society is unusual in its dismissal of the value of childhood fairy tales.
B) show how modern science has altered modern parents' views of fairy tales.
C) demonstrate what might happen if a child is not exposed to fairy tales.
D) show the contrast between fairy tales now and then.

6. The psychologist Piaget claims that children cannot comprehend abstract ideas until late adolescence. If valid, what effect does this have on the author's arguments in the passage?

A) It weakens the claim that fairy tales are not effective in furthering development once a child gets older.
B) It weakens the claim that adults who were never exposed to fairy tales will permanently escape into a fantasy world.
C) It strengthens the claim that a child is not able to understand scientific explanations.
D) It strengthens the claim that fairy tales are a significant aspect of psychological development.

CARS PRACTICE PASSAGE 6

Any incident is comic that calls our attention to the physical in a person when it is the moral side that is concerned.

Why do we laugh at a public speaker who sneezes just at the most pathetic moment of his speech? Where lies the comic element in this sentence, taken from a funeral speech and quoted by a German philosopher: "He was virtuous and plump"? In the fact that our attention is suddenly recalled from the soul to the body. A speaker whose most eloquent sentences are cut short by the twinges of a bad tooth; one of the characters who never begins to speak without stopping in the middle to complain of his shoes being too small, or his belt too tight, etc. A person embarrassed by his appearance is the image suggested to us in all these examples. Excessive stoutness is laughable probably because it calls up an image of the same kind. This too is what sometimes makes bashfulness somewhat ridiculous. The bashful man rather gives the impression of a person embarrassed by his body, looking round for some convenient cloak-room in which to deposit it.

This is just why the tragic poet is so careful to avoid anything calculated to attract attention to the material side of his heroes. No sooner does anxiety about the body manifest itself than the intrusion of a comic element is to be feared. On this account, the hero in a tragedy does not eat or drink or warm himself. He does not even sit down any more than can be helped. To sit down in the middle of a fine speech would imply that you remembered you had a body. Napoleon, who was a psychologist when he wished to be so, noted that the transition from tragedy to comedy is effected simply by sitting down. "She received me in tragic fashion, continuing in a way most embarrassing to me. Finally, to make her change her style, I requested her to take a seat. This is the best method for cutting short a tragic scene, for as soon as you are seated it all becomes comedy."

Let us now give a wider scope to this image of the body taking precedence of the soul. We shall obtain something more general—the manner seeking to outdo the matter, the letter aiming at ousting the spirit. Is it not perchance this idea that comedy is trying to suggest to us when holding up a profession to ridicule? It makes the lawyer, the magistrate and the doctor speak as though health and justice were of little moment—the main point being that we should have lawyers, magistrates and doctors, and that all outward formalities pertaining to these professions should be scrupulously respected. The means substituted for the end, the manner for the matter; no longer is it the profession that is made for the public, but rather the public for the profession. Constant attention to form and the mechanical application of rules here bring about a kind of professional automatism analogous to that imposed upon the soul by the habits of the body, and equally laughable. Numerous are the examples of this on the stage.

Here we have the first illustration of a law which will appear with increasing distinctness. When a musician strikes a note on an instrument, other notes start up of themselves, not so loud as the first, yet connected with it by certain definite relations, which coalesce with it and determine its quality. These are what are called in physics the overtones of the fundamental note. It would seem that comic fancy, even in its most far-fetched inventions, obeys a similar law. For instance, consider this comic note: appearance seeking to triumph over reality. If our analysis is correct, this note must have as its overtones the body tantalizing the mind, the body taking precedence of the mind. No sooner, then, does the comic poet strike the first note than he will add the second on to it, involuntarily and instinctively. In other words, he will duplicate what is ridiculous professionally with something that is ridiculous physically.

Adapted from H. Bergson, "Laughter: An Essay on the Meaning of the Comic." © 1914 by The MacMillan Co.

1. Which of the following statements made in the passage is NOT supported in the passage by example or explanation?

A) The stage offers numerous examples of laughable automatism.
B) Bashfulness may be laughable in certain circumstances.
C) Comic moments occur when the focus unexpectedly shifts from soul to body.
D) Sitting down is the best technique for ending a tragic episode.

2. The analogy to music serves in the passage to:

A) offer a counterpoint to the law the author articulates.
B) draw an analogy between the tragic poet and the musician.
C) illustrate the far-fetched inventions of comic fancy.
D) support the author's discussion of the multilayered nature of comic moments.

3. Suppose accounts written by Napoleon's personal secretary revealed that Napoleon always stood when receiving diplomatic guests. Based on this and information from the passage, the author would most likely assert which of the following about Napoleon?

A) He sought to demonstrate power over the individuals he dealt with.
B) He chose to give his soul precedence over his body.
C) He wished to avoid one source of levity in affairs of state.
D) He had not yet come to understand that sitting produces a comic situation.

4. When the author refers to the "outward formalities" (paragraph 4) of the professions of lawyers, magistrates, and doctors, he most nearly means:

A) the formal, rule-bound approach those positions require.
B) the comically formal appearance of people uniformed for work in those professions.
C) the respect owed to those who pursue such intellectually strenuous careers.
D) the professional courtesy of not mocking professions that contribute positively to society.

5. If a literary scholar uncovered a version of Euripides's ancient Greek tragedy *Medea* that included a scene in which Medea, the heroine, is sitting at dinner as she discusses her plan to murder her children, this discovery would have which of the following relationships to the arguments presented in the passage?

A) It would support Napoleon's assertion that sitting shortens a tragic scene.
B) It would further illustrate the author's point about manner substituting for matter.
C) It would be inconsistent the author's conception of the tragic poet.
D) It would weaken the German philosopher's proposed relation between plumpness and virtue.

6. The author would most likely disagree with which of the following statements?

A) A cough may draw attention to the body.
B) An artist may choose to play overtones as well as tones.
C) Referring to excessive tallness probably calls up a laughable image.
D) A tragic hero is unlikely to be found brushing his teeth.

CARS PRACTICE PASSAGE 7

The notion that memory can be "distorted" assumes that there is a standard by which we can judge or measure what a veridical memory must be. If this is difficult with individual memory, it is even more complex with collective memory, where the past event or experience remembered was truly a different event or experience for its different participants. Moreover, whereas we can accept with little question that biography or the lifetime is the appropriate or "natural" frame for individual memory, there is no such evident frame for cultural memories. Neither national boundaries nor linguistic ones are as self-evidently the right containers for collective memory as the person is for individual memory.

I take the view that, in an important sense, there is no such thing as individual memory, and it is well for me to make this plain at the outset. Memory is social. It is social, first of all, because it is located in institutions rather than in individual human minds in the form of rules, laws, standardized procedures, and records, a whole set of cultural practices through which people recognize a debt to the past (including the notion of "debt" itself) or through which they express moral continuity with the past (tradition, identity, career, curriculum). These cultural forms store and transmit information that individuals make use of without themselves "memorizing" it. The individual's capacity to make use of the past piggybacks on the social and cultural practices of memory. I can move over great distances at a speed of 600 miles per hour without knowing the first thing about what keeps an airplane aloft. I benefit from a cultural storehouse of knowledge, very little of which I am obliged to have in my own head. Cultural memory, available for the use of an individual, is distributed across social institutions and cultural artifacts.

As soon as you recognize how collective memory, and even individual memory, is inextricable from social and historical processes, the notion of "distortion" of the truth becomes problematic. As the British historian Peter Burke writes, "Remembering the past and writing about it no longer seem the innocent activities they were once taken to be. Neither memories nor histories seem objective any longer. In both cases, this selection, interpretation and distortion is socially conditioned. It is not the work of individuals alone." Distortion is to some degree inevitable, rather than representing an aberration from a norm. Memory is distortion since memory is invariably and inevitably selective. A way of seeing is a way of not seeing, a way of remembering is a way of forgetting, too. If memory were only a kind of registration, a "true" memory might be possible. But memory is a process of encoding information, storing information, and strategically retrieving information, and there are social, psychological, and historical influences at each point.

Contest, conflict, controversy—these are the hallmark of studies of collective memory, rather than the concept of distortion.

Discovering the attitudes and interests of the present therefore becomes of much greater concern than the legitimate claims of the past upon them. However, a focus on distortion still makes sense in studies of collective or cultural memory. Even the most ardently relativist scholars among us shiver with revulsion at certain versions of the past that cry out "distortion." The most famous example is the flourishing fringe group of Holocaust revisionists who deny that there was ever a plan to exterminate the Jews or that such a plan was ever set in place. The question of what content of the past is not or cannot or should not be subject to latter-day reinterpretation haunts the papers at a 1990 conference at U.C.L.A. on "Nazism and the 'Final Solution': Probing the Limits of Representation." The fascination with conflicting versions of the past and the excitement over legitimately revisionist interpretations of once settled and consensual accounts come precisely from the fact that even trained historians (or perhaps especially trained historians) retain strong beliefs in a veritable past. If interpretation were free-floating, entirely manipulable to serve present interests, altogether unanchored by a bedrock body of unshakable evidence, controversies over the past would ultimately be uninteresting. But in fact they are interesting. They are compelling. And they are gripping because people trust that a past we can to some extent know and can to some extent come to agreement about really happened.

Adapted from M. Schudson, "Dynamics in Distortion of Collective Memory," in *Memory Distortion: How Minds, Brains, and Societies Reconstruct the Past*, edited by Daniel L. Schacter, Cambridge, Mass.: Harvard University Press, Copyright © 1995 by the President and Fellows of Harvard College.

1. With which of the following statements would the author most likely agree regarding the nature of individual memory?

   A) It is a fiction created to explain collective memory.
   B) It causes conceptual problems when considering approaches to understanding distortion.
   C) It is entwined with and dependent on social institutions that perpetuate it.
   D) It is distinct from collective memory in several important ways.

2. In the last lines of the final paragraph, the author notes that controversies over the past are in fact interesting. How is this claim related to the author's argument in this paragraph?

A) It is a side note used to conclude the discussion, but has little relevance to the argument as a whole.
B) It is of historical importance regarding the underpinnings of distortions that periodically occur.
C) It supports the overall argument by implication, as the contrary notion would undermine it.
D) It is an exception noted to anticipate arguments to the contrary.

3. In the first paragraph, the author says that "there's no such evident frame for cultural memories." This most likely means that:

A) the fact that the human race has no natural lifespan implies a continuity of institutional memories for the race as a whole.
B) cultural memories are a property of a group and are thus not shared with other groups.
C) cultural memories are not directly accessible to individuals, whose memories have natural frames.
D) national and linguistic boundaries, not an individual lifespan, define the nature of collective memories.

4. The author's claims regarding the nature of individual memory would be most *undermined* if which of the following were to become evident?

A) The relationship of seemingly persistent cultural memories to any particular individual depends largely on that individual's personal history and perceptions.
B) Individuals can demonstrably memorize information in a standard memory task.
C) Cultural forms are exceptionally consistent within certain linguistic realms.
D) Small, isolated populations carry little institutional memory, yet thrive within their environments.

5. The author argues that memory is inevitably distortion. Which of the following, if true, would most support this point of view?

A) We selectively choose the memories we report to others.
B) The majority of participants in memory tests are able to successfully recall most items in a list.
C) Numerous mental faculties have been shown to be integral to the process of memory storage and retrieval.
D) Studies show that human attention is limited and that little sensory information is retrievable later in time.

6. The author says toward the end of the passage that "people trust that a past we can to some extent know and can to some extent come to agreement about really happened," while stating elsewhere in the passage that there is no such thing as individual memory. These claims are:

A) not inconsistent, because they refer to discussions of different aspects of memory.
B) consistent, because the claim regarding the possibility of agreement supports the claim regarding individual memory.
C) somewhat contradictory, because it is difficult to justify the notion that controversies over the past are gripping given the absence of individual memories.
D) strongly at odds, because the claim regarding the non-existence of individual memory undermines the claim regarding coming to agreement about the past.

7. Suppose a psychological study were performed in which participants in a group setting were asked to come to a consensus regarding the value of recording certain (real or hypothetical) historical facts and ignoring others. If in the study it was observed that certain dominant individuals had a much greater influence on the process of selecting the salient facts to report (e.g., one or a few were able to alter the views of the majority on many issues), what effect would this have on the author's claim in the first sentence of the third paragraph?

A) It would have little bearing on the issue, as dominant individuals have always had inordinate influence on documented facts.
B) It would tend to support the author's claim, as it would show a particular mechanism via which distortions of collective memory might proceed.
C) It would tend to weaken the author's claim, as it would show that distortion of memories is a fairly ordinary event in social settings.
D) It would tend to weaken the author's claim, as it would explain the ultimate origin of most distortions of collective memory.

CARS PRACTICE PASSAGE 8

The noble portico of the Perkins House in Windham, Connecticut (1832), the elliptical arches of the facade of the Rider House in Rensselaersville, New York (1823), the intricate parapets of the Norris House in Bristol, Rhode Island (1810), and hundreds of other equally striking details all attest to the fact that builders throughout the United States were not only thinking about architecture, but were also enjoying it.

Such builders have often been criticized for not finding that elusive median between convention and invention or for being either slavishly imitative or indulgently original. This criticism has often focused on their use of the Greek temple front. On the one hand, [it was claimed that] it had become too much of a standard; it was applied indiscriminately to house, bank, tavern, or store. On the other hand, it was rarely designed according to precedent. American builders quickly learned that a wood column supporting only a light load could be much thinner than a stone member holding up a heavy pediment. Such attenuation not only seemed awkward to critics who knew the history of the orders, but it was also symptomatic of a tendency to place expediency over a concern for the culture of architecture.

Although many examples can be found to validate this criticism, the same point can also be used to illustrate the positive qualities of the period's architecture. The temple front may often have been used indiscriminately, but the flaunting of this iconic element served a purpose that was deeper than functional appropriateness. Its persistent use was a statement about republicanism; it was an affirmation of that system of government and an acknowledgment of a common set of values. Similarly, the custom adopted in this period of painting all buildings white, even older structures, has often been called an insensitive response to local circumstances and a manifestation of a worrying tendency toward conformity. But this convention also showed that architecture had become an important medium of expression, one which Americans could use to show their shared identity as citizens of a new nation.

A similar interpretation can be made of many gestures which have often been called ungainly and ungrammatical. They can be thought of as attempts to find an appropriate local or regional realization of basic classical themes. The temple front may frequently have been used unthinkingly, but it was often artfully adapted to a specific location. It could serve the narrow house lots of Charleston, South Carolina, as well as the ample frontages of the gridded towns of the Ohio valley; it was applicable equally to the hot and humid climate of the Mississippi plantation house and the cold winters of the Nantucket whaler's residence; it could be made of stone to give presence to a prominent urban building and of wood as was appropriate for a modest country house. Similarly, the formal front did not necessarily lie about what happened behind. The

New England farmhouse of this period may have had a portico which led to a sequence of house, shed, barn, and outbuildings, all of which were frequently joined together and straggled into the backyard. Yet the front and the back each encapsulated a significant aspect of the life and dreams of the inhabitants of these buildings. Although different, the two can be read as complementary parts of an unaffected whole.

By 1814 a few Americans were already claiming a special affinity between the American and Greek republics. When the Greeks went to war with the Turks in 1821, the Greek temple front became the symbol of republicanism. As the portico proliferated, architects often decried such an unthinking adaptation of form to function. Nevertheless, they also championed Greek architecture, or specific versions of it, for less than idealistic reasons. Many favored the Doric order, not out of any sense of appropriateness, but because it was easier and cheaper to build. Robert Mills, for example, emphasized commodity and firmness because he understood that these were qualities which most directly appealed to his clients. Mills knew all too well his country's "tastes and requirements." Probably no one understood these problems better than Thomas Jefferson. He shunned Greek architecture and remained committed to what he thought were the more complex and subtle Roman orders. But he did not make his living from architecture. Had he done so, he might have had to reflect more deeply on his experience with the Virginia State Capitol, the scope of which was drastically reduced by a recalcitrant legislature.

Adapted from D. P. Handlin, *American Architecture.* © 1985 by Thames and Hudson.

1. The author would most likely agree that the Greek temple front was all of the following EXCEPT:

A) used at times in unusual ways.
B) a manifestation of American architectural philosophies.
C) a manifestation of American political and economic ideologies.
D) overused.

2. Which of the following best expresses the main idea of the passage?

A) American builders in the 1800s weathered criticism in order to use architecture to help establish an American system of values and government.

B) 19th century American builders had different ideas about architecture than those in the rest of the world, ideas which at first garnered criticism but that also altered and reshaped the discipline, making it more adaptable and creating new possibilities for future generations.

C) Early Americans needed the arts to help them create a national identity different from anything in existence at that time; some 19th century American builders contributed to this effort by using classic elements, such as the Greek temple front, in innovative ways.

D) Although some critics characterized the approach as inappropriate, some 19th century American builders' use and revision of the Greek temple front enabled them to usefully represent the people's values and to fulfill their needs.

3. In this passage, the word "republicanism" is used to describe:

A) the Greek system of government.
B) a government based on common values.
C) government by representation.
D) minimalist government.

4. The author mentions the war between Greece and Turkey in order to:

A) explain the origin of a phenomenon discussed in the third paragraph.
B) justify the architects' criticism of the overuse of the portico.
C) demonstrate the similarity between the United States and Greece.
D) defend Thomas Jefferson's dislike of Greek architecture.

5. Craig Whitaker, in his book *Architecture and the American Dream*, writes "that Americans treat the front of their buildings (as a public or presentational face) much differently than the rear of their buildings (as a private or more functional face)." This perspective if valid:

A) calls into question the author's claim that American architecture is similar to that in other parts of the world.
B) calls into question the author's claim that the front of American buildings was consistent with what occurred behind them.
C) supports the author's claim that the front of American buildings was consistent with what occurred behind them.
D) supports the author's claim that the formal front was incompatible with the sometimes haphazard structure behind it.

6. The author's reference to the contemporary custom "of painting all buildings white" in the third paragraph functions as all of the following EXCEPT:

A) a comparable example to that of the Greek temple front.
B) support for the main idea of the paragraph.
C) support for republicanism.
D) an illustration of the simultaneously negative and positive aspects of some architectural practices.

Chapter 41
Solutions to CARS
Practice Passages

SOLUTIONS TO CARS PRACTICE PASSAGE 1

1. **D** This is a Retrieval question.

   A: No. The Internet is mentioned as a factor in the change, but the emergence of the Internet wasn't the (or even a) frozen moment. It was the availability of the publishing tools that allowed regular folks to communicate and produce news about September 11th (paragraph 3).

   B: No. Roosevelt's death is mentioned at the beginning of the passage, but the news coverage was the traditional radio coverage, supplemented by in-depth newspaper and magazine coverage. After his death, news continued to be disseminated in the same way.

   C: No. Kennedy's assassination is mentioned after Roosevelt's death, and there is a "newer medium" with the use of television, but detail and context were still provided by newspapers and magazines. There was no major change after the event in how news was produced.

   D: Yes. The passage says that the attacks "followed a similarly grim pattern" but then goes on to say, "but something else, something profound, was happening" and explains the major changes in how the news was created and reported by "regular people" (paragraph 3).

2. **C** This is an Inference question.

   A: No. The author says that these are the people "who already get so little attention from Big Media" (paragraph 8). Therefore, they do *not* have a strong voice in today's current model, and the author believes that their voice should be stronger than it is.

   B: No. The author says that serious journalism is "a victim" of the consolidation of media companies.

   C: Yes. The communication network is currently a medium for the voices of those who "can afford to buy multimillion-dollar printing presses," to the detriment of serious journalism (paragraphs 4 and 6).

   D: The author mentions the pamphleteer as part of a metaphor for the possible consequences of the unraveling of today's media model, not as someone who actually exists or is a part of the news production today.

3. **A** This is a New Information question.

   A: Yes. This is an example of the new trend toward citizen journalists getting information out more quickly than Big Media. Toward the end of the passage, the author uses the phrase in this answer choice to refer to the citizen journalists who are "educated enough to take part in the wired conversation, who have the technical skills, and who...have the time and equipment" (paragraph 8).

   B: No. The author uses this phrase (paragraph 7) as a metaphor for the unreliable information spread by those who are unreliable. While a blogger is not necessarily reliable, this particular situation deals with a blogger who got accurate and relevant information to consumers.

   C: No. This is the exact opposite of the correct answer. This phrase (paragraph 4) refers to those in Big Media, who were the ones who were late to the story.

   D: No. This phrase refers to the serious journalists who were doing "big investigative projects, backed by deep pockets" until Big Media began to shift away from that type of journalism. While the author hopes that the system will move toward more voices with more information, bloggers are not yet that "principal voice," which the author indicates by asking, "Who will serve as [that] voice" (paragraph 7)?

4.   **B**   This is a Main Idea question.

    A: No. While the author of the passage does discuss the role of financial issues in the world of Big Media, he never discusses the financial considerations of citizen journalists, or the advertisers' role in those considerations.

    B: Yes. The author's main point is that the rise of the Internet and social media sites has given consumers many more options for accessing information, and this is causing a significant change in the established order of the news world. This change is possible because the business model of news production has shifted in a way as to open up places for and create a demand for consumer-produced news.

    C: No. The main point of the passage concerns broad shifts in the media landscape, not questions of how a particular journalist may or may not be successful.

    D: No. The author has a largely positive attitude toward "citizen journalism"; he identifies Big Media, not bloggers, as the cause of the problem.

5.   **B**   This is an Inference question.

    A: No. In the text, the author says that "hollowing-out syndrome" involves cutting the amount and quality of the journalism in order to raise profits. There is no mention of laying off any employees.

    B: Yes. The author explains that the "demands of Wall Street and the greed of investors have subsumed the 'public trust' part of journalism" (paragraph 6).

    C: No. There is no discussion of the actual logistics of publishing the paper. There is no mention of cutting the length of stories in order to make room for ads.

    D: No. The phrase cited in the question stem is in reference to the quality of news being put out by Big Media. It does not refer to consumers.

6.   **D**   This is an Inference question.

    A: No. This choice is too extreme. While the author does spend some time discussing problems with Big Media, he also says that "anarchy in news is not my idea of a solution" and that consumers "need, and want, trusted sources" (paragraph 7).

    B: No. While it could be true that finding credible information is difficult, the author never suggests that bloggers convey misinformation. Furthermore, the author describes news anarchy as a future concern, not as a present reality.

    C: No. The "always" in this answer choice is problematic. Bloggers may have good information, but the author never suggests that they are always the best option.

    D: Yes. In the fifth paragraph, the author discusses how those at the edge of the communication networks can be harsh critics for politicians and business people, but then he goes on to say that "they can also be fervent and valuable allies."

7.   **A**   This is a Strengthen question.

    A: Yes. The author explains that "in order to raise profits," those in charge of producing the news have found they can cut "the amount and quality of journalism." He goes on to say that "serious journalism continue[s] to be a victim" of the increasing consolidation of media companies (paragraph 6). In this situation, there is a lack of quality and reporting.

    B: No. This is an advantage of citizen journalism, but it has nothing to do with Big Media or its business plan.

    C: No. This is about a new model of news production, not Big Media's current business plan. Also, there is nothing about the negative effect of the plan on journalism.

    D: No. This is a consequence of a faulty business plan for publications, but it doesn't have anything to do with the quality or amount of journalism.

SOLUTIONS TO CARS PRACTICE PASSAGE 2

1. **B**   This is an Inference question.

   A: No. This is an example of the aetiological function of a particular myth to which the passage alludes, but it is only one example of it, not a definition of the term itself.

   B: Yes. The author uses the phrase "explanatory function" later in the same paragraph to also describe myths. The examples in the passage show myths can give causal explanations for everyday situations.

   C: No. This explanation is appealing, because it is the most common dictionary definition of aetiology, but it is not relevant to the passage. The author does not suggest that myths give actual empirical or factual causal explanations. Furthermore, this would be an example of one type of explanation, not a definition of the term itself.

   D: No. This is the right answer to the wrong question. Promoting social cohesion is something Eliade claims that myths do (paragraph 3), not a definition, in the context of the passage, of the word *aetiological*.

2. **C**   This is an Inference question.

   A: No. This statement is similar to Campbell's view of myth (see paragraph 4), but not to Bidney's.

   B: No. This statement is part of Eliade's point of view, not Bidney's (see paragraphs 2 and 3).

   C: Yes. In the first paragraph, Bidney defines myth as a form of "religious expression" which will be "gradually superseded," that is, outgrown, with "the advancement of truth and the growth of human intelligence," that is, the advancement of civilization itself. It should also help that it's the only one that suggests a negative attitude toward myth, which Bidney demonstrates.

   D: No. This statement aligns most closely with Campbell's concept of the psychological function of myth (paragraph 4), not Bidney's concept of myth (paragraph 1).

3. **A**   This is an Inference question.

   A: Yes. The passage says that the fourth function, which is the psychological one, is the most important because it supports the other three, including the sociological and the mystical (see paragraph 4). Note that the author lists the four functions in the middle of the paragraph, and then discusses each in the same order.

   B: No. While this is one aspect of the psychological function (paragraph 4), it is not why Campbell thinks the psychological function is the most important of the four. Remember that "part right equals all wrong." The correct reference ("psychological") is not enough to make this the credited response; the choice must also accurately reflect Campbell's reasoning.

   C: No. In this statement, the reference ("sociological") is wrong, even though the description does align with the psychological function.

   D: No. While this statement is an accurate description of the sociological function, this (sociological) is not what Campbell considers to be the most significant function of myth.

4. **D** This is an Inference question.
   A: No. While Campbell might agree with this statement (see paragraphs 4 and 5), there is no evidence in the passage that Eliade does. Eliade's view that myth "provides human beings with models and patterns of behavior thought to be divinely established" (paragraph 2) and that "myths put [people] in touch not only with themselves but with the entire cosmos" (paragraph 3) is not enough to support the claim that myths provide complete understanding of ourselves.
   B: No. While the first part of this statement corresponds to the statement in the third paragraph that "myths provide safe passage into reality," there is no evidence in the passage that Eliade believes that myths are not, or cannot be, true.
   C: No. This statement corresponds to Campbell's view (paragraph 4), but there is no evidence in the passage that Eliade would concur about a specifically psychological function.
   D: Yes. This statement aligns with the observation in paragraph 3 that "this explanatory function [of myth] must be understood...as an attempt to understand the question of how all things came, fundamentally, to be the way they are."

5. **B** This is a Structure question.
   A: No. The discussion in the third paragraph leading into the quote is about myth's function, according to Eliade, of providing some explanation (although not necessarily a factual one) of the way things are in reality. Eliade suggests that myths do in fact have relationship to truth; they "provide safe passage into reality" and put people "in touch not only with themselves but with the entire cosmos." Therefore, neither the quote nor the paragraph in which it appears is questioning if myth represents reality.
   B: Yes. This statement expresses the idea discussed in the sentences directly adjacent to the quote, which is the only evidence we have for the author's understanding of the quote: the "explanatory function [of myth] must be understood ontologically, as an attempt to understand the question of how all things came, fundamentally, to be the way they are." Note that by stating "This cannot be denied" and by using the phrase "They tell, surely..." the author is indicating agreement with Eliade's ideas discussed in this part of the passage.
   C: No. This answer choice would require your own interpretation of the quote and/or the play from which it comes, rather than being based on and supported by the passage. There is no discussion of the value of life in the passage.
   D: No. This concept comes up at the end of the passage, where the author suggests that the claim that myth has disappeared from Western history is itself a myth. There is no direct relationship between this statement and the quote from Hamlet.

6. **C** This is a New Information question.
   A: No. Plato's statement does not disagree with Eliade's perspective—even Eliade is not arguing that myths are a literal reality, but only that they provide a functional value.
   B: No. The author does not discuss for which kinds of people (based on level of education) myth may or may not be relevant. This choice misrepresents the author's argument by bringing in an issue that is never raised in the passage.
   C: Yes. Plato's view of myth as a construct with a functional value is consistent with the author's concept that the root of all myth is human truth and that some myth still exists with us. The phrase "myth of demythologization" suggests that myth is in fact present in the history of the Western world—both Plato and the author acknowledge that myths still exist and have some purpose.
   D: No. There is no evidence in the passage that the author believes that myths are not literally true. The only statement in the passage on that topic is from Bidney (paragraph 1), and the author is critical of Bidney's claims.

SOLUTIONS TO CARS PRACTICE PASSAGE 3

1. **C** This is a Main Idea question.
   A: No. At the end of the passage, the authors indicate that psychological truth, not psychology itself, can be an art. Furthermore, even if this were fully supported by the passage, it would be too narrow to be the main point.
   B: No. This is a specific claim made in the passage (paragraph 5), but it does not does not capture the overall theme of the passage as a whole, which is about the value of psychology in general as a means of understanding a work.
   C: Yes. This answer choice addresses more of the concerns of the passage than do the other options. The passage as a whole discusses how we should distinguish between the "mental structure of the poet" (paragraph 2) and the work itself, and what role looking at the author's psychology within the process of creation should play.
   D: No. While both poets and painters are mentioned in paragraph 2, the author does not discuss psychological differences between them. Furthermore, as in choice A, even if this were supported by the text, it would be too narrow to be the main point of the entire passage.

2. **D** This is a Structure question.
   A: No. this answer is overly negative in tone. In paragraph 5 the authors do state that this analysis has been "overrated" and that the study of other elements like revisions has more to offer (and, in paragraph 6, that none of this is necessary to an understanding of the work). However, the authors don't go so far as to say that the study of early drafts is useless. Finally, this is not directly relevant to the discussion of Feuillerat's study, which looks at later revisions and corrections.
   B: No. This answer, as with choice A, has the wrong tone. In the discussion of Feuillerat in paragraph 5, the passage suggests that it is in fact possible to make such an assessment of Proust's creative process.
   C: No. This choice is too negative. While the authors state in paragraph 6 that this type of analysis is not necessary to an understanding of the text (because you can get the same understanding by looking at other alternatives as well), they do not discount the value of it in and of itself. Furthermore, while the authors state that study of the early stages of a work is overrated (paragraph 5), they do not apply the same judgment to studies of revisions and corrections in the process of composition (like Feuillerat's study), which has "more which is literarily profitable."
   D: Yes. The author cites Feuillerat as an example of when a study of the creative process is "illuminating" (see sentences preceding, including, and following Feuillerat's name).

3. **D** This is an Inference question.
   A: No. The authors say this in paragraph 4. Although the contrast "may be exaggerated," it can be easily made.
   B: No. This is a paraphrase of the final sentence of paragraph 2: "every impression is shaped by his art."
   C: No. This statement is in the final paragraph of the passage: "psychology is only preparatory to the act of creation."
   D: Yes. The authors assert the opposite in paragraph 4: "the critical theories of classicism and romanticism differ more violently than the creative practices of their best writers."

4. **A** This is a Retrieval question.

    A: Yes. See paragraph 3. James is included in the list of authors "given to thinking and writing analytically about their art."

    B: No. James is included in a list of authors, and there is no suggestion that he was also a psychologist. Note the transitional phrase "and then we have" leading into the mention of psychologists in paragraph 3. This distinguishes the list of "authors" from the discussion of psychologists.

    C: No. The authors do not make this connection; the passage does not state that psychologists have studied James.

    D: No. The authors do not make a value judgment about James' work.

5. **B** This is a New Information question.

    A: No. See paragraphs 5 and 6. The authors do not place much importance upon the significance of drafts in relation to the final work. They also claim in paragraph 6 that other approaches, including imagining an alternative not actually written by the author, are equally valid.

    B: Yes. See paragraph 6. The authors say that it is just as meaningful to consider other alternative works as it is to see the different works or versions considered by an author.

    C: No. While the authors state that an examination of revisions is not *necessary* to understanding a work, they do not go so far as to say that it is irrelevant (paragraph 6). This choice (including the strong word "scornful") is too extreme.

    D: No. The authors do not discuss who should or should not interpret art. While the passage does discuss the possibility of taking a psychological approach, it does not claim that actual psychologists, not literary scholars, should carry out such interpretations.

6. **C** This is a Retrieval question.

    A: No. This choice is out of scope. The authors do not discuss the relevance of the author's time to the author's work.

    B: No. This choice is out of scope. The authors do not discuss the psychological health of artists.

    C: Yes. This is found in the first sentence of paragraph 4: "Any modern treatment of the creative process will chiefly concern the relative parts played by the unconscious and the conscious mind" (note the word "chiefly").

    D: No. While the authors admit that looking at revisions can be of some value, they do not believe it to be necessary. Therefore, the authors do not consider this to be of *primary* importance (see paragraph 6).

SOLUTIONS TO CARS PRACTICE PASSAGE 4

1. **C** This is an Inference question.

    A: No. The passage criticizes scholars of dance but makes no suggestions about how ballet itself should be altered.

    B: No. The author emphasizes the resemblance of ballet to other dance forms, and it is critical of scholars who portray Western dance as distinct or superior.

    C: Yes. The last three paragraphs argue that ballet is "ethnic;" that is, particular to this specific culture and representative of a Western worldview. Therefore, ballet should not be understood as transcending or separated from Western culture.

    D: No. Although the author does state that ballet includes these themes and that this, in part, is a characteristic of Western culture, the author never states that other dance forms (including other Western dance forms) do not include themes of love and suffering.

2. **D**   This is a Specific Inference/Tone question.
    A: No. The author argues that these dance scholars are incorrect in their approach to ballet. In paragraph 3, these scholars set themselves up as false authorities.
    B: No. This is reversed. The scholars reject the idea that ballet is an ethnic dance form, while the author argues the opposite.
    C: No. The author's criticism of the dance scholars is based on their miscommunication with anthropologists. The scholars do not consider anthropology.
    D: Yes. In the first paragraph, the author refers to a miscommunication between anthropologists and dance scholars. The next two paragraphs clarify the problem and in the third paragraph, you see that dance scholars incorrectly "set themselves up as authorities."

3. **B**   This is a Structure question.
    A: No. Immediately before the example, the author makes the claim that ballet has a distinctive appearance. There is no discussion of whether or not it incorporates other perspectives.
    B: Yes. The author presents the example as proof of the previous claim: that ballet has an extremely distinctive look.
    C: No. The author does not describe any difference or give any particulars about Hopi dance. Look at the text introducing the example to interpret the author's purpose in presenting it.
    D: No. This is reversed. In this paragraph the author is arguing that ballet is ethnological, in the sense of being particular to Western culture.

4. **A**   This is an Inference question.
    A: Yes. In the final sentence of paragraph 3, the author criticizes Sorell for the attitude that contemporary Western dancers do not share characteristics with primitive dancers. Ballet is, in the passage, the principal example of contemporary Western dance.
    B: No. Sorell and the other dance scholars use stereotypes to describe primitive dance. This choice represents the author's point of view, not Sorell's.
    C: No. There is no claim concerning what contemporary dancers should do. The debate is over dance scholarship.
    D: No. The author's criticism of Sorell in paragraph 3 is based on his use of stereotypes. Unlike the anthropologists in the preceding paragraph, Sorell is unlikely to recognize the varieties of primitive dance.

5. **B**   This is a Retrieval question.
    A: No. In paragraph 2, the author states that primitive (non-Western) dance comes in a variety of forms.
    B: Yes. In paragraph 5, the author describes a difference between Western and more "ethnologic" dance experts. The "ethnologic" ones make claims only about their own traditions, unlike the Westerners who "set themselves up as authorities" in various dance traditions.
    C: No. The author rejects the idea that primitive dances are frozen as part of the double myth. There is no information about which form of dance involves more change.
    D: No. Although the author rejects the notion that primitive dances are frozen, there is no evidence in the passage for this comparison. Note that just because two answer choices are opposites, this does not imply that one of the two must be correct.

6. **C** This is a New Information question.
   A: No. In paragraph 2, the author states that anthropologists no longer claim (and should not claim) to have knowledge about the origin of primeval dance.
   B: No. As with choice A, this answer contradicts the author's statement that we know nothing about the "dance of primeval man" (paragraph 2).
   C: **Yes. In paragraph 2, the author says, "I will not add another origin theory for dance, because I don't know anyone who was there." The author is arguing that anthropologists and dance scholars have no direct evidence for making claims about the origins of dance and so should not make overarching claims on the subject. The anthropologist in the question stem violates this stricture.**
   D: No. Although the author does emphasize that no evidence is available about the origin of *primeval* dance, the author does, in the second paragraph, discuss the category of *primitive* dance as one which anthropologists study and about which they have a great deal of useful information. When a passage draws a distinction between similar sounding terms, be careful not to pick an answer that confuses them with each other.

SOLUTIONS TO CARS PRACTICE PASSAGE 5

1. **C** This is an Inference question.
   A: No. In paragraph 5, it says that someone who has not been able to read fairy tales as a child will escape into a fantasy world, not that fairy tales provide this escape.
   B: No. Even though the passage states that fairy tales provide fantasy and excitement (paragraph 1), these are not the *most* important benefit of reading fairy tales.
   C: **Yes. In paragraph 3, the author states "This is where the fairy tale provides what the child needs most: it begins exactly where the child is emotionally, shows him where he has to go, and how to do it." Therefore, inspiration is what the child needs most from fairy tales.**
   D: No. This choice takes words from the passage out of context. In paragraph 5, the author describes how a child deprived of true fantasy "may later, as an adolescent *no longer under the emotional sway of his parents*, come to hate the rational world and escape entirely into a fantasy world, as if to make up for what was lost in childhood [emphasis added]." Independence is not given as a result of exposure to fairy tales or true fantasy.

2. **C** This is an Inference question.
   A: No. Just because the Victorians encouraged their children to read fairy tales (paragraph 1), this does not mean that they preferred these stories to any others. This is too extreme.
   B: No. The contrast made in paragraph 1 is not that modern parents are worried about the proper development of their children while Victorians were not. The only information given about the Victorians is that they encouraged the enjoyment of fairy tales.
   C: **Yes. "Even our Victorian ancestors...not only permitted but encouraged their children to enjoy...fairy tales." This choice is consistent with the depiction of Victorians in paragraph 1.**
   D: No. This choice takes words from the passage out of context. The author states in paragraph 1, "Even our Victorian ancestors, despite their emphasis on moral discipline and their stodgy way of life, not only permitted but encouraged their children to enjoy the fantasy and excitement of fairy tales." Therefore, the author states that the Victorians encouraged reading of fairy tales despite the value they placed on morality, not because of it.

3. **B** This is a Main Idea question.

    A: No. This is the main idea of the first paragraph, not the entire passage. This choice is too narrow.

    B: **Yes. This statement best summarizes all of the ideas in the passage. The author, after introducing the theme of fairy tales in the first paragraph, discusses why scientific explanations are not useful to children (paragraph 2), and why the very different kind of information offered through fairy tales is much more valuable for a child's emotional development (paragraph 3). The author continues this theme through the last two paragraphs by discussing the value of "free floating fantasy" as offered by fairy stories, and the harm done to children who are deprived of it.**

    C: No. This is the main idea of the third paragraph, not the entire passage. This choice is too narrow.

    D: No. This choice is not supported by the passage; the author never indicates that people of all ages enjoy fairy tales.

4. **C** This is a Retrieval Roman numeral question.

    I: **True. Paragraph 5 states: "If a child is told only stories "true to reality," then he may conclude that much of his inner reality is unacceptable to his parents. Many a child thus estranges himself from his inner life...."**

    II: False. Paragraph 3 says that without fairy tales, "the child cannot invent stories on his own...." Therefore, a realistic story will not enable the child to do so.

    III: **True. Paragraph 2 states: "realistic explanations are usually incomprehensible to children."**

5. **A** This is a Structure question.

    A: **Yes. The example is provided to show that even though Victorians "emphasized moral discipline" and were "stodgy," they still encouraged the enjoyment of fairy tales, as opposed to modern parents who are less strict, yet disregard the importance of fairy tales today.**

    B: No. The passage never makes the claim that modern science is what changed the parents' view of fairy tales. The author himself questions why modern parents' discourage fairy tales.

    C: No. The Victorians do expose their children to fairy tales; they even "encourage" it.

    D: No. The passage never describes fairy tales as being different from one time to another.

6. **C** This is a New Information/Strengthen-Weaken question.

    A: No. This choice is out of scope; this claim is never made in the passage.

    B: No. The fact that children cannot process abstract ideas until adolescence is not relevant to this particular claim, and therefore it does not weaken it.

    C: **Yes. Paragraph 2 states: "realistic explanations are usually incomprehensible to children, because they lack the abstract understanding required to make sense of them." The fact that a child is incapable of processing abstract ideas until late adolescence would strengthen this idea.**

    D: No. The idea that children cannot process abstract ideas until late adolescence does not do anything to the claim that fairy tales are important to psychological development.

SOLUTIONS TO CARS PRACTICE PASSAGE 6

1. **A**   This is a Structure question.

   A: **Yes. Remember, you're looking for the claim for which the author *doesn't* offer any specific support or explanation. Although the author makes this claim in paragraph 4, he does not offer any examples or explain why plays and/or stage shows particularly exemplify this point.**

   B: No. The author explains this statement in paragraph 2 after addressing why excessive stoutness is laughable, saying, "This too is what sometimes makes bashfulness somewhat ridiculous. The bashful man rather gives the impression of a person embarrassed by his body."

   C: No. In paragraph 2 the author writes, "Where lies the comic element in this sentence...? In the fact that our attention is suddenly recalled from the soul to the body." Several examples follow, such as the speaker cut short by a painful tooth.

   D: No. This statement, made by Napoleon (paragraph 5) is explained immediately after: "for as soon as you are seated it all becomes comedy."

2. **D**   This is a Structure question.

   A: No. The analogy to music is consistent with the author's explicit argument, rather than serving as a counterpoint or contrast.

   B: No. The tragic poet avoids striking a comic "note" so as to avoid bringing in unwanted overtones (paragraph 3), while in the analogy to music the author discusses how when one note, musical or comic, is struck, another inevitably follows. Therefore, there is a contrast rather than an analogy drawn between a tragic poet and a musician.

   C: No. This choice includes some words from the relevant paragraph (paragraph 5), but the meaning is different. The "far-fetched inventions" of comic fancy are extreme cases that still obey the rule; the author's analogy to music does not specifically serve to illustrate those extreme cases.

   D: **Yes. In paragraph 5, after explaining the musical effect whereby "other notes start up of themselves," the author writes, "These are what are called in physics the overtones of the fundamental note. It would seem that comic fancy, even in its most far-fetched inventions, obeys a similar law." His purpose in describing the effect in music is to support his analysis that comedy operates in the same fashion. "No sooner, then, does the comic poet strike the first note than he will add the second on to it, involuntarily and instinctively. In other words, he will duplicate what is ridiculous professionally with something that is ridiculous physically." This description of one tone or "note" adding on to another supports the descriptive word "multilayered" in this choice.**

3. **C**   This is a New Information question.

   A: No. There is no indication that this is about demonstrating power, either from the new information or from the passage. This choice is out of scope.

   B: No. This choice is tempting, as the author says that sitting gives the body precedence over the soul (paragraph 4). However, there is no evidence that this was considered by Napoleon. The only evidence we have of his awareness of the significance of sitting relates to the "transition from tragedy to comedy."

   C: **Yes. The author states in paragraph 3 that Napoleon "had noticed that the transition from tragedy to comedy is effected simply by sitting down" and supports this assertion with a quote from Napoleon: "...for as soon as you are seated it all becomes comedy." The author indicates that Napoleon was aware that sitting in *any* situation would produce comedy, so by not sitting, the author would most likely say that he was consciously avoiding one source of comedy.**

D: No. If Napoleon never sat when receiving guests, this suggests that he attached some importance to standing. Therefore, you cannot infer that he did *not* understand that sitting was comic (if anything, it suggests that he may in fact have already understood this).

4. **A**   This is an Inference question.

   A: **Yes. The "outward formalities" of the professions of lawyers, magistrates, and doctors are the things that make their jobs ridiculous, as they speak "as though health and justice were of little moment" (paragraph 4). He further explains, "Constant attention to form and the mechanical application of rules" (paragraph 4) are what is laughable about these professions.**

   B: No. The author does not address their uniforms or clothing. This is a misinterpretation of "outward formalities."

   C: No. The author does not indicate that these are intellectually stimulating careers. Be careful not to use outside knowledge or opinion.

   D: No. The author does not mention these professions positively contributing to society. Again, be careful not to use outside knowledge or your own opinion.

5. **C**   This is a New Information question.

   A: No. There is no indication that a tragic scene has been shortened here.

   B: No. There is no indication that manner (Medea's behavior) has substituted for matter (the tragic content of the play).

   C: **Yes. The new information describes a writer of tragedy, Euripides, who allowed his heroine to both sit and eat. This is inconsistent the author's assertion in paragraph 3 that the tragic poet presents his heroes in a certain way because he fears the comic element in drawing attention to the body. "On this account, the hero in a tragedy does not eat or drink or warm himself. He does not even sit down any more than can be helped." (You may not be sure whether Euripides might be called a tragic *poet* or not, but the theme of tragedy itself makes this relevant to the passage.)**

   D: No. Neither plumpness nor virtue is addressed in the new information. Also, the issue of the author's reference to the speech quoted by the German philosopher is that of a relationship between a mention of plumpness and comedy, not of some generalized relationship between plumpness and virtue.

6. **B**   This is an Inference question.

   A: No. A cough would be similar to a sneeze, which the author says in paragraph 2 could draw attention to the body. So, the author is unlikely to disagree with this claim.

   B: **Yes. Remember, you're looking for the statement the author would *disagree* with. The final paragraph indicates that "When a musician strikes a note on an instrument, other notes start up of themselves." Later in that paragraph the author, in the context of the analogy, states that "No sooner, then, does the comic poet strike the first note than he will add the second on to it, involuntarily and instinctively" (emphasis added). So, the author does not believe the artist "may choose to play" overtones, and therefore the author is most likely to disagree with this statement.**

   C: No. Referring to excessive tallness, like the author's example of excessive stoutness in paragraph 2, probably calls up a laughable image. Therefore, the author is unlikely to disagree with this statement.

   D: No. The author would be likely to agree that brushing one's teeth is a similar kind of physical action (touching one's mouth) to eating or drinking, two activities he says tragic poets are unlikely to depict their heroes doing. So, the author would likely agree rather than disagree with this statement.

SOLUTIONS TO CARS PRACTICE PASSAGE 7

1. **C** This is an Inference question.

   A: No. This choice is too extreme. The author suggests that in some important sense there is no such thing as individual memory, but he is stressing the interdependence of individual and collective memory, not the complete absence of the former. There is also no suggestion that the idea of individual memory was constructed as a way of explaining collective memory.

   B: No. This answer may be tempting for those who don't check back to the passage, as the author says that there is no such thing as individual memory, and that the concept of distortion becomes problematic once one dispels the notion that individual memory is independent of collective memory. However, you don't know, based on the text, that the nature of individual memory itself causes problems in considering distortion. That is, the concept of individual memory may be problematic, but the author does not suggest that individual memory causes conceptual problems.

   C: Yes. The author makes this point in a number of places in the second paragraph, especially in the last line when he notes that "cultural memory…is distributed across social institutions."

   D: No. This is the opposite of what the passage suggests. The author stresses the dependence of individual memory on collective institutions. That is, individual memory doesn't really exist because "memory is social" (paragraph 2). The author's point is not that they are two different things, but rather that they are one and the same thing.

2. **C** This is a Structure question.

   A: No. The statement in question does have a bearing on the overall argument. If the controversies did not exist, it would suggest that collective memories might be entirely unstable and therefore of no use in judging how much we might come to agreement about what really happened.

   B: No. The statement is not in itself of historical importance, as far as we know. That statement is, rather, about some aspect of history.

   C: Yes. This statement, when examined along with the prior sentence, is used by the author to point out that memory is not so entirely open to interpretation that it is a matter of pure fiction. The passage states: "If interpretation were free-floating, entirely manipulable to serve present interests, altogether unanchored by a bedrock body of unshakable evidence, controversies over the past would ultimately be uninteresting. But in fact they are interesting. They are compelling. And they are gripping because people trust that a past we can to some extent know and can to some extent come to agreement about really happened." If controversies were uninteresting (the contrary notion), it would suggest that there is no foundation at all for agreement, which would be inconsistent with the author's argument in this paragraph.

   D: No. It is not an exception, but instead a statement of fact according to the author. Furthermore, it is not used to anticipate opposing arguments; rather, it is used to directly support the author's claim that it makes sense to study distortions of widely accepted historical interpretations.

3. **A** This is an Inference question.

   A: Yes. This is a rather oblique way of referring to something the author says nearby in the first paragraph, that "the biography of a lifetime is the appropriate "natural" frame for individual memory." Given this fact and the statement mentioned in the question stem, you can conclude that the fact that "there's no…evident frame" means that the ongoing "lifespan" of the human race, still around, obviates any snapshot of race memory as representative of the whole.

B: No. The author never suggests that there is no sharing of experience or memory between different cultures.

C: No. This contradicts the passage, as individuals certainly have access to common cultural memories and in fact depend on this access to survive (see paragraph 2).

D: No. This is the opposite of what the author states in the first paragraph: "Neither national boundaries nor linguistic ones are as self-evidently the right containers for collective memory as the person is for individual memory."

4. **A** This is a Weaken question.

A: **Yes. When answering a Weaken or Strengthen question, don't evaluate whether or not the answer choice is true; rather, take each choice as a true statement and judge whether or not it has the required effect on the author's argument. The author's main view of individual memory is that it's partly illusory, since it reflects so many aspects of cultural knowledge carried over from generation to generation and vested in various institutions. This choice would weaken this claim, as it would indicate that social memories are changeable and do not necessarily persist outside the individual.**

B: No. The fact that people can memorize information is not inconsistent with the author's argument about the nature of memory. By saying that memory is inherently social, the author is not literally arguing that individuals cannot remember things.

C: No. This would strengthen the argument, if anything, as it would support the notion that memories reside chiefly in institutions rather than individuals.

D: No. This choice is not strong enough to "most undermine" the passage. While this statement doesn't support the author's claim that institutional memory is advantageous (paragraph 2), it doesn't significantly weaken the author's argument as a whole, especially as compared to choice A. It relates only to a small and probably non-representative sample, rather than to individual and institutional memory as it functions more generally.

5. **D** This is a Strengthen question.

A: No. The author says that the choice of what we recall and the consequent distortion is "socially conditioned" (third paragraph), implying that it's unconscious. If we were to purposefully and consciously choose to withhold certain information and report other information, it wouldn't affect the underlying issue of what was available for the recollection of the individual.

B: No. This would have no effect on the author's claim, as it would show a capability on a particular task, but it would not affect the unconscious biases in storage and retrieval the author is interested in.

C: No. This might support the failure of the mental hardware to store or retrieve certain items of memory, but it wouldn't have much effect on the issue of socially conditioned memory distortions.

D: **Yes. The author's point is that memory is inherently distorted, as it involves selecting what to pay attention to and what to ignore. If the brain is inherently limited in its ability to notice and store memories, then the individual must inevitably choose what to notice and what to ignore, as the author argues in paragraph 3.**

6. **A** This is an Evaluate question.

A: **Yes. The statement regarding agreement about the past is a statement about what may be derived from collective memory, institutions, and the like. The statement about individual memories is generally unrelated to the idea of coming to some agreement about what has actually happened in the past.**

B: No. While the statements are consistent (see explanation of choice A), it is not because the second claim in the question stem supports the first. An argument might be made that the first claim supports the second, if weakly, but not the other way around.

C: No. Difficulties in judging whether controversies over the past are gripping or not are irrelevant, as you are told directly by the passage that they are gripping. Furthermore, the author does not literally argue that individual memories do not exist, but rather that individual memory is inherently conditioned by social institutions and practices.

D: No. The relationship stated in this answer choice is not supported by the passage. The idea that individual memories are inextricably linked to cultural memories is not inconsistent with the idea that we can come to some agreement about what's occurred in our collective past.

7. **B** This is a New Information question.

A: No. The fact that dominant individuals have inordinate influence would go directly to the heart of issue of why certain cultural memories are emphasized and others are downplayed.

B: Yes. If dominant individuals can influence large groups to change their opinions about what is most relevant and what is less so, then their influence would have a direct bearing on "social and historical processes" and therefore on the author's claim that the notion of distortion is problematic.

C: No. That distortions are fairly ordinary would tend to strengthen rather than weaken the author's claim.

D: No. The second half of this answer ("explain the ultimate origin") is too extreme. This choice also incorrectly states that the situation described would weaken the author's claim, when in fact it would support it.

SOLUTIONS TO CARS PRACTICE PASSAGE 8

1. **D** This is an Inference EXCEPT question.

A: No. The author would agree with this statement. The author states in paragraph 4 that the temple front was "often artfully adapted to a specific location." So, even though the author essentially disagrees with the negative evaluation of the critics cited in paragraph 2, he agrees with one aspect of their claims: that "it was rarely designed according to precedent" (that is, that it took on different, unorthodox forms).

B: No. The author would agree with this statement. The author argues in paragraph 3 that painting buildings white "showed that architecture had become an important medium of expression, one which Americans could use to show their shared identity as citizens of a new nation." Because the author draws an analogy between using the temple front and the practice of painting buildings white, and because the author argues that use of the temple front "was an affirmation of that system of government and an acknowledgment of a common set of values" (paragraph 2), you can infer that the use of the temple front also illustrated this same architectural philosophy. Furthermore, later in the passage the author states in reference to the use of the temple front: "Yet the front and the back each encapsulated a significant aspect of the life and dreams of the inhabitants of these buildings. Although different, the two can be read as complementary parts of an unaffected whole" (paragraph 4). This can also be seen as a manifestation of American architectural principles.

C: No. The author would agree with this statement. The third paragraph describes the Greek temple front as "an affirmation of that [republican] system of government and an acknowledgment of a common set of values"; in the fifth paragraph, it is literally a "symbol of republicanism." This connects the temple front to political ideologies. The final paragraph connects it to economic ideologies via the reference to Mills, who, we are told, used it because of its economy—that is, its cheapness—which he knew to be one of the "qualities which most directly appealed to his clients" and one of "his country's 'tastes and requirements.'"

D: Yes. While the second paragraph indicates that builders were criticized for overusing the Greek temple front, the author does not indicate agreement on that matter. The author only states that they "*may* often have been used indiscriminately" (third paragraph) and that they "*may* frequently have been used unthinkingly" (fourth paragraph), but his tone about the use of Greek temple fronts is positive. That is, overall, the author would not agree they were used too often (see paragraphs 3 and 4).

2. **D** This is a Main Idea question.
   A: No. This choice states that architecture helped *establish* an American system of values and government, but the passage only indicates, in the third paragraph, that architecture helped affirm the system of government and acknowledge and demonstrate the system of values. Paragraph 5 suggests the same; use of the temple front showed (rather than created) the affinity felt between the American and Greek republics.
   B: No. First, the passage is largely about the significance of the adoption of a Greek model by American builders. Even though this model was adapted to local contexts (paragraph 3), this suggests a similarity rather than a contrast between American and classical Greek builders. Furthermore, although there is a suggestion that the temple front was used to reflect an American identity (paragraph 3), there is no explicit discussion of a contrast between the architectural ideas of American builders and those elsewhere. Finally, there is no discussion in the passage of the impact of this particular influence on the field of architecture as a whole.
   C: No. The reference to "the arts" in this choice goes beyond the scope of the passage: other arts besides architecture are not mentioned. Furthermore, there is no suggestion that Americans "needed" the arts, including architecture, to create a unique national identity. Just because something contributes to a result does not show that the result could not have occurred without it.
   D: Yes. The criticism is described in paragraph 2, and paragraphs 3–5 show how use of the temple front reflected needs and values (including a shared identity, people's "life and dreams," republicanism, and economy).

3. **A** This is an Inference question.
   A: Yes. This question asks you to define the word as it is used in the passage, so your definition needs to have support in the passage text rather than being based on outside knowledge. The only mentions of republicanism in this passage appear in the third paragraph and in the last one. All that the author indicates of republicanism in the third paragraph is that it is a system of government affirmed by the persistent use of the Greek temple front; all that he indicates in the last paragraph is that America and Greece are republics, and the temple front symbolizes republicanism. Note: although one could also infer from the passage that republicanism is the American system of government, the answer does not have to include everything to which the term could be said to refer (and, "American system of government" is not an answer choice).

B: No. This choice confuses the two separate ways in which the author describes the temple front in the third paragraph: as "an affirmation of *that* system of government [republicanism] and an acknowledgment of a common set of values" (emphasis added). The passage never indicates that the two are one and the same.

C: No. This choice tempts you to use outside knowledge. Although republicanism is in fact government by representation, this is never mentioned in the passage.

D: No. This choice also tempts you to use outside knowledge, and also to confuse republicanism (as a system of government) with Republicanism (as an ideology attached to the American Republican Party). While minimalist government is an ideal of some modern Republicans in the United States, there is no discussion of it in the passage.

4. **A** This is a Structure question.

    A: Yes. What the passage does say about the war is that the Greek temple front became symbolic of republicanism at the same time. That idea—of "a statement about republicanism" is discussed in the third paragraph. Note: don't eliminate choices only because they refer to a different paragraph than the location of the information in the question stem. Sometimes issues reoccur, and paragraphs may be linked to each other thematically.

    B: No. While the author does mention the architects' critique of the use of the temple front in the same paragraph (paragraph 5), he does not agree with or justify the architects' criticism. This choice mistakes the author's tone; although earlier in the passage he says that "many examples can be found to validate this criticism" he goes on to say that "those same points can also be used to illustrate the positive qualities of the period's architecture" (paragraph 3).

    C: No. The previous sentence does tell us that some Americans claimed an *affinity* between Greece and the United States, but there is no suggestion that this affinity was based on going to war in general, or in going to war with the Turks in particular.

    D: No. This choice may be tempting because it appears in the same paragraph. However, it refers to a different issue; there is no connection drawn between Jefferson's views on architecture and the war between Greece and the Turks. Also, the author does not indicate agreement with (or defense of) Jefferson's views.

5. **B** This is a New Information question.

    Note: Choices B, C, and D all relate to the same issue: the consistency of the front of American buildings with their rear or back. The issue of consistency comes up in paragraph 4 of the passage, where the author writes: "Similarly, the formal front did not necessarily lie about what happened behind. The New England farmhouse of this period may have had a portico which led to a sequence of house, shed, barn, and outbuildings, all of which were frequently joined together and straggled into the backyard. Yet the front and the back each encapsulated a significant aspect of the life and dreams of the inhabitants of these buildings. Although different, the two can be read as complementary parts of an unaffected whole." Thus, the author's argument is that front and back were tied together as a part of one consistent whole.

    A: No. This new information has no impact on the author's claim, since the quote from Whitaker's book gives no information about other parts of the world.

    B: Yes. Whitaker argues that front and rear are treated "much differently," as if they are in clear contrast with each other. This would call the author's argument for compatibility into question.

C: No. Whitaker explicitly contrasts Americans' treatment of the front of their buildings from that of the rear, so this quote cannot support the author's claim about consistency in paragraph 4.

D: No. According to paragraph 4, the front and back are compatible, not incompatible. This choice misrepresents the author's argument.

6. **C** This is a Structure EXCEPT question.

A: No. This is a function of the reference. The Greek temple front functions as "an acknowledgment of a common set of values." "Similarly...the custom adopted in this period of painting all buildings white...also showed that architecture had become an important medium of expression, one which Americans could use to show their shared identity as citizens of a new nation."

B: No. This is a function of the reference. The main idea of paragraph 3 is that the architecture of the period, in particular the use of the temple front, has positive qualities. Painting buildings white is given as an example; it "showed that architecture had become an important medium of expression, one which Americans could use to show their shared identity as citizens of a new nation." The author draws an analogy between the temple front and white paint, and uses the analogy to support his overall argument about the value of using the temple front.

C: **Yes. This is NOT a function of the reference. While the use of the temple front is in part "a statement about republicanism," there is no such claim made about the meaning of painting buildings white. The author only says that this practice "showed that architecture had become an important medium of expression, one which Americans could use to show their shared identity as citizens of a new nation." The two (republicanism and shared identity), while perhaps related, are not equated with each other in the passage. Furthermore, the author does not himself support or argue for republicanism anywhere in the passage. He simply describes it as a system of government that was affirmed at the time.**

D: No. This is a function of the reference. The author appears to accept the criticism that painting buildings white may be "an insensitive response to local circumstances and a manifestation of a worrying tendency toward conformity." But he goes on to say that "this convention *also* showed that architecture had become an important medium of expression, one which Americans could use to show their shared identity as citizens of a new nation" (emphasis added). The word "also" in particular suggests that the author is not refuting the criticism, but rather is arguing that there is a positive as well as potentially negative aspect to this practice.

PASSAGE PERMISSIONS INFORMATION

NOTES

NOTES

NOTES

NOTES

NOTES

NOTES

NOTES

NOTES

NOTES

NOTES